A Scenic Driving Tour of the Roanoke Valley

D0125828

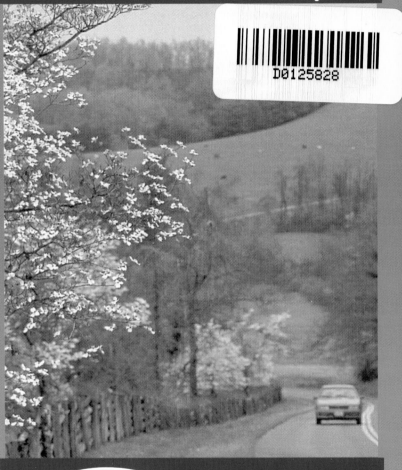

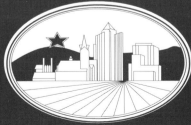

The
Roanoke Valley
Convention and
Visitors Bureau

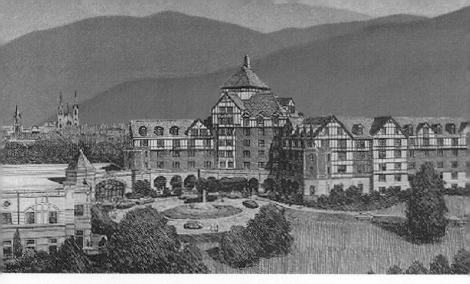

There are 100's of reasons for visiting Roanoke.

Start with these 6.

1. Market on the Square is the historic 188 year old farmers market that offers a culinary arcade of American and international cuisine.

2. Smith Mountain Lake is the largest lake in Virginia and offers some of the best boating and fishing in the East.

3. Virginia Museum of Transportation lets you relive railroad's golden past and be taken to the future.

4. Cruise along the Blue Ridge Parkway and experience the spectacular views that Virginia is famous for.

5. Golf anyone? The Roanoke Valley offers a wide variety of public and private golf facilities which our guests are welcome to enjoy.

6. The Hotel Roanoke & Conference Center offers our guests luxurious rooms and unsurpassed personal service.

For reservations, see your travel professional or call 540-985-5900.

THE HOTEL ROANOKE & CONFERENCE CENTER

A DOUBLETREE HOTEL

800-222-TREE

Inspired by the past. Created for the future.

In partnership with Virginia Tech
110 Shenandoah Avenue, Roanoke, VA 24016

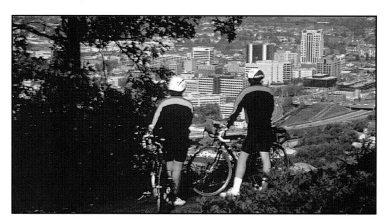

A Scenic Driving Tour of the Roanoke Valley

Experience the best and brightest of the Roanoke Valley. Whether you have an afternoon or just an hour, select a route and enjoy the valley's terrific sights and impressive mountain vistas.

Venture up Mill Mountain, one of the only mountain ranges within a city limit east of Phoenix, Arizona, for a breathtaking view of the entire Roanoke Valley. There you have a closer look at Roanoke's 100 foot star, a landmark erected in 1949. **Mill Mountain Zoological Park** adjoins the star within a ten acre park exhibiting over 43 species of animals, including "Ruby" the Siberian tiger.

To get there, from the **Visitor Information Center** (located on 114 Market Street), take a left on Salem Avenue and another left on Jefferson Street. Follow the blue directional signs to Walnut Avenue and turn left. It is just a short 12 minute drive.

Next, take the four-mile scenic loop up to the top of **Roanoke Mountain.** It has seven magnificent overlooks with panoramic and rural views of the Valley. Follow the Blue Ridge Parkway signs from Mill Mountain and turn north to milepost 120. You will pass Roanoke Mountain Campground, a perfect area for seasonal picnics or primitive camping. A convenient five minute drive to the Parkway. (Note: This loop closes at dusk.)

Just ten minutes from Roanoke Mountain is **Virginia's Explore Park** the valley's newest attraction. The park is both educational and fun. It interprets the area's history in the 1800's depicting a Blue Ridge Settlement and Town. Visit the park Saturday through Monday in the months of April through October. The exit for the Park is off the Parkway at milepost 115, just 5 miles north of Roanoke Mountain.

Retracing your drive back to the

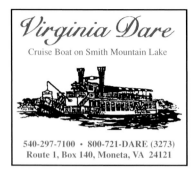

foot of Mill Mountain on Walnut Avenue, be adventurous and turn right on Piedmont Avenue and another right on Riverland Road to the sixth block. There you will see **Miniature Graceland**, one couple's hobby of recreating a miniature scale of Elvis Presley's domain. A life size statue of Elvis is just to the right of the collection. This statue was dedicated to the children killed in the March 1995 Oklahoma City bombing. The attraction has become a popular and unique Roanoke landmark.

Return to Walnut Avenue via Piedmont Avenue turning just toward downtown and cross Jefferson Street to enter the **Old Southwest Historic District** an Neighborhood. The neighborhood was established over 200 years ago in 1771 when King George III of England granted 150 acres to James Alexander. Until the end of World War II "Old Southwest" was considered one of the premier neighborhoods in the city with the largest concentration of Victorian homes. Today, many of the homes have been refurbished including the **Mary Bladon House Bed & Breakfast**, an 1890's Victorian Home, in the heart of Old

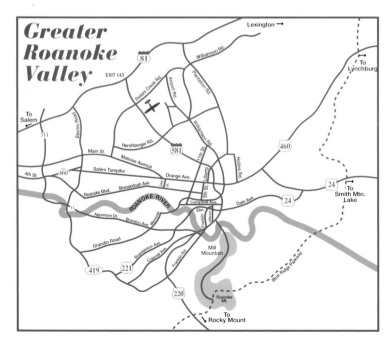

Greater Roanoke Valley

ROANOKE VALLEY

Attractions

Virginia Museum of Transportation Downtown Roanoke (540) 342-5670

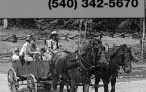

Virginia's Explore Park Milepost 115 on The Blue Ridge Parkway (540) 427-1800

Dixie Caverns & Pottery Salem, VA (540) 380-2085

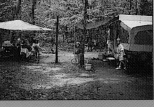

Mill Mountain Zoo Three miles off the Blue Ridge Parkway (540) 343-3241

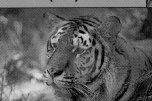

George Washington & Jefferson National Forests (540) 265-6054

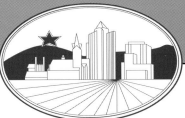

Festivals
Recreation

Culture
Excitement

"The Capital of the Blue Ridge"

114 Market Street, Roanoke, VA 24011-1402 800-635-5535
Roanoke Valley Visitor Information Center Open 9am-5pm daily

Southwest, at 381 Washington Avenue.

Follow Franklin Road (220 North Business) to downtown and turn left on Third Street toward the **Virginia Museum of Transportation** at 303 Norfolk Avenue. The Transportation Museum contains one of the largest collections of rolling stock in the East and a variety of modes of transportation in a restored freight station.

Follow the blue and green directional signs from the Transportation Museum to the **Historic Farmers Market**. The Historic Farmers Market is the oldest working market of its kind in Virginia, featuring stalls filled with colorful fresh produce and flowers. The market is surrounded by specialty shops, antique galleries and fine restaurants. You will pass **Center in the Square** on

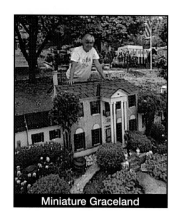

Miniature Graceland

Campbell Avenue. Center in the Square houses museums of art, history, and science. It is also home to Mill Mountain Theatre, Hopkins Planetarium, and the Arts Council of the Blue Ridge.

As you drive through the Market (turning right off Campbell Avenue

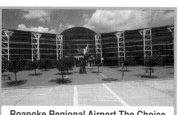
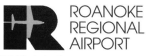
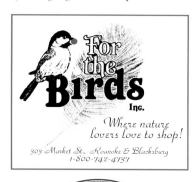
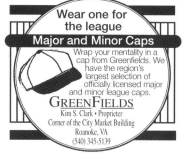

SHOPPING

BOOKS STRINGS &THINGS

Books • Cards • Magazines
Compact Discs • Tapes
202 Market Square
(540) 344-5511
Open Evenings

WERTZ'S COUNTRY STORE

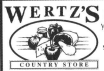

For over 100 years, Wertz's has been synonymous with the freshest produce and quality food products from the Blue Ridge Region. "The Wine Cellar", located on the store's lower level, offers a broad range of regional and international wines.

215 Market St. SE, Roanoke, VA 24011
703-342-5133 or 800-767-3110

Lä Dē Dä

Fantastical Frocks for Women
Young... & Young at Heart

Corner of Church & Market on the Historic Roanoke City Market
10-6 Monday-Saturday
(540) 345-6131

HOUSE UNIQUE Galleria Inc.

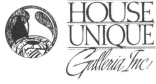

Fine Art, Crafts, Gifts for the home & office

112 Market St.
540-345-0697   1-800-889-1076

GALLERY 3

Fine Out, American Crafts,
Custom Framing

213 Market Square
(540) 343-9698

We're giving Roanoke a great new look.

Watch for exciting new changes in store for you at

TANGLEWOOD MALL

Routes 220 & 581S
at Franklin Road Exit
10am to 9pm Monday through Saturday,
1pm to 6pm Sunday

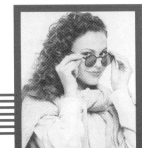

Expect the Unexpected in Downtown Roanoke!

Discover the options and offerings in Downtown Roanoke with restaurants, shops, cultural attractions, entertainment, Historic City Market and more.
It All Comes Together in Downtown Roanoke.

DOWNTOWN ROANOKE

Call 540-342-2028

ACCOMMODATIONS

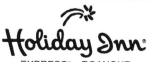
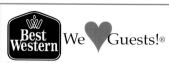
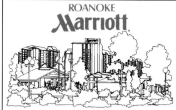
and right on Church Avenue) **Fire Station Number One** is on your left. This station was built in 1906 and modeled after Independence Hall in Philadelphia. Lee Plaza, a War Memorial, remembers all of those who served in the armed forces and died in wars past. This memorial is four blocks further on Church Avenue (west).

For a look at an old-fashioned college town brimming over with charm, the City of Salem is 20 minutes from Downtown via U.S. 220

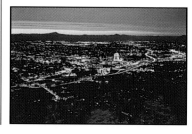

South (an extension of I-581 South) to Route 419 at Tanglewood Mall. Along the way, don't miss **To The Rescue**, located in the upper level of Tanglewood Mall. This interactive museum, chronicles the history of the volunteer rescue squad movement and emergency medical services. Heading toward Salem take advantage of the shopping, dining and movie theater possibilities. Continue on Route 419 to Route 460 West which leads into Main Street in **Downtown Salem**. While downtown, you can shop for antiques or produce at the **Salem's Farmer's Market**. Visit the historic **Roanoke College** campus, the **Salem Museum** or **Longwood Park**, a popular recreational sight for families and college students. For a change of pace, experience **Dixie Caverns and Pottery**.

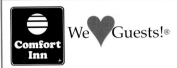

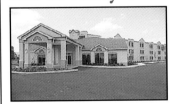

RESTAURANTS

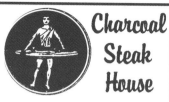

Charcoal Steak House

PRIVATE ROOMS AVAILABLE - COCKTAILS
1-800-446-9253 DIAL (540)336-3710
5225 Williamson Road Roanoke, Virginia
Open: Mon. - Fri. 11 am., Sat 4 pm.

Voted Roanokes Best
Italian Restaurant

The Italian Gourmet
Est. 1986

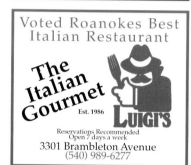

LUIGI'S

Reservations Recommended
Open 7 days a week
3301 Brambleton Avenue
(540) 989-6277

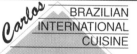

Carlos
BRAZILIAN
INTERNATIONAL
CUISINE

Brazilian • French
Spanish • American
food at it's best.

Lunch 11:00-2:00 Mon.-Sat.
Dinner 5:00-9:30 Mon.-Thurs.
5:00-11:00 Fri.-Sat.

312 Market St.   (540) 345-7661

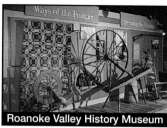

Roanoke Valley History Museum

Located just a few miles further on south U.S. 11, these caverns are particularly unique in that the tour guide takes you up, instead of down into the mountain. As you head north on I-81 take I-581 South and complete you tour at the **George Washington & Jefferson National Forests Information Center** located off Exit 2N (Peters Creek Road) and take a left into Valleypointe Industrial park at the first stoplight.

From interstates to leisurely

Voted Best Market Restaurant

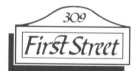

309
First Street

309 Market Street
Downtown Roanoke
(540) 343-0179

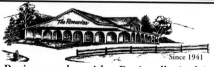

THE Roanoker RESTAURANT
Since 1941

Begin your day with a Regionally Acclaimed Southern Breakfast.
Give us an hour notice and we'll prepare our homemade Box
Lunch, Fried Chicken, Ham Biscuits, Potato Salad & Apple Pie
perfect while touring the area.
*Serving Breakfast, Lunch, Dinner, Daily Specials & Reasonable Prices
with Virginia Mountain Hospitality.*
Colonial Ave. at I-581 and Wonju 540-344-7746

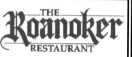

back roads, rest assured your driving tour will include beautiful views, historic sites and a wide variety of recreational opportunities. Contact the **Roanoke Valley Convention & Visitors Bureau** for additional information on attractions, dining and accommodations. (114 Market Street, Roanoke, VA 24011-1402) **(540) 342-6025 or (800) 635-5535.**

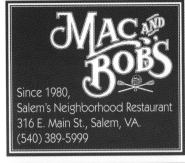
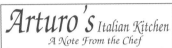
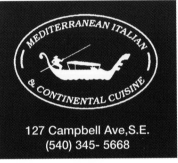
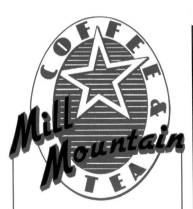
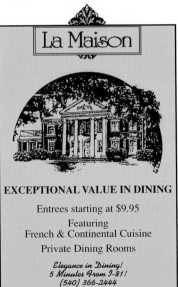

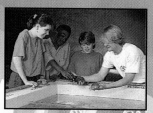
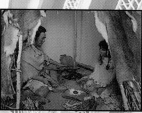
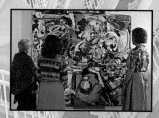
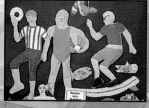
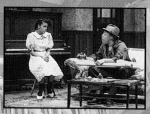

the fattest ducks in the world hold court over bread crumbs and crackers. This place gives a whole new meaning to the cliché "Lucky Duck," and is the most popular stroll on campus.

Christiansburg

Visual Arts

NEW RIVER VALLEY ARTS COUNCIL
(540) 381-1430
This active organization publishes an arts directory, a lively magazine and calendar of local artists. It's a rich source of information on the arts in the region.

PALETTE ART GALLERY
Roanoke Rd., just off
U.S. 11/460   (540) 382-8861
For more than 30 years, Palette Art Gallery has provided a showcase for Southwest Virginia artists at its rambling building. Begun by Vance Miller, an 84-year-old Impressionist painter, the Palette is chock-full of art, quaint and conservative. The gallery has no indoor plumbing, and a coal stove provides the heat. You'll find many of Miller's paintings in Virginia Tech offices. In addition to being a great source of art, the Gallery has returned nearly $100,000 to the community for charitable causes since opening in 1961.

Museums

THE MONTGOMERY MUSEUM
AND LEWIS MILLER
REGIONAL ART CENTER
300 S. Pepper St.   (540) 382-5644
A Valley-wide project to promote Montgomery County's rich history and arts, this center is in a mid-19th century home of American and Flemish bond brick made from local materials, with hand-hewn oak beams and rafters. A curious aspect of the manse portion of the house is a step-up feature in the back rooms, thought to be a carry-over from Colonial days when some people believed that evil spirits bearing illness traveled the night air along floors. The house contains both historic and contemporary works, including exhibits and shows of Southwest Virginia artists and crafters. It also houses a genealogical research area, historic small-press library and archives.

The Center is open 2 to 5 PM weekends May through October or by appointment.

Floyd

Visual Arts

OLD CHURCH GALLERY
U.S. 221   (540) 745-4849
In this 1850 Greek Revival building, art exhibits are adjacent to the history room. A century-old copper still used to make moonshine whiskey is on display. The gallery has an active quilter's guild, a monthly literary group, an arts and crafts workshop and children's programs in the summer.

NEW MOUNTAIN MERCANTILE
HERE AND NOW GALLERY
114 N. Locust St.   (540) 745-4278
For art and crafts definitely out of the ordinary, don't miss New Mountain Mercantile and its Here and Now Gallery. The gallery, in one corner of the 100-year-old Boyd Store building, 6 miles off Mile 165.2 of the Blue Ridge Parkway, highlights the work of a different artist each month. What looks like an ordinary building on the outside is extraordinary inside. It's just down the block from Cockram's General Store.

The store and gallery are open 10 AM to 6 PM Tuesday through Saturday and noon to 5 PM on Sunday.

Theater

FLOYD THEATRE GROUP
Floyd   *No phone*
This group started with Skit Night for locals and ended up with an enthusiastic collection of folks who present outstanding plays. Skit Night is still an annual event, joined by productions that enjoy tremendous community support and participation — yet another facet of cultural activities in Floyd County.

Other Cultural Attractions

COCKRAM'S GENERAL STORE
S. Locust St.   *(540) 745-4563*
The culture of mountainous Floyd County doesn't get any better than this! At 7 PM Friday night, folks start showing up with fiddles, harmonicas, banjos and guitars, and what follows is a Floyd County tradition. The flat-footing begins, old-timers reminisce, and the music that is the lifeblood of Floyd County mountain spirit soothes the wounds of the work week. This gathering is an endangered cultural species that is personally financed by Freeman Cockram, who believes Floyd Countians need such a place to gather. Don't miss this New River Valley landmark.

MABRY MILL
Mile 176, Blue Ridge Pkwy.   *(540) 745-4329*
Undoubtedly the most scenic and most-photographed place on the Blue Ridge Parkway, Mabry Mill has been called one of the most picturesque water mills in the United States. It still grinds flour for buckwheat cakes and produces some of the most delicious cornmeal you can buy for Southern-style cornbread. Mabry Mill also is a workshop of live crafts (many for sale), music and exhibits that shows a way of life a century ago. The site has a restaurant.

Giles County

Visual Arts

THE MOUNTAIN LAKE SYMPOSIUM & GALLERY
Mountain Lake   *(540) 626-7121*
In the rarefied air on the second-highest mountain in Virginia, Mountain Lake provides the picturesque setting each year for the Mountain Lake Symposium, begun by the Virginia Tech Department of Art and Art History. The event has gained national recognition as an art criticism conference. Supported by the Virginia Museum of Fine Arts, it is yet another jewel in the cultural crown of the Blue Ridge. While at Mountain Lake, also check out its Gallery, the home of the popular, whimsical Bob Evans Knobbits.

NEW RIVER VALLEY ARTS AND CRAFTS GUILD
U.S. 460, Pembroke   *(540) 626-3309*
Handmade treasures in the mountain tradition are both made and sold in the New River Valley Arts and Crafts Guild in the heart of Pembroke. There's usually a quilt in the making, as well as rug weaving and other activities going on among the 60 artists who display and sell here.

Hours are 10 AM to 5 PM Tuesday through Saturday an 1 to 4 PM Sunday.

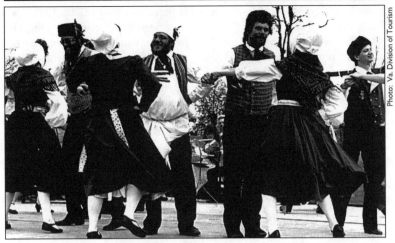

Traditional German dancing entertains visitors at the Museum of American Frontier Culture.

ANDREW JOHNSTON MUSEUM & RESEARCH CENTER

Main St., Pearisburg   (540) 921-5000

This restored brick house next to the Post Office is home to a genealogy library and historic Giles County displays. It is open by appointment.

Radford

Visual Arts

FLOSSIE MARTIN GALLERY

Radford University   (540) 831-5754

This modern facility occupies 2,000 square feet on the beautiful Radford University campus. The combination gallery/museum features rotating exhibits of both regional and nationally known artists. The gallery's roster has included the avant-garde John Cage, environmental artist Christo and Dr. Jehan Sadat (wife of the former leader of Egypt), who displayed her own personal Egyptian art collection.

Hours are 10 AM to 4 PM Monday through Friday, noon to 4 PM on Sunday

and extended hours of 6 to 9 PM on Thursday during fall and winter.

Theater

THE LONG WAY HOME OUTDOOR DRAMA

Ingles Homestead
Amphitheater   (540) 639-0679

For 23 years now, the only outdoor theater drama in Virginia has been wowing audiences with the Earl Hobson Smith historic epic, *The Long Way Home*. This exciting drama focuses on local history: the heroic adventure of Mary Draper Ingles.

Ingles was captured after fleeing from a 1755 attack by Indians on the north fork of the Roanoke River, where she saw her mother and infant nephew murdered by the Shawnees. Forced to travel west 800 miles to make salt for the tribe, the story tells of her courageous escape and long trek back to Radford to warn of an upcoming attack.

This saga is re-enacted in the Ingles Homestead Amphitheater at the heroine's homesite and grave — a must-see event for theater and history buffs.

Performances are given Thursday through Sunday, June through Labor Day. Tickets are $7 for adults and $3.50 for children ages 1 to 12.

Other Cultural Attractions

RADFORD UNIVERSITY COLLEGE OF VISUAL AND PERFORMING ARTS
(540) 831-5141

The university offers the public solo music performances, theater, art exhibits, classical ballet, Big Band music, jazz and modern dance. Call the university for a schedule.

Pulaski County

Visual Arts

THE FINE ARTS CENTER FOR THE NEW RIVER VALLEY
21 W. Main St.   *(540) 980-7363*

This facility is the cultural hub of the New River Valley, featuring contemporary works, music shows, private collections and amateur and professional artists. It is housed in a storefront building considered a prime example of Victorian commercial architecture. Built in 1898, the Center has been designated a Virginia Historic Landmark.

Other Cultural Attractions

HISTORIC OLD NEWBERN & WILDERNESS ROAD REGIONAL MUSEUM
New River Historical Society   *(540) 674-4835*

Nineteen original 1810 buildings comprise part of the 57 properties of the Old Newbern National Historic District, a neighborhood originally planned by early settlers. Newbern served as Pulaski

County's seat from 1839 to 1893, when the courthouse was destroyed by fire. This interesting tour takes you through the historic buildings, some already renovated and some in the process, including a slave cabin, old jail, rose garden, pre-Civil War church, buggy shed and small weather-boarded barn. The museum is filled with Civil War artifacts and sponsors a Civil War Re-enactors' Boot Camp and Civil War Weekend (Pulaski County is the site of the famous Battle of Cloyd's Mountain) to flea markets, dinners and holiday events.

Nearby are some great shops and restaurants, including Valley Pike Inn, Granny Swain's Country Store and PJ's Carousel Village, the world's largest manufacturer of carousel horses and animals.

Museum hours are 10:30 AM to 4:30 PM Tuesday through Saturday; 1:30 to 4:30 PM Sunday.

Alleghany Highlands Region

Visual Arts

ALLEGHANY HIGHLANDS ARTS & CRAFTS CENTER
439 E. Ridgeway St.
Clifton Forge   *(540) 862-4447*

The galleries' changing exhibits feature works by Alleghany Highlands artists and those from other areas. Among the fine regional art and hand-crafted products of juried quality on sale here are pottery, wooden ware, jewelry, stained glass, quilts and fiber arts.

The center is open 10 AM to 4:30 PM Monday through Saturday during May, June, July and August and Tuesday through Saturday October through April during the same hours.

THE HIGHLAND
COUNTY ARTS COUNCIL

P.O. Box 175
Monterey 24465   *No phone*

The Highland County Arts Council has provided children's programs, as well as artists in residence who go into the schools. Other projects are a Maple Festival crafts booth, Highland-style dance classes and storytelling.

Museums

BATH COUNTY
HISTORICAL SOCIETY MUSEUM

Courthouse Square   *(540) 839-2543*

Artifacts of Bath County and the Indian and Civil wars — books, apparel and photographs — are prominent here. It also has a genealogy library and has published a history of the county. The museum is open 8:30 AM to 4:30 PM Monday and Wednesday through Friday May through November. Tuesday hours are noon to 8 PM.

MAPLE MUSEUM

U.S. 220, Monterey   *(540) 468-2550*

In the land of maples is a museum celebrating old-time sugaring. See a replica of a sugar house, where you can watch sugar- and syrup-making demonstrations. Tools and equipment used by sugar makers throughout the years are displayed. Old-timers who can't otherwise get to the real sugar camps will find this especially interesting. It is open daily.

Music

GARTH NEWEL MUSIC CENTER

Hot Springs   *(540) 839-5018*

From among the giant hemlocks, the hills of Bath County come alive with the sound of music. The importance of the Garth Newel Center to the culture of the Alleghany Highlands and western Virginia cannot be underestimated. Musicians, students and awe-inspired audiences come together in this unspoiled mountain area to hear music by the likes of Mozart, Haydn and Dvorak, in an enchanting mountain setting.

The Center features the Garth Newel Chamber Players and Garth Newel Piano Trio. It provides an intensive residential Chamber Music Study Program for serious young musicians, who receive full scholarships. The architecture and acoustics of Herter Hall provide the perfect ambiance for chamber music and create a unique sense of being outdoors while actually indoors! Before the performance, many visitors have made it a tradition to join friends for a picnic on the grounds.

Garth Newel also sponsors holiday weekends that are a feast for lovers of chamber music, with gourmet meals, fine wine and convivial company.

Other Cultural Attractions

BEAR MOUNTAIN OUTDOOR SCHOOL

U.S. 250, Hightown   *(540) 468-2700*

Bear Mountain Outdoor School, on a 600-acre mountain farm at 4,200 feet in Highland County, at the headwaters of the Potomac River, merges practical experience with a refreshing vacation break from the fast track. Workshops, seminars and retreats are primarily week-long and weekend offerings from April through October, and include a variety of outdoor and rural pursuits. For example, the Building Skills and Rural Living Skills workshops/seminars are hands-on sessions for do-it-yourselfers; the Mountain Ecology and Family Retreats stress environmental responsibility and apprecia-

Alleghany Highlands
Region Profile:

Stewart H. Bostic

Imagine yourself on a steam excursion 40 years ago. The air is crisp and the leaves are just beginning to show fall colors as you steam through the mountain passes in the railroad coach of the Chesapeake & Ohio, one of America's great passenger trains.

Listen to the echo of the big steam locomotive's chime whistle as it rounds a bend in the track that snakes through the breathtaking Alleghany Highlands. Waiting for you at the historic Clifton Forge Railroad station is a day of fun.

Days gone by?

Not really, thanks to Stewart H. Bostic, a rail fan supreme who makes history come alive each year with excursions and events through the Chesapeake & Ohio Historical Society Archives and Rail Facilities. The group is one of the largest organizations in the world dedicated to the study of a single railroad, which traces its roots back to 1836.

The Societies publish a monthly magazine and have a collection of historic passenger and freight cars covering the period of the 1920s to the 1950s. The collection includes more than 100,000 ink-on-linen engineering and mechanical drawings, 50,000 photos and thousands of publications about the railroad that made the sleepy Alleghany County town of Clifton Forge boom and bustle long ago. Much of the credit for this vast railroad treasure trove belongs to Bostic, who worked for the C&O from 1944, at the age of 17, until his retirement in 1985.

In between, he served his country in the U.S. Army Air Corps from 1945 to 1947 and stayed in the Army Reserves through 1958. Not one to stay away from railroads for long, however, Bostic then served as a railway consultant from 1987 to 1992.

Over many years, Bostic, 68, not only helped establish the C&O Railroad Historical Society but also has served as archives building manager, assistant archivist, operations officer for COHS passenger cars and assistant to the COHS president.

His latest endeavor is helping to restore the old C&O Freight House and developing a railroad museum, passenger car shop and display area for the coaches the Society already has restored. In 1994 Bostic's group worked on fitting a combination car with display cases for programs for school children and for use as a traveling museum. This year's project is finishing up a caboose and Kanawha club car.

Bostic's wife, Ida Marie, a native of nearby Ronceverte, West Virginia, says her husband is never happier than when he's "tinkering and sweating" on restoring a bedraggled old railroad car with his friends. Although that's sometimes difficult for Ida Marie to understand, it's nevertheless a romance that many others share. The C&O Railroad Historical Society now has 2,500 members in 49 states.

Lest anyone think, however, that Bostic's interests are strictly historical, one need only look at his many other civic endeavors to enhance the quality of life in Alleghany County. He is a deacon at Temple Baptist, a Shriner and a member of the American Legion.

Alleghany Chamber of Commerce director Michelle Wright calls Bostic one of the county's "most active, best-known, tireless supporters for tourism." Chairman of its Ambassadors Committee, Bostic even arranged to have a railroad caboose donated to the Chamber for its promotional efforts.

For some, trains are a hobby. For others, trains are their life. Stewart Bostic says trains have been both a joy and an education for him. In 1994 Bostic discovered he has lymphomic cancer. However, he says his treatments have progressed well and that he's optimistic that the cancer will soon be in remission. He hasn't let it interfere with the important work at hand, restoring a former way of life that he wants to share with future generations. Sharing that love of the history of the iron horse has made the Alleghany Highlands a better community for thousands of residents and visitors.

tion. Qualified instructors who are experts in their fields lead the workshops

The Lodge, rustic cabins and outdoor teaching areas draw guests from around the country who share a common interest. Meals focus on natural foods, and evening activities heighten the enjoyment of this mountain top vacation. All programs include lodging, meals and instructional materials. Bear Mountain can design custom programs for organized groups by special arrangements. Call Thomas Brody, owner/director, for a schedule.

CHESAPEAKE & OHIO HISTORICAL SOCIETY

312 E. Ridgeway St.
Clifton Forge   *(800) 453-2647*

This international railroad historical society deals with the history of the Chesapeake & Ohio Railway. Its predecessors and successors operated in Virginia, West Virginia, Kentucky, Ohio, Michigan, Indiana and Ontario. The organization's archives division has one of the largest institutional collections devoted to a single railway, including more than 100,000 ink-on-linen original engineering drawings, 50,000 mechanical drawings and 50,000 photographic images, dating from the 1870s to 1980s. A library contains thousands of books, magazines and pamphlets devoted to railroad history in general and C&O history in particular. The Society also owns 19 pieces of historic original C&O railroad equipment, some of which is open for display by appointment, and some in storage awaiting restoration. Several passenger cars have been restored and are used to interpret the railway experience at special events in Clifton Forge and over several states. The premier restored passenger car is the dining car Gadsby's Tavern. The Society, which has more than 2,700 members in 50 states, produces the annual Chessie Calendar, carrying on an unbroken tradition begun by the railway in 1934.

The archives and gift shop are open 9 AM to 5 PM Monday through Saturday year round.

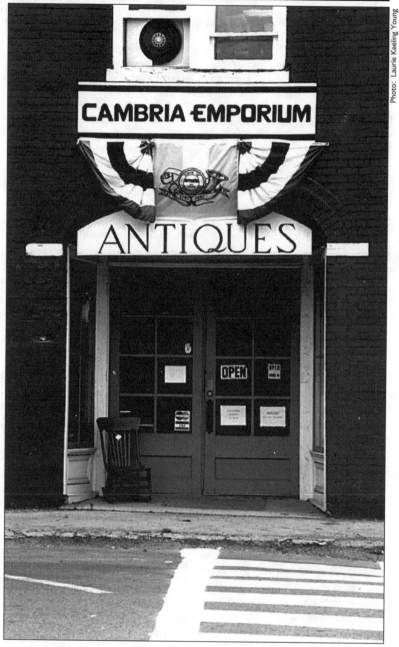

Antique lovers can take advantage of the multitude of antique shops throughout the Blue Ridge.

Inside
Shopping

Whether you're looking for antiques, handcrafts or outlet malls for bargains in clothing and housewares, the Blue Ridge region has it all. Of course, there are the usual shopping malls, Wal-Marts and Kmarts. But most towns in the Blue Ridge have at least one quaint little antique shop and a place that sells the work of local craftsmen.

Some fine furniture makers in the region, such as E.A. Clore in Madison or Suter's in Harrisonburg, sell directly to the consumer. You must visit their showrooms to see what they make, because you won't find their beautiful furniture elsewhere.

This is also true for the shops selling fine handcrafts. Places such as the Blue Ridge Pottery on U.S. 33 near Skyline Drive and Limeton Pottery in Front Royal specialize in ceramics that are crafted literally right next door. Other shops, such as Forever Country in New Market and the Handcraft House in Madison, represent dozens of artisans whose creations also cannot be found in department stores.

Charlottesville is known for its fine downtown shops that sell crafts and other objets d'art from around the globe. There, you can just as easily find an African mask as a bar of American soap.

If you're visiting from out of state and want a made-in-Virginia souvenir, there are plenty of shops specializing in such products. Virginia Born and Bred in Lexington is one fine example, selling beautiful brass and silver items as well as folk art, woven goods, peanuts, jams and jellies. Virginia Made in Staunton is another.

The following is a description of some of our favorite shops in the cities, towns and rural areas we've covered in this guidebook. This is in no way a comprehensive listing, and we may have inadvertently missed your favorite shop. Also, in the retail world, shops come and go, so call ahead if you have your heart set on a particular store. This seems especially true in the antiques trade. We've given you the businesses' phone numbers here — something *Insiders' Guides*® typically do not include in chapters such as this — to save you possible disappointment at the end of a long drive.

Drop us a line and give us your Insider's perspective if you know of a top-notch place we've missed.

Shenandoah Valley Region

Winchester

One of the finest places in the region to find handcrafted jewelry, clothing, ceramics and home furnishings is **Winchester's Handworks Gallery**, (540) 662-3927, in the Loudoun Street Mall (for pedestrians only). Around the corner on W. Piccadilly Street is the beautiful **Colonial Art and Craft Shop**, (540) 662-6513, which sells fine china, crystal and silver, elegant lamps and picture frames. **Kimberly's Antiques and Linens**, (540) 662-2195, is not too far away on N. Braddock Street. Housed in Civil War general Sheridan's headquarters, Kimberly's sells 19th-century artwork, antique quilts and crochet spreads, and fine bed linens. **Claire's**, (540) 662-0344, is one of several shops in Creekside Village, a Williamsburg-style shopping development on U.S. 11 south of Winchester. Claire's carries women's clothing, and the other shops' wares vary from dolls to pewter carvings.

Strasburg

Strasburg considers itself the antique capital of Virginia. We don't necessarily endorse this claim, but we do agree that very fine antiques can be found here at fair prices. Whether you're a serious collector or someone who just likes to drool at beautiful things, you must visit the **Strasburg Emporium**, (540) 465-3711, a 65,000-square-foot downtown building that houses more than 100 antique and art dealers. The building, right on N. Massanutten Street, used to be a silk mill. Along with high quality formal and country furniture, you'll find a lot of unusual items at the Emporium, such as old carousel horses, hobby horses, carriages, stoneware and iron beds. The Strasburg Emporium is open daily and has plenty of free parking.

Bits, Bytes & Books, (540) 465-4200, on W. King Street, has a vast collection of old and new mysteries, westerns, science fiction and children's books, locally

crafted gifts and glass collectibles. The **Cedar Creek Relic Shop**, (540) 869-5207, a couple of miles away in downtown Middletown, claims to have the largest collection of authentic Civil War relics for sale in the Shenandoah Valley. If you're hankering for a sword, bayonet, musket or an artillery shell from that bloody war this shop has it.

Front Royal

If you follow U.S. 522 S. from Winchester toward Front Royal on a weekend, you'll find that traffic slows to a crawl at a big outdoor flea market where you can find almost anything. On Commerce Street in Front Royal, a smaller weekend flea market is a fun place to browse, and you can make some good finds among the array of books, T-shirts, tools and other items.

In downtown Front Royal, the **Limeton Pottery** studio and gallery, (540) 636-8666, features locally made stoneware and earthenware pottery, along with note cards, baskets and other handcrafted items. **Simonpietri's Gift Shop**, (540) 635-3558) on U.S. 522 S. at the edge of town has a kitschy mixture of tourist items and crafts. The **Royal Oak Bookshop**, (540) 635-7070, on S. Royal Avenue, has a wonderful selection of new and used books. It's open seven days a week, but if you stop by after hours, you can sort through a selection of free books to get you through the night. Across the street is **J's Gourmet**, (504) 636-9293, where you can purchase Virginia wines, exotic coffees and spices, breads, meats and cheeses. Across from the visitors center on Main Street is **Valley Crafters**, (540) 635-4699, a shop selling baby doll clothes, quilts and country crafts.

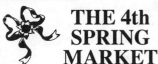
Luray

In downtown Luray, **Mama's Treasures**, (540) 743-1352, has an extensive collection of colorful glassware and old costume jewelry, along with some antique furniture and quilts. **Zib's Country Connection**, (540) 743-7394, on E. Main, offers a collection of unique Victorian greeting cards, handcrafted gifts, collectibles and some antiques. Five miles east of Luray on Va. 211, at the entrance to the Shenandoah National Park, sits the **Pine Knoll Gift Shop**, (540) 743-5805. This old-time store is crammed with Elvis and Hank Williams souvenirs, knives, quilts, baskets, coonskin caps, Native American moccasins and jewelry, jams and jellies, fireworks, great fudge and peanut brittle.

New Market

New Market's downtown **Paper Treasures**, (540) 740-3135, is a fascinating place to browse through old books, magazines and prints. The store sells old copies of *Collier's Weekly*, *The Saturday Evening Post*, *Ebony*, *Life* and old Civil War maps and books. It also carries a good selection of children's literature.

Shenandoah Valley Crafts and Gifts, (540) 740-3899, on Congress Street (U.S. 11), has a great mix of country furniture, fireworks, hand-loomed rugs, quilts and Virginia hams — and don't miss the Rock Shop. Also on Congress Street is the **Christmas Gallery**, (540) 740-3000, which sells handmade crafts, wreaths, snow babies and hundreds of ornaments.

Woodstock-Edinburg

Seven Bends Gallery, (540) 459-5525, in downtown Woodstock displays and sells original watercolors and photographs of the valley, along with stoneware pottery, hand-woven coverlets, stained-glass lamps, '50s collectibles and other handcrafted items. Woodstock is also home to an **Aileen Stores Inc.** outlet, (540) 459-3077, that sells women's sportswear for up to 70 percent off retail.

Every Saturday and Sunday, a huge flea market takes place between

Woodstock and Edinburg, offering antiques and collectibles both inside and outdoors. To get to **The Flea Market**, (540) 984-8771, take Exit 283 from I-81. It's off U.S. 11 on Landfill Road.

Richard's Antiques, (540) 984-4502, a mile south of Edinburg on U.S. 11, specializes in fine country and formal antiques and paintings.

Harrisonburg and Rockingham County

ANTIQUES

Nearly two dozen antique shops can be found throughout this area, which includes not just the thriving university city of Harrisonburg but also the little towns of Mt. Crawford, McGaheysville, Dayton and Elkton.

Chalot's Antiques, (540) 433-0872, is a mecca for lovers of fine old furniture. Right on Main Street in tiny Mt. Crawford, in a building nearly 200 years old, the shop deals in high quality 18th- and 19th-century furniture. There are hundreds of pieces of flow blue China in this shop, along with Victorian bric-a-brac, primitive accessories and old glassware.

The Antique Mart, (540) 289-MART, in McGaheysville is a restored old bank building that houses 25 shops of furniture and other collectibles. Farther east, in Elkton, is one of the area's finer antique shops, the **Curiosity Shop**, (540) 298-1404, where you'll find antique furniture, folk art, primitives, quilts and old tools for the most discriminating buyer.

Jeff's Antiques, (540) 879-9961, in Dayton specializes in oak and walnut furniture and also carries pottery, primitives, toys and oil lamps.

In the Dayton Farmer's Market you'll find **Log Cabin Antiques**, (540) 434-9885, among an array of shops.

Downtown Harrisonburg has several shops selling antiques and collectibles, most notably **James McHone Antique Jewelry**, (540) 433-1833. Here you will find exquisite estate and antique jewelry, sterling flatware and oil paintings. **Villager Antiques**, (540) 433-7226, sells painted country glassware and pottery, along with oak and walnut formal furniture.

HANDCRAFTS

The Mennonite-operated **Gift and Thrift Shop**, (540) 433-8844, in downtown Harrisonburg takes you around the globe with its selection of gorgeous weavings, ceramics, clothing and other crafts made in about 35 developing nations. Many of the craftsmen are refugees, disadvantaged minorities or people with physical disabilities. The proceeds go to the Mennonite Central Committee, the relief and development wing of the church. The prices are great, and spending money here helps people in need.

Suter's, (540) 434-2131, at 2610 S. Main Street has been around since the early 1800s, when Daniel Suter, a skilled Mennonite cabinetmaker and carpenter, settled in the Harrisonburg area and began making furniture. Today, William Suter and his daughter, Carol, carry on the family tradition of quality craftsmanship. The company makes gorgeous Colonial reproductions in cherry, mahogany and walnut, using the finest techniques. They have showrooms here and in Richmond, or you can send for a color catalog.

Tucked away in the **Skyline Village Shopping Center** on E. Market Street is an unexpected place to find unique handcrafted porcelain jewelry, pottery, wooden ware, rugs and other crafts. **The**

Bay Pottery, (540) 432-1580, also has a store in nearby Broadway on S. Main Street.

It's definitely worth driving to the little town of Dayton, just south of Harrisonburg, for the **Dayton Farmer's Market**, (540) 879-9885, a place where the merchants are incredibly friendly. Inside the indoor market on Va. 42, peddlers sell fresh poultry, seafood, beef, home-baked goods, fresh fruits and vegetables, cheeses, nuts and other dried goods. Specialty shops carry Early American tin lighting, pottery, quality antiques and handcrafts, clothes and even grandfather clocks. You can have a hearty, delicious lunch at **Huyard's Country Kitchen** inside the market. Nearby in Dayton is the **Clothes Line**, (540) 879-2505, a fabric shop that also sells brilliantly colored hand-woven rugs and quilts. There's a hitching post out front where buggy-riding Mennonites tie their horses while they shop.

East of Harrisonburg in McGaheysville is the **Country Goose Gift and Craft Shop**, (540) 289-9626, that sells fine crafts made in the Shenandoah Valley. It's a short drive from Massanutten Resort on Va. 996. Here you will find salt-glazed pottery, handmade country furniture, folk art, baskets, benches, pillows, quilt racks, weavings and much more.

OTHER UNUSUAL SHOPPING SPOTS

The central business district has some specialty shops worth a visit, such as **Touch the Earth**, (540) 434-2895, with its Native American clothing, African jewelry and other exotic gifts.

North of Harrisonburg near Timberville, is a great place to partake of the region's sweetest crop of all: apples. **Showalter's Orchard and Greenhouse**, (540) 896-7582, on Va. 881, has its own cider mill and sells freshly pressed cider and many varieties of apples from late September through December 1. **Ryan's Fruit Market**, (540) 896-1233, on Va. 613 northwest of Timberville, sells apples, peaches, sweet cider and pumpkins from the first of September to mid-November.

Locals flock to the **Green Valley Book Fair**, (540) 434-4260, which is held several weekends in the spring, summer, fall and winter at a warehouse near Mt. Crawford. Every spring and fall there is also a record fair, lasting only a single weekend. New books and records are sold at cut-rate prices.

Staunton and Augusta County

ANTIQUES

Historic downtown Staunton is full of interesting boutiques, including many antique shops — so many, that Staunton has a brochure just for antique shopping! Staunton has a treasure trove of architectural delights packed into five National Historic Districts, offering numerous places to hunt for antiques. Twenty-two shops are listed in the new brochure, many within walking distance of one another. **Rose Street Interiors**, (540) 886-0578, at 2209 N. Augusta, sells some exquisite furniture but mostly curios, lamps, pillows, crafts, gifts and custom frames.

In the renovated Wharf Area is **Depot Antiques**, (540) 885-8326, a lovely shop featured in *Southern Living*, where you'll find country formal furniture, folk art and gifts. Across the street, you can get lost in the **Jolly Roger Haggle Shop**, (540) 886-9527, a collector's paradise with coins, jewelry, china, old money, weapons, Civil War and Native American artifacts and much more. Another great place to buy antiques is the **Belle Grae**

Inn, (540) 886-5151, at 515 W. Frederick Street, where you can also stay overnight and dine in the inn's fine restaurant.

Just north of Staunton, **Dusty's Antique Market**, (540) 248-2018, houses more than a dozen dealers of oak and walnut furniture, tools, quilts, primitives and other old things, and the nearby **Rocky's Antique Mart**, (540) 234-9900, is headquarters for dozens of dealers selling everything from brass beds and china presses to gorgeous estate jewelry and sterling silver.

Also north of Staunton is the **Verona Flea Market**, (540) 0248-3532, which is open Thursday through Sunday. Thirty dealers sell a large variety of oak, pine, cherry, walnut and other antique furniture, along with quilts and linens, old books, china and more.

HANDCRAFTS

The **Virginia Made Shop**, (540) 886-7180, off Exit 222 on I-81, has an extensive collection of foods, wines, handcrafts and other souvenirs from the Commonwealth. It's right next to the **Bacova Guild**, (800) 544-6118, famous for silk-screened handcrafts and Rowe's Family Restaurant, an excellent place to sample down-home regional cooking and a favorite hangout for the Statler Brothers. The cookies here are big, homemade and delicious, as are the pies.

Silver Linings on W. Beverley, (540) 885-7808, in the downtown is a popular shop with tourists and locals. You'll find jewelry, including exotic and hard-to-find beads, and folk art from around the world, along with clothes, pocketbooks and funky bric-a-brac. Across the street is the fascinating **Once Upon a Time Clock Shop**, (540) 885-6064, which sells antique wall clocks of every variety. It's "open by chance or by appointment."

Elder's Antique and Classic Autos, (540) 885-0500, on New Street, has a big window through which you can see sleek old Rolls Royces and other beauties.

OTHER UNUSUAL SHOPPING SPOTS

A brochure, "The Gift Connection," highlights 15 unique shopping experiences in the historic downtown district. Get your copy by calling the visitors center at (800) 332-5219.

The first block of E. Beverley in downtown Staunton is a fun place to browse through shops and have lunch. The **Pampered Palate**, (540) 886-9463, sells gourmet sandwiches and also has an unusually good selection of Virginia, French and Italian wines. They do gift baskets too. Next door, **Grandma's Bait Clothing Store**, (540) 886-2222, carries fine clothing for infants and children, and the **Golden Tub Bath Shop**, (540) 885-8470, sells everything for the bath, including elegant soaps, towels and accessories. **Holt's China**, (540) 885-0217, at 16 E. Beverley, specializes in beautiful china, Madam Alexander dolls, fine glassware, special occasion gifts and children's books. **The Emporium**, (540) 885-1673, 101 E. Beverley, features a large selection of toys and gifts. **Arthur's**, (540) 885-8609, at 3 E. Beverley, has a dazzling collection of lamps, Colonial Williamsburg reproductions and brass, pewter and silver items. And fanciers of odds and ends will want to browse through **Collector's Choice**, (540) 885-8572, at 18 W. Beverley. The downtown emporium has a wonderful selection of sculptures, dolls, toys, collector's plates and figurines, among other curios.

And book lovers can get their fill of best-sellers and all types of new books at **The Bookstack**, (540) 885-2665, 1 E. Beverley Street. The shop also carries gift items, T-shirts and stationery.

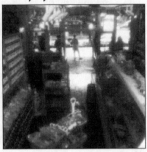
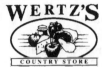
Waynesboro and Stuarts Draft

The **Waynesboro Village Factory Outlet Mall**, (540) 949-5000, right off I-64, houses dozens of specialty shops carrying discounted brand-name clothing, shoes, luggage, home furnishings, lingerie and more. Liz Claiborne, Corning/Revere, Bass Shoes, Van Heusen, Barbizon, Leather Loft, L'eggs/Hanes/Bali and Bugle Boy are but a few of the stores at this attractively designed outdoor mall. Arts and crafts vendors often sell quality merchandise in the center area of the mall. Every Wednesday is Gallery Night, a time for music and art.

The **Virginia Metalcrafters** outlet in the mall will probably stir your curiosity enough to make you fight for a parking place at their foundry, showroom and retail store, (540) 949-9432, downtown at 1010 E. Main Street. Through an observation window, you can watch craftsmen use the age-old technique of pouring molten brass into sand molds, then grinding, sanding and polishing the rough castings into faithful reproductions of 17th-and 18th-century brass objects. The foundry reproduces candlesticks, lighting fixtures, fireplace tools and other pieces from historic places such as Colonial Williamsburg, Charleston, Newport, Monticello, Winterthur and Old Sturbridge Village.

Another special find in Waynesboro is **The Christmas Store**, (540) 943-6246, at 326 W. Main Street. It carries Christmas collectibles, Snow Village, Heritage Village, Radko, figural ornaments, antique Santa reproductions and American Christmas folk art.

A number of Mennonite-operated businesses make shopping a real pleasure in the Stuarts Draft area. **Kinsinger's Kountry Kitchen**, (540) 337-2668, on Va. 651, sells breads, cookies, cakes and pies made from scratch. The hummingbird cake and cheese herb bread are out of this world. About a half-mile away on Va. 608 is **The Cheese Shop**, (540) 337-4224, an Amish-Mennonite family business since 1960. The store sells more than 30 varieties of cheese at great prices, along with nuts, dried fruits and other dry foods in bulk. The Cheese Shop is closed on Sundays.

The Candy Shop, (540) 337-0298, on Va. 608 near U.S. 340, sells a complete line of Hershey products, including reproductions of early tins and glass. There are no tours at the nearby Hershey plant in Stuarts Draft, but some of the items made there include Reese's Pieces, Whatchmacallits and Bar None. The Candy Shop also carries quilts, which they will custom make, along with handmade furniture.

In downtown Waynesboro at 328 W. Main St. is the **Valley Framing Studio and Gallery**, (540) 943-7529, which claims it has the Shenandoah Valley's largest inventory of frame supplies, limited edition prints and bronzes, as well as ceramics and other gifts. The white building next door at 326 W. Main is the **Christmas Store**, (540) 943-6246, which year round peddles the spirit of the yuletide season along with other arts, crafts and interesting curios.

Lexington

ANTIQUES

The **Lexington Historical Shop**, (540) 463-2615, in College Square Shopping Center, is the only shop of its kind in Virginia. It specializes in Confederate-related original materials — autographs, documents, books, prints, soldiers' letters, flags, belt buckles, uniforms and more — to awe any Civil War buff. Owner Bob Lurate also offers Virginia-related histories, maps and other documents, along with antique quilts and other collectibles. A catalog is available.

One of the finest antique stores in the Rockbridge County region is **Old South Antiques Ltd.**, (540) 348-5360, in the charming village of Brownsburg, 15 minutes north of Lexington via U.S. 11/710

or Va. 39/252. Old South specializes in New England, Pennsylvania and Southern antiques in original paint and refinished cherry, walnut and pine. The shop is recommended by American Country South for its country-style wares and known for its large selection of American Country furniture and accessories.

Braford Antiques, (540) 291-2217, on Va. 130, is another exquisite shop down the road from Natural Bridge. The Brafords have a fine collection of 19th-century American furniture and pieces from Asia.

GENERAL STORES

Enjoy a step back in time with the Lexington area's two real general stores, **The General Store**, (540) 261-3860, 2522 Beech Avenue in Buena Vista, and the **Olde Country Store**, (540) 348-1300, on Va. Byway 39 in historic Rockbridge Baths. Both have been in business 100 years and in many ways actually are working museums. Don't miss the made-in-Virginia items and country crafts. Maury River even offers you the once-in-a-lifetime opportunity to visit an old-fashioned working outhouse! And next door is a swinging bridge across the river — a rare find these days. In Buena Vista, visitors love The General Store, with its early farm and transportation exhibit and century-old display cases. Aromas waft through the old building, where you can find a bit of everything, including blue jeans, bulk seed, fabric and kitchenwares.

HANDCRAFTS

Artists in Cahoots, (540) 464-1147, is a cooperative gallery of local artists and crafters downtown at 1 Washington Street. You'll find oil and watercolors, pottery, metalwork, hand-blown glass, photography, sculpture, hand-painted silk scarves and porcelain jewelry.

OTHER UNUSUAL SHOPPING SPOTS

Downtown shopping is a panorama of boutique-type shops that will keep you browsing all day. For gifts, try **Fantasies**, (540) 463-7222, at 21 Nelson Street, for the new, subtle and dazzling. **Virginia Born and Bred**, (800) 437-2452, at 16 W. Washington Street, is a sophisticated shop chock-full of Old Dominion handcrafts, wine, fine brass work, linens and more. For sleek or funky dresses and exotic jewelry and accessories, don't miss **Pappagallo**, (540) 463-5988, at 23 N. Main. If new and used books are your idea of a perfect afternoon of browsing, go to the **Second Story**, (540) 463-6264, in College Square Shopping Center, or **The Best Seller**, (540) 463-4647, on Nelson Street.

T.G.I.F., (540) 463-9730, 30 S. Main, is a popular destination for Washington & Lee students, with its seconds from J. Crew, Tweeds and other fashionable clothing manufacturers.

If you're hankering for chocolate, head down to **Cocoa Mill Chocolates**, (540) 464-8400, on W. Nelson Street. Hand-dipped, scrumptious confections are sold individually or by the box, and the owners also have a mail-order service.

In Rockbridge County, on Va. 606 at Racine, Don Haynie and Tom Hamlin welcome you to the wonderful world of herbs in a big way. They are the darlings of the local garden club set for the way they have renovated **Buffalo Springs Herb Farm**, (540) 348-1083, an extraordinary 18th-century stone house and garden open for herbal teas, luncheons and tours. These two perfectionists have a huge following for their herb workshops that always feature flawless food (such as hand-pressed herbal cookies) and decor. There is a gorgeous gift shop in a big red barn that sells herbal products, dried flowers and garden books. Their display gardens look like something out of Williamsburg. You'll see a culinary garden, springhouse tea garden and four-square heirloom vegetable and herb garden.

To make a wonderful trip even better, Buffalo Springs is next to historic **Wades Mill**, (540) 348-1400, a working water-powered flour mill that is listed on the National Register of Historic Places. The mill is open from April to mid-December and produces and sells all kinds of bread flours, cornmeal, cereal and bran. They also sell gift boxes.

Botetourt County, Troutville and Fincastle

ANTIQUES

Many a Roanoker loves to take a trip out to the cool, crisp countryside in autumn, buy apples from the county orchards and go antiquing. The opportunities are numerous on U.S. 11 heading into Troutville and U.S. 220 on the way to historic Fincastle. Both towns have more than their fair share of terrific little antique shops. In Troutville, the **Troutville Antique Mart**, (540) 992-4249, beside the Troutville Fire Station, provides the best opportunity for browsing under one roof. Here, a dozen dealers display fine antiques and collectibles, and the prices are some of the lowest you'll find. How about a first-class 1890s leather and wooden trunk for $100? You may find it here.

HANDCRAFTS

A real unexpected gem in a rural area, in the same building as a swimming pool store and monument designer, **Amerind Gallery**, (540) 992-1066, U.S. 220 N., Daleville, specializes in artwork of Native American and western artists. It is a member of the Indian Arts and Crafts Association and guarantees the authenticity of every Native American handmade item in the gallery. A visit here is a veritable education in American art forms and cultures, expressed in superb original works, including a wide selection of the same beautiful silver jewelry you would find in New Mexico.

Across town, in Troutville, there's a breath of fresh air in every gift at Al and Rachael Nichol's **Apple Barn**, (540) 992-3551, off U.S. 11 on a working apple farm. You can browse through country collectibles sipping a complimentary cup of hot, spiced cider and buy or pick your own bag of apples before you leave the picturesque orchard setting. The store is an exclusive outlet for Cat's Meow collectibles and is its No. 1 dealer. Rachael also has a new store in Buchanan, a town with a growing Main Street program. All the latest Roanoke Valley collection can be found in these shops.

ORCHARDS

Botetourt County is apple orchard country. There's nothing more beautiful than the acres of delicate apple blossoms that signal the coming of spring in the Blue Ridge. The county has quite a few orchards, large and small. Probably the biggest and best-known are **Ikenberry**, (540) 992-2448, and **Layman's**, (540) 992-2687, both on U.S. 220 in Daleville. In addition to apples of every kind, you can buy such seasonal specials as pumpkins, sweet corn and peaches. As each year goes by, more and more orchardists are selling off their vast spreads to meet the demand for developable land. How long this area will be known for its orchards is questionable.

Craig County

Whatever your need, you'll find it at **New Castle Mercantile**, (540) 864-5560, at 325 Main Street. In this tiny mountain community, New Castle Mercantile fills the bill for seeds, animal feed, hardware, housewares and toys. If you grew up in the country, this place will bring back memories of the stores your grandparents took you to on trips into town.

Roanoke

ANTIQUES

The Roanoke Valley is a treasure chest of top-notch, low-cost antiques. When movie star Debbie Reynolds' daughter, actress and author Carrie Fisher, came to visit at her mom's Roanoke home, antiquing was the first thing she wanted to do — and she spent all day! What you'll find is a tremendous variety downtown. **Trudy's Antiques**, (540) 343-2004, 12 Wells Avenue N.E., specializes in old prints and advertising, dolls, jewelry and glassware. **Sandra's Cellar**, (540) 342-8123, 120 Campbell Avenue S.E., is a nostalgic trip through vintage clothing, furniture and toys. **Bob Beard Antiques**, (540) 981-1757, is open "by chance or appointment" at 105 Market Street, and it's a source of unexpected finds. The slogan at **Russell's Yesteryear**, (540) 342-1750, 117 E. Campbell Avenue, is "When you visit the Market, stop in and see us. If you don't, we both lose money." Lovers of Civil War antiques will want to visit historian Howard McManus' shop, **Magic City Station**, (540) 344-2302, at 11 S. Jefferson Street, to see his collection of memorabilia. McManus is an expert on the Battle of Cloyd's Mountain in Pulaski County and the war in Southwest Virginia. For a complete list of antique shops in the Valley, call (540) 342-6025.

HANDCRAFTS

If fine handcrafts are what you're seeking, look no farther than the historic **City Market**. You will find the perfect gift and probably end up buying something for yourself, as well. **Gallery 3**, (540) 343-9698, 213 Market Street, offers the epitome of art for the kitchen, wood, glass, gifts and clothing. Gallery 3 is a favorite shopping spot for corporate art collectors too, who will find works by both local and nationally known artists. On the first Friday of each month, Gallery 3 offers Art By Night, featuring local artists and their work. Custom framing also is available.

Also located on the Market, at 206 Market Square, is **Studios on the Square**, (540) 345-4076, a second-floor studio where 18 working artists demonstrate and sell wares that include pottery, paper, fiber, wood, textiles, jewelry, baskets, stained glass, photography and fine paintings. The climb upstairs to this treasure house of arts and crafts stores is well worth it. You'll think you're in a loft in New York, and chances are you won't leave empty handed. *V Magazine* offices are also up here, and Editor Jim Cubby would love the chance to talk to you about all the nightlife and goings on throughout the Blue Ridge.

OUTLETS

On U.S. 220 S., hunters and those who like the camouflage look can track down bargains at **Trebark Outfitters**, (540) 774-9007, 3434 Buck Mountain Road. Jim Crumley, the inventor of Trebark camouflage, lives in Roanoke and offers good deals at his store. Hunting and fishing lovers and fans of the sporting life will also enjoy the **Orvis Factory Outlet**, (540) 344-4520, downtown at 21-B Campbell Avenue. Summers are an especially good time to shop, since you can get discounts of up to 80 percent on winter

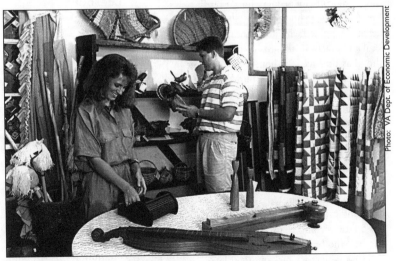

Photo: VA Dept. of Economic Development

Shoppers in the Blue Ridge can find an array of mountain crafts and gifts.

items offered in their national catalog and in the Orvis Retail Store just a block away.

Tremendous buys in hand-made pottery can be found at the **Emerson Creek Pottery** outlet, (540) 342-7656, at 108 Market Street. Also downtown, but a little more difficult to find, is **Design Accessories**, (540) 344-8958, on First Street, an outlet store for custom-made Austrian crystal jewelry. Again, you can find discounts of 70 percent or more on watches, jewelry and accessories featured in national bridal magazines. For household items, go to **Crossroads Mall** on Williamson Road to **Waccamaw Pottery**, (540) 563-4948.

SPECIALTY STORES

Specialty stores and boutiques abound throughout the Roanoke City Market. In the Market Building, which anchors the popular shopping area, you can buy surplus Army gear at **Sam's On the Market**, (540) 342-7300, 304 Market Street. **Greenfields**, (540) 345-5139, specializes in better-quality sports jerseys and sports caps. A shop just for people who like birds, **For the Birds**, (540) 345-9393, 303 Market Street, is filled with items both whimsical and practical, all bird-oriented. The shop has bird feeders, houses and seed, books and tapes, binoculars, bird-themed clothing and gifts and a large selection of garden items (bird baths, fountains and little critters for your garden).

Several popular Blacksburg stores in the New River Valley have branches here, including **Books, Strings & Things**, (540) 342-5511, 202 Market Square, a great place to browse among tapes, CDs, books, cards and calendars. Its children's corner has a little rocking chair, which endears parents who bring their prodigy to read and rock while they pick out their favorite oldies. **House Unique Galleria**, (540)

345-0697, is another remarkable shop here. Fine arts, crafts and gifts for the home and office, children's toys and other delightful finds are displayed beautifully.

And **La De Da**, (540) 345-6131, a whimsical boutique for women's clothing, caters to the young and young-in-spirit with flowing clothing that look like it came straight out of a dreamy TV commercial.

Printer's Ink, (540) 774-3445, a full-service bookstore at 4917 Grandin Road Ext., carries all kinds of books, magazines, Hallmark cards and gift items and Dept. 56 items. Another good place to buy books and magazines is **Ram's Head Bookshop**, (540) 344-1237, in the Tower Shopping Mall on Colonial Avenue.

The major malls in the area — Crossroads, Tanglewood and Valley View — also have some specialty stores.

East of the Blue Ridge Region

Leesburg and Loudoun County

You won't find any monolithic mega-malls in beautiful Loudoun County, but that doesn't mean there's no place to shop. Grab your wallet and head for historic downtown Leesburg (intersection of U.S. 7 and U.S. 15), where more than 100 specialty retailers do business along Market and King streets. The city's colorful Market Station, at the corner of Loudoun and Harrison streets, offers another 100 or so shops, and, if you still haven't had enough, more than 250 stores stretch along the U.S. 7 corridor up to the Fairfax County line. This route will take you through the communities of Ashburn, Sterling and Sterling Park.

West of Leesburg on U.S. 7 in Round Hill is **Hill High's Country Store**, (540) 338-7173, where you can shop for handmade crafts and rest from your shopping labors with a deli sandwich or a wedge of hot fruit pie.

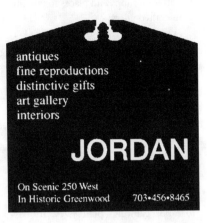

antiques
fine reproductions
distinctive gifts
art gallery
interiors

JORDAN

On Scenic 250 West
In Historic Greenwood   703•456•8465

Middleburg

At the southern edge of Loudoun County is Middleburg, the capital of Virginia's Hunt Country. Washington Street (U.S. 50), the town's main artery, is lined with antique, clothing, saddle, book and jewelry shops — more than 60 stores in the historic district alone. Wander down the cobbled side streets to find more antiques, riding clothes, home furnishings, handcrafted gifts, clothing and art.

The Finicky Filly, (540) 687-6841, carries very upscale women's clothing, accessories and gifts. The **Middleburg Antiques Center**, (540) 687-5551, has a selection of period antiques, rugs, silver and estate items on consignment. Be sure to check out the **White Elephant**, (540) 687-8800, another consignment shop, which handles everything from antiques to clothing. It's not unusual to find treasures such as a pair of barely used Gucci shoes — and even more fun to speculate as to what Middleburg celeb might have worn them. Washington Street's **Dominion Saddlery**, (540) 687-6720, and the **Tack Box**, (540) 687-3231, on Federal Street cater to the equestrian crowd and have delightful Hunt Country gifts. **The Fun Shop**, (540)687-6590, on Washington Street has an interesting array of gifts.

Several exceptional art galleries here include **Red Fox Fine Art**, (540) 687-6301, behind the Red Fox Tavern; and **The Sporting Gallery**, (540) 687-6447, on Washington Street, the town's oldest gallery. Both have paintings and bronzes of the calibre you'd expect in a major city.

Warrenton and Fauquier County

Like Leesburg, Warrenton's exterior is choked with malls and fast-food places, but the historic center of town is still a fun place to shop. Among the many antique stores are three on Main Street: **Courthouse Antiques**, (540) 349-9275, which has furniture ranging from the early 18th century to the 20th century; **Loveladies Antiques**, (540) 349-8786, which has a 16,000-item inventory ranging from textiles, art glass, fine china and sterling to estate jewelry and furniture; and **Antiques and Accents**, (540) 349-8021, a charming shop with beautifully displayed items from primitive to formal, including hand-painted furniture.

Washington

This tiny community of fewer than 200 residents in Rappahannock County boasts a number of sophisticated galleries, antique shops and places to buy fine handcrafted gifts.

Peter Kramer, (540) 675-3625, at Gay and Jett streets has been making beautiful furniture for 25 years in this lovely old town. Each of his creations is one-of-a-kind, a hand-crafted creation made from native American wood. Some of the furniture is rather whimsical, while other pieces are more classical and austere.

The **Rush River Company,** (540) 675-1136, a crafts gallery on Main Street, displays and sells works of more than 20 artists. You'll find furniture, fabrics, photographs, paintings, pottery, jewelry, baskets and clothing here.

The **Earth Gallery,** (540) 675-1610, carries a fine collection of minerals, fossils and crystals, as well as music, art, jewelry, books and more. Another eclectic shop is **Rare Finds,** (540) 675-1400, with collectibles and decorating items ranging from bridal gifts to oriental carpets.

Sperryville

Just south of Washington, in Sperryville, you'll find scores of antique and craft shops, including the **Sperryville Emporium,** (540) 987-8235, a series of connecting buildings where you can find everything from antiques and apples to country hams and honey.

Faith Mountain Herbs and Antiques, (540) 987-8547, sells flowers, herbs, crafts and fashions for women, with many items priced well below retail. **Elmer's Antiques,** (540) 987-8355, handles walnut, cherry and oak antiques and also sells apples and presses its own cider in season. **Country Manor,** (540) 987-8761, is the last shop on Va. 211 W. before you get to Skyline Drive. Here you can browse for hours among carvings and

baskets, including white oak ones woven locally and grape vine ones woven by the Manor's owner, Phyllis Swindler.

Culpeper County

In Culpeper, **Springhouse Antiques,** (540) 825-6643, on Main Street specializes in country pine and oak antique furniture, quilts, linens and kitchen collectibles.

Madison County

ANTIQUES AND HANDCRAFTS

In Madison the **Bleak-Thrift House,** (540) 948-3645, is a restored old home, c. 1838, where you will find antique furniture, glassware, primitives, lace and linens. English boxwoods surround the home, which is in downtown Madison on Main Street (U.S. 29 Business). You can enjoy a spot of English tea and scones in the tea room Thursday through Sunday.

Madison is headquarters for **E.A. Clore Sons Inc.,** (540) 948-5821, makers of simple but handsome furniture since 1830. "We don't make any fancy furniture," says company president Edward Clore, "but we try to make it last . . . and, by golly, it does." Nestled in a hollow three-tenths of a mile from Va. 637, E.A. Clore specializes in handmade Early American furniture from walnut, cherry, oak and mahogany. Clore sells directly from its factory to the consumer, and its showrooms are right next door.

The **Little Shop of Madison,** (540) 948-4147, at 320 S. Main Street, is a quilt-making supply shop and a decorating business specializing in window treatments.

Just to the north, in the tiny mountain

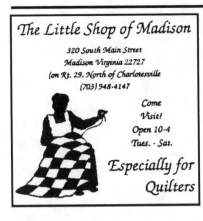

antique furniture, old silver and pewter, Chinese imports, prints and paintings, primitives, folk art, imported tiles and French medieval-style tapestries.

Orange County

ANTIQUES

At one time, Orange County was the largest Virginia county ever formed, stretching to the Mississppi River on the west and the Great Lakes to the north. Today, its territory is more modest, but it's packed with historical landmarks and shops with period pieces. North of Orange on U.S. 15 is **Carousel Antiques**, (540) 825-1558, which carries a nice variety of old treasures. It's closed Wednesday and Thursday.

Across from the post office in Barboursville is **Elsie's Antique Shop**, (804) 985-2778, open weekends only until 3 PM and offering an ever-changing array of items.

At the end of Orange's Main Street, in the old hardware building, is **Main Street Antiques**, (540) 672-5517, which carries

town of Criglersville, sits the **Mountain Store**, (540) 923-4349, open only on weekends. It's a truly wonderful place that offers books, hand-made crafts and an interesting selection of children's toys and jigsaw puzzles.

Two miles south of Madison on U.S. 29, called the "antique corridor" by locals, are several shops worth visiting. **Eunice & Fester Antiques**, (540) 948-4647, is a humorous landmark with sophisticated items for the serious collector. It has a fine selection of American furniture from Colonial to art deco. Accessories with design merit are emphasized. Reupholstered vintage furniture is a specialty. **Handcraft House**, (540) 948-6323, situated on U.S. 29, sells very fine crafts made by more than 300 artisans from across the nation. They feature Cat's Meow houses, rubber stamps and accessories, Byer's Choice Carolers and Yankee candles.

About 7 miles south of Madison on U.S. 29 is **Country Garden Antiques**, (540) 948-3240, a unique antique shop that also specializes in garden ornaments imported directly from England and antique period mantles. Items in this eclectic collection include American and English

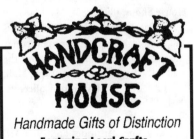

Handmade Gifts of Distinction
Featuring Local Crafts
Over 200 artisans and craftsman
Rt. 29 Madison, VA • (703) 948-6323

everything from glass bottles to furniture. It's a great place for browsing.

HANDCRAFTS

The Somerset Shop (540) 672-2511, in Somerset at the crossroads of Va. 20 and Va. 231 south of Montpelier, features high quality handcrafted items from more than 150 artisans, many of them local. Amidst the pleasant smell of potpourri, you can choose from hand-woven rugs and placemats, dried flower arrangements, jams and jellies, baskets, folk dolls, pottery, wreaths and wooden accessories.

Other places where you're likely to find handmade objects are the **Old Town Gift Shop** (540) 672-5123, on Main Street in Orange; or **Darby Needlecraft and Gifts,** (540) 672-5822, also on Main Street. **The Country Mouse,** (540) 672-5336, on Church Street in Orange, carries herbs, lotions and herb books, some of which are by Virginia writers.

Greene County

When U.S. 29 arrives in Ruckersville, it intersects with U.S. 33 and forms a crossroads that bustles with activity for antique lovers. The three-story **Greene House Shops,** (804) 985-2438, houses at least 50 dealers of antiques, crafts, quilts and all kinds of gifts. It's open every day and even accepts credit cards. Across the road is the **Country Store Antique Mall**, (804) 985-3649, and **Antique Collectors**, (804) 985-8966, which offers Victorian furniture, china, crystal and sterling.

Early Time Antiques and Fine Art, (804) 985-3602, also in Ruckersville, has a good reputation for its 18th- and 19th-century furniture, oil paintings and accessories.

Farther west on U.S. 33 is a popular stop called the **Blue Ridge Pottery,** (804) 985-6080, housed in what was once the Golden Horseshoe Inn, c. 1827. The Inn, which sits along the old Spotswood Trail, used to serve travelers making the difficult climb over the mountains. Gen. Stonewall Jackson reportedly stayed here during the war, using the inn as his temporary headquarters only a few weeks before he was killed. Alan Ward and his family throw their stoneware pottery in a little studio right next door to Blue Ridge Pottery and welcome visitors. Ward's pottery, which is modeled after traditional Valley styles but painted with modern, vibrant glazes, is sold in the shop, along with locally made crafts, Virginia wines, apple butter and jams and Christmas decorations.

Closer to Stanardsville is the **Edgewood Farm Nursery,** (804) 985-3782, which stocks one of the largest selections of herbs and perennials in the state. You can walk to the nursery from Edgewood Farm, an elegant, hospitable bed and breakfast inn run by Eleanor Schwartz. Norman Schwartz, her husband, operates the nursery.

Charlottesville and Surrounding Area

ANTIQUES

The Charlottesville area has more than two dozen antique stores, not counting the dozens of mini-shops that share a single roof.

On U.S. 250 W. is an exclusive shop, **1740 House Antiques,** (804) 977-1740, which sells American and English furniture and fine art. Another on the same road is **Jordan,** (540) 456-8465, 16 miles west of town, which carries elegant period antiques arranged in lifestyle room settings with all the accessories. Sales personnel will serve you cappuccino to sip while you shop, and be sure to see the **Jordan Art Gallery**, which showcases the work of local, national and international artists.

DeLoach Antiques, (804) 979-7209, at 1211 W. Main Street, is a charming place to find stylish and unusual decorative objects and antiques at very good prices. An eclectic selection of Neoclassical, French, English and American pieces are displayed throughout a elegantly decorated townhouse that was built by one of Thomas Jefferson's master craftsmen in 1817.

If you're interested in either antique or new rugs from the villages of the Middle East, stop by the **Sun Bow Trading Company**, (804) 293-8821, on Fourth Street. Saul, the owner, has many a tale to tell about these tribal textiles and nomadic Oriental rugs and his journeys to find them.

The **Greenwood Antique Center**, (540) 456-8465, is about 15 miles west of Charlottesville on U.S. 250. It sells fine old furniture, primitives, glassware, Chinese porcelain, works of art and jewelry. **Whitehouse Antiques**, (540) 942-1194, in nearby Afton, has American period pieces, from country to formal. The shop also caters to the dealer trade and has new inventory weekly. **Afton House Antiques**, (540) 456-6759, offers fascinating collections of antique furniture, arts, crafts, dolls and home furnishings.

If you're looking for out-of-print books, the **Daedalus Bookshop**, (804) 293-7595, on Fourth Street has 80,000 books on three floors. The **Heartwood Bookshop**, (804) 295-7083, has two locations on Elliewood. At No. 5 is a large used book collection, while No. 9 has an impressive rare book collection, with an emphasis on Americana and literature.

Finally, for a trip back in time, you must not miss **Tuckahoe Antique Mall**, (804) 361-2121, on Va. 151 at Nellysford, near Wintergreen Resort. You could spend an entire day looking through the 50 shops — 10,000 square feet — of quality antique furniture, including oak, walnut and pine, plus collectibles, art and glassware. The mall is open Thursday through Sunday.

HANDCRAFTS

Charlottesville is known for having an abundance of shops selling exquisite crafts from around the world. Many of the shops seem more like galleries, and some function as both.

The historic Downtown Mall is a good place to start exploring such stores. On the west end, close to the Omni, **The Nicholas & Alexandra Gallery**, (804) 295-4003, stocks dolls, rugs, toys, artwork and other crafts made in republics of the former Soviet Union. Right next door is **Renaissance Gallery**, (804) 296-9208, an unusual shop selling rugs, pottery, masks and other items from Africa, South America and Asia. If you need spinning and weaving supplies, look no farther than **Stony Mountain Fibers**, (804) 295-2008, a stone's throw away.

Artworks, (804) 979-2888, centrally located on the mall, is another gallery of contemporary crafts that sells jewelry, pottery, art pieces and hand-printed clothing. **Paula Lewis**, (804) 295-6244, on Fourth Street and E. Jefferson, also has a splendid collection of old and new quilts, along with country folk art, Pueblo Indian pottery, quilting supplies and books.

The McGuffey Art Center, (804) 295-7973, is a renovated elementary school within walking distance of the Downtown Mall housing a contemporary gallery, as well as workshops and studios where more than 40 artists and crafts makers create their works. A number of these

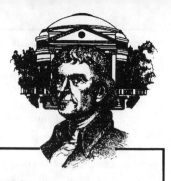
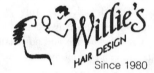
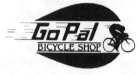
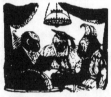
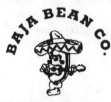
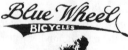
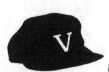

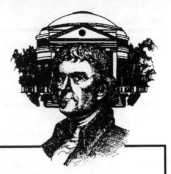
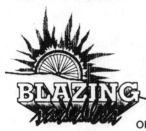
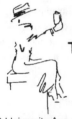
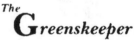
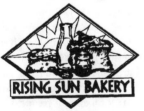
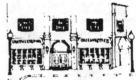
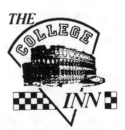
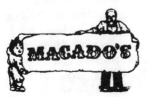

gifted artists at work here are represented by galleries in New York City and other major cities. A small gift shop sells some of their creations. You'll find pottery, photography, prints, stained glass, sculpture, jewelry and much more.

The Crafter's Gallery, (804) 295-7006, 9 miles west of Charlottesville on U.S. 250, sells contemporary crafts, glassware, pottery, ironware, silver and weavings.

Lewis Glaser Inc., (804) 973-7783, at 1700 Sourwood Place, specializes in hand-cut Colonial-style goose quill pens. Internationally known quill maker Nancy Floyd is the exclusive producer of quill pens used by the U.S. Supreme Court.

Just a short drive into the countryside, in downtown Nellysford in Nelson County, you'll find **Valley Green Art and Craft Co-op**, (804) 361-9316, a gem of a store displaying the works of many fine Virginia artisans. Pieces include paintings, photography, jewelry, stained glass, porcelain dolls, furniture and wearable fiber art fashions.

UNIVERSITY CORNER SPECIALTY SHOPS

"On the Corner" is the local term for a tight little neighborhood of shops, cafes and restaurants only a half-block from the Rotunda and the original UVA campus. A number of specialty shops make the corner an interesting place to browse.

Derek's U-Spirit, (804) 977-1606, 104 14th Street, sells UVA sweatshirts, pants, hats, fraternity and sorority items and other college souvenirs. A short walk away on 14th Street is **Innovations**, (804) 971-8088, a hair salon catering to the university and professional crowd. Some say you have to be a magician to get through four rigorous years at the demanding University of Virginia. No wonder **Magic Tricks**,

(804) 293-5788, at 101 14th Street, is nearby, selling a wide assortment of amusing tricks, gags, games and novelties.

Arnette's, (804) 977-8451, at University and Elliewood avenues, has three floors full of unique gifts, cards, clothing and accessories. There's something for everyone in this charming family-run store — even a science and nature shop for kids.

Barr-ee Station, (804) 979-7981, on University Avenue is a great outlet store that sells brand-name, high-quality clothing for men and women at cut-rate prices.

The Phoenix, (804) 296-1115, on 14th Street is a unique women's boutique that sells exquisite and funky dresses, unusual T-shirts, exotic earrings, belts and other accessories. **The Garment District**, (804) 296-1003, on University Avenue caters to university women with its cute, fashionable clothing at reasonable prices.

For traditionalists, **Eljo's**, (804) 295-5230, at 3 Elliewood Avenue, has been selling preppie clothes for more than 40 years, offering the best of Ralph Lauren, Southwick, Corbin and Gitman.

On the athletic front, the **"Go Pal" Bicycle Shop**, (804) 295-1212, on 14th Street and 198 Zan Road, specializes in mountain and road bikes, with a wide selection of Trek and Bianchi models. They are also licensed to repair all kinds of bikes. **Blue Wheel Bicycles**, (804) 977-1870, at 19 Elliewood Avenue, sells fine bicycles at competitive prices, along with a good selection of accessories. This bike shop has been around for more than 20 years. **Ragged Mountain Running Shop**, (804) 293-3367, on Elliewood Avenue, has a great selection of running and aerobic shoes at very competitive prices.

Freeman-Victorious Framing, (804) 296-3456, at 1413 University Avenue, not only does framing, but also sells antique prints and posters, mirrors, and other fine gifts.

Heartwood Bookshop, (804) 295-7083, at 5 Elliewood Avenue, also has a great collection of secondhand scholarly and popular books in both hardback and paperback. You'll find cookbooks, histories, literature, mysteries, nature, science fiction, an antiquarian collection and more (see the earlier entry under Antiques for more information.)

Mincer's, (804) 296-5687, at University Avenue and Elliewood, is open seven days a week and has been selling university sportswear for more than 40 years.

Also on University Corner is **Willie's Hair Design**, (804) 295-1242.

HISTORIC DOWNTOWN MALL

We've already described some of the shops in the downtown pedestrian mall that specialize in exquisite handcrafts. There are also other delightful specialty shops, most of which are owner-operated.

One of the most interesting places to browse is the **Old Hardware Store**, (804) 977-1518, a block-long building that houses a restaurant and soda fountain, several specialty food bars and shops selling just about everything: gold and silver jewelry, games, wrought iron and more. The Old Hardware Store is aptly named; it operated from 1895 to 1976 and was once the premier hardware store in central Virginia. Not only did it sell rope and tools and other hardware, but you could also find fine china and silver there, along with everyday crockery and eggs and other staples. Just like the old days, the Old Hardware Store still has something for everyone. You can even get your hair trimmed and your shoes shined here.

Other outstanding specialty shops on the Downtown Mall include **Palais Royal**, (804) 979-4111, which has the finest in French designer linens, robes, towels and blankets, and **The Jeweler's Eye**, (804) 979-5919, an eclectic collection of jewelry dating from the 1700s through the 1900s.

Pewter Corner, (804) 971-3788, at 421 E. Main Street, claims it has the largest selection of pewter in the United States.

The Mall has two fine Oriental rug shops: **Purcell Oriental Rug Co. Ltd.**, (804) 971-8822, and **T.S. Eways**, (804) 979-3038, right next door.

The **Williams Corner Bookstore**, (804) 977-4858, just a couple of doors down from the Old Hardware Store, is considered by some to be the best bookstore in town.

Market Street Wineshop and Gourmet Grocery, (804) 296-3854 or (800) 377-VINE, at 311 E. Market Street, is a gathering place where everybody seems to know everyone else, but if you're a first-time visitor you'll receive the same friendly welcome as the regulars. The store has one of the state's largest selections of wine and beer, from the old and rare to the good and cheap.

BARRACKS ROAD SHOPPING CENTER

At Barracks Road and Emmet Street is a unique shopping enclave made up of dozens of delightful specialty shops and a few department stores within walking distance (just watch the traffic).

For a vast selection of ladies' shoes, check out **Scarpa**, (804) 396-0040, where the styles go from collegiate casual to formal in all the top brands. At nearby **Talbot's**, (804) 296-3580, you'll find a premier selection of classic apparel and accessories in a comfortable, home-like atmosphere. (Roanoke has a Talbot's too.) This store is especially popular with the community and UVA population. **Les**

Fabriques, (804) 296-0757, with its designer and bridal fabrics, buttons and other accessories, also sells top-brand sewing machines.

Speaking of youngsters, **Shenanigans**, (804) 295-4797, is a great place to find children's books, toys, stuffed animals, dolls from around the world and children's music, including sing-along videos. True to its name, **Whimsies**, (804) 977-8767, has fanciful and spunky children's wear, including clothes for infants to pre-teens. It's next door to Shenanigans.

The Book Gallery, (804) 977-2892, has a great selection of children's books, along with other books on topics ranging from Thomas Jefferson and Virginia history to home decorating and sports.

For those who answer to the call of the wild, head to **Blue Ridge Mountain Sports**, (804) 977-4400, for camping, backpacking, hiking and outdoor outfitting needs.

Virginia's best is showcased in **The Virginia Shop**, (804) 977-0080, located on the Island behind Ruby Tuesdays Restaurant. A great selection of gifts, food, wine, books, music and much more — all with the Old Dominion mark of quality — is for sale here seven days a week.

Nature by Design, (804) 977-6100, is a fascinating shop for folks of all ages, selling such variety as polished rocks for less than a dollar and driftwood water fountains at $1,300. Jewelry, bird feeders, garden accessories, chimes, agate bookends, puzzles, games and more all have a touch of nature.

Keller & George, (804) 293-5011, is where you'll find the popular Jefferson cup, along with fine jewelry and distinctive and unusual gifts.

Plow & Hearth, (804) 977-3707, sells beautiful outdoor ornaments and furniture made of wrought iron, cedar and other sturdy materials.

For women's clothing, **Krissia**, (804) 295-9249, sells exquisite lingerie, fine hosiery and slippers for day and evening wear. **Levy's**, (804) 295-4270, sells gorgeous, sophisticated sportswear and bathing suits downstairs and formal wear and snappy business suits on the upper level.

Nearby **Seminole Square**, (804) 296-4141, is an exquisite furniture store that has been furnishing homes in Central Virginia since 1926. **Gilmore, Hamm and Snyder Inc.**, (804) 973-8114, sells quality furniture by such manufacturers as Henkel Harris, Brown Jordan, Pennsylvania House, and Hickory Chair, along with hand-woven Oriental rugs, lamps, pictures, mirrors and window treatments.

Lynchburg

ANTIQUES

A phenomenal array of antique stores — nearly 20 in all — bring collectors and browsers to this historic and cultural city. For a list of them all, contact the visitors center at (804) 847-1811.

For a whirlwind tour of downtown shops, visit **Redcoat Antiques**, (804) 528-3182, 1421 Main Street, and **Sweeney's Curious Goods**, (804) 846-7839, 1220 Main Street. There's also a concentration near River Ridge Mall off Candlers Mountain Road, beside Liberty University.

HANDCRAFTS

Virginia Handcrafts Inc., (804) 846-7029, part of the Farm Basket shopping complex at 2008 Langhorne Road, will keep you wandering around all day. It's a casual shop where browsers and their chil-

SHOPPING

dren are welcome. The spacious store features a collection of American crafts, including kaleidoscopes, game boards, pottery and jewelry. These are displayed among paintings, planters, fountains, lamps, rugs and much more than can possibly be described here. One room is devoted to crafts made by Virginians. The atmosphere is just plain fun!

Adjoining it is the **Farm Basket Shop**, (804) 528-1107, where you can browse through rooms of carefully chosen gift items from around the world. Children can entertain themselves with an imported wooden train in a toy department that also overflows with stuffed animals, dolls and baby gifts. You can create custom invitations and announcements by computer. A mail-order catalog is available. If hunger strikes, stop for a cucumber sandwich at the complex's restaurant, which has some of the best home-style food in the area. The Farm Basket's fruit is locally grown in their own mountain orchards. This is a Lynchburg landmark not to be missed!

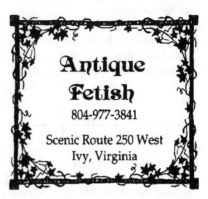

Antique Fetish
804-977-3841

Scenic Route 250 West
Ivy, Virginia

OUTLETS

Lynchburg has 14 terrific outlets and discount stores. A complete list is available from the visitors center, (804) 847-1732.

The granddaddy of them all, the first shoe company south of the Mason-Dixon line (founded 1888) and the most famous, is **Craddock-Terry Shoe Factory Outlet**, (804) 847-3535, at 601 12th Street. You can choose among 300,000 pairs of shoes in stock from the national Masseys catalogs and — the best part — get up to a whopping 70 percent off. You'll see the billboards with the gigantic plastic pairs of red high heel pumps as you come into town on major roads. The store special-

izes in hard to find sizes and widths. Shoe lovers will recognize national brand names, such as Rockport and American Gentleman. It's worth an overnight stay for an average family just to buy seasonal shoes and see the sights of Lynchburg at the same time. Another fine shoe outlet is **Consolidated Shoe Store**, (804) 237-5569, 10200 Timberlake Road.

For clothes and accessories, there's **Carolina Hosiery**, (804) 846-5099, at 525 Alleghany Avenue, and **Tultex Mill Outlet**, (804) 385-6477, at Forest Plaza West Shopping Center. For the largest Tultex collection, known worldwide, go to Martinsville, home of Tultex. It borders the Blue Ridge and also has furniture outlets.

SPECIALTY SHOPS

For both specialty shopping and terrific eating, go to the **Community Market**, (804) 847-1499, Main at 12th Street, established in 1783. You'll find homemade crafts, Virginia-made goods and baked goods. Something is always going at the Market, the hub of Lynchburg activity since the days of Thomas Jefferson, who scared local citizens by biting into a tomato, long thought to be a poisonous fruit. This market and the one in Roanoke are centerpieces of Blue Ridge life and a joy to behold.

For best-sellers, regional histories, travel guides, children's books and everything kind of book in between, stop in at **The Bookstore**, (804) 384-1746, in the Boonsboro Shopping Center, 4925 Boonsboro Road.

Smith Mountain Lake

GENERAL AND SPECIALTY STORES AND SERVICES

Smith Mountain Lake has two major shopping areas: **Bridgewater Plaza** on Route 122 at Hales Ford Bridge, home of the official Smith Mountain Lake Partnership Visitors Center, and **Village Square**, at Va. 122/655, Moneta.

Hales Ford is the very center of lake life. Here you'll find enough interesting little shops to see while the kids play miniature golf at **Harbortown Golf**, (540) 721-1203, or play games at the arcade. On summer weekends, live entertainment draws crowds, and, during the rest of the year, the steady seasonal stream of boats and visitors from around the world are often entertainment enough.

Bridgewater Plaza's anchor, in addition to the miniature golf course, is **Bridgewater Marina and Boat Rentals** and **Bridgewater Para-Sail**, (540) 721-1639.

Lovers of fine art will enjoy **The Little Gallery**, (540) 721-1596, where you can find one-of-a-kind treasures and see the works of well-known artists, as well as emerging local ones.

Gifts Ahoy, (540) 721-5303, will delight children and has the lake's most unique collection of gifts and greeting cards. The Plaza also has the refreshing **Ice Cream Cottage**, (540) 721-1305, where your family can get such cooling fare as flavored shaved ice or your favorite ice cream in a waffle cone.

At Village Square there's **Village Accents**, (540) 297-7751, a collector's showcase that includes such items as clown figurines such as Emmett Kelly Jr. and Native American sculpture. **Smith Mountain Flowers**, (540) 297-6524, has gifts, candy, fruit and flowers for any occasion.

Beyond these two centers, other shops are either general or specialized and far flung. **Classic Collections**, (540) 297-2804, on Va. 122, north of Hales Ford bridge, has quilts, pottery, baskets, customer designed flags, teddy bears, bird carvings and oak rockers. The **Old Hales Ford Country Store**, (540) 721-5504, nearly 4 miles north of Hales Ford bridge, has souvenirs and just about anything else you need while enjoying the lake.

Bedford County

ANTIQUES

Bedford County has nearly 20 antique stores within a close radius of each other. In downtown Bedford, at 201 N. Bridge Street, is **Bridge Street Antiques**, (540) 586-6611, specializing in furniture, tools, silver and primitives. Books, toys and Virginia antiques can be found downtown at **Hamiltons**, (540) 586-5592, at 155 W. Main. Farther out of town, you'll find **Old Country Store**, (540) 586-1665, a mile west of Bedford on Va. 460. Twelve dealers do business at **The Peddler Antiques** (804) 525-6030, on Va. 854 between routes 811 and 221. You'll find many shops between Lynchburg and Bedford. For a complete list, call the Bedford Area Chamber of Commerce at (540) 586-9401.

OUTLETS

If you love pottery and seeing how it's made, it's worth a trip to Bedford to visit **Emerson Creek Pottery's** factory in Bedford County. The company's product line is sold in all 50 states and is becoming widely collected as a fine art. The retail shop, (540) 297-7884, provides tour schedules and directions to their stores. If you're going just to shop, the seconds shop is in an 1825 log cabin next to the factory on Va. 727 E., 10 miles from Bedford. A showroom houses a permanent display of the pottery's 14-year-old private collection. Emerson Creek Pottery is known for its designs of fields of wildflowers dancing in a spectrum of pastel and vibrant hues. Each pot is hand-decorated. The line consists of earthenware pottery, including vases, coffee mugs, pitchers, lamps, creamers and sugars, flowerpots and lotion bottles in more than a dozen colors and patterns.

Franklin County

GENERAL STORES

Don't leave Franklin County without a visit to **Boone's Country Store**, (703) 721-2478, a few miles from the intersection of Va. 122 at Burnt Chimney and Va. 116 at Boone's Mill, the winding mountain road to Roanoke. Run by German Baptists, the store has the most heavenly sticky buns, pies, cakes, rolls and homemade entrees this side of Amish country. The store also sells country items and piece goods. If you want to take home an authentic reminder of German Baptist country, don't miss Boone's.

HANDCRAFTS

For a tremendous buy on hand-smocked children's items and clothing, as well as good quality children's con-

signment clothing and juvenile accessories, travel the main road between Roanoke and Rocky Mount, U.S. 220, and stop at **Kids Kastoffs**, (540) 483-2496. You'll find the same quality as in specialty stores, at about a third of the cost. Downtown Rocky Mount is the location of **From the Heart**, (540) 489-3887, 178 Franklin Street, a store with a unique assortment of gift items, local art, toys, pottery, linen and antiques.

OUTLETS

Southern Lamp & Shade Showroom, (540) 483-4738, on U.S. 220, near Wirtz, has a great selection of lamps and shades at below retail prices. It's well worth visiting if you're shopping for lighting. In Rocky Mount, **Virginia Apparel Outlet**, (540) 483-8266, 721 N. Main Street, has a fine selection of clothing for the entire family at outlet prices.

New River Valley Region

Blacksburg

ANTIQUES

Antique stores are spread out all over the New River Valley, especially in the Blacksburg area. Downtown, there are **Grady's Antiques**, (540) 951-0623, at 208 N. Main Street; **Other Times LTD**, (540) 552-1615, at 891 Kabrich Street; and **Heirloom Originals**, (540) 552-9241, 609 N. Main. They each have a good selection of collectibles and decorative antiques.

OUTLETS

Blacksburg's downtown has two good clothing outlets catering to the Virginia Tech crowd. **T.G.I.F. Outlets**, (540) 951-3541, on N. Main, sells returns and overstock for clothing catalogs with sporty apparel. You'll find J. Crew, Clifford & Wills, Smythe & County and Lands End. On S. Main, in the Blacksburg Square Shopping Center, you can shop at **Virginia Apparel Outlet**, (540) 961-2889, which manufactures and retails for major catalog companies including L.L. Bean, Vanity Fair, Bugle Boy and Botany 500.

SPECIALTY SHOPS

In the downtown, a very special store that started out as a hole in the wall several decades ago has since grown to be one of the most popular art supply and overall neat-stuff stores in western Virginia. Everyone in the know in the New River Valley knows this is **Mish Mish**, (540) 552-1020, which probably should be renamed Hodge Podge. It's at 204 Draper Road. Shoppers of any age could spend the entire day there looking at everything from the finest art supplies and watercolors to a rainbow of Silly Putty.

You'll want to stop at **Printer's Ink**, (540) 552-5676, at University Mall, for all your books, magazines, greeting cards and gift items from Hallmark and other popular designers.

Sixty specialty shops and **Peebles Department Store** are among the stores at **New River Valley Mall**, (540) 381-0004, 782 New River Road off U.S. 460 in Blacksburg. The specialty stores, along with Peebles, really are a cut above those you find in other western Virginia shopping malls. The mall also wins your heart with free wheelchairs, high chairs in the food court, strollers and special programs.

Christiansburg

ANTIQUES

Cambria Emporium, (540) 381-0949, at 596 Depot Street in Christiansburg, is the best place in Montgomery County to find tiny antique treasures and surprises. The big, red, three-story building in the historic Cambria area of the county is a landmark in itself, constructed in 1908 and renovated several years ago as an antiques mall housing 20 dealers. Here, among 20,000 square feet of space, you

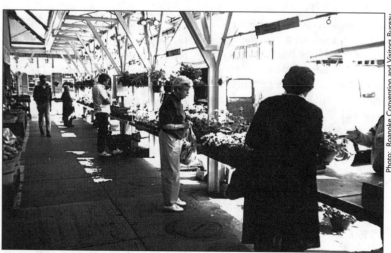

The Historic Farmers Market in Roanoke.

Photo: Roanoke Convention and Visitors Bureau

can find every antique imaginable in a pleasant, old-time setting. It's open, airy and uncluttered. You'll find broad categories of glassware, furniture, dishes, quilts, vintage clothing and fine china. Along with those, you'll run across small reminders of the past that will make you ooh and ahh! For the antique lover, Cambria Emporium is definitely worth an overnight in this charming town. The Oaks bed and breakfast inn nearby is the perfect place to stay. Don't forget to go upstairs to see **Casey's Country Store**, a room laid out like a general store of the 1900s. A counter sign reads, "If it ain't priced, it ain't for sale, folks!" That's the spirit of Cambria Emporium.

OUTLETS

You can get great savings in both irregular and first quality chic Donkenny women's fashions at the **Donkenny Fashion Outlet**, (540) 382-8538, on N. Franklin Street. Think of it — irregulars for up to $6.25 and regular clothing for up to $45. For castoffs of every kind, stop at **Big Lots**, (540) 381-5124, at the Northgate Village Shopping Center at 1695 N. Franklin on U.S. 460. It's one of a chain packed with discontinued merchandise and overstocks from insurance claims, buy-outs and bankruptcies. You can get unreal prices if you hit the store at the right time, so constant vigilance pays off!

Floyd County

GENERAL STORES

Without a doubt, counterculture-flavored Floyd County has the most diverse, interesting shopping of any area in the New River and, some might say, the entire Blue Ridge. **Cockram's General Store**, (540) 745-4563, is the essence of that idea. For more than 75 years,

Cockram's has been the center of Floyd County entertainment, nightlife and culture. It has become famous not only for its merchandise but for its famous Friday Night Flatfooting Jamboree (see our Arts and Culture chapter). Owner Freeman Cockram's landmark store was rescued from debt several years ago by the community that cherishes it as its cultural center, in a move reminiscent of old-fashioned note burnings and barn raisings. As a general store, Cockram's offers a plethora of merchandise, including potted possum and bib overalls, sold from an old-fashioned candy counter.

Down the road a piece is another interesting general store, **Poor Farmers Market**, (540) 952-2670, a combination grocery store, deli and gift shop, on U.S. 58 in Meadows of Dan, just off the Blue Ridge Parkway. This hub for locals and tourists alike got its start when owner Felecia Shelor told a local farmer she'd buy his produce and then peddle it wholesale. The business boomed, and the store has grown 10 times its original size since 1983. Its deli serves great lunches, with such favorites as fried apple pies and the Hungry Hillbilly sandwich. The owner's life story is as interesting as the store: She rose from a life of poverty as a bride of 15 to a store owner with 15 employees. You'll love this place, and the prices are great!

HANDCRAFTS

When you're traveling the Blue Ridge Parkway looking for a unique Blue Ridge gift, don't miss **New Mountain Mercantile**, (540) 745-4ART, a shop at 114 Locust Street, 6 miles from Milepost 165.2 in Floyd. It's filled with many hand-made items. Browse through stunning tie-dyed and batik clothing, dolls, pottery, jewelry, American Indian handcrafts, perfume made of essential oils, candles (both herbal and decorative), stained glass, quilts, field guides and books on subjects such as herb gardening and gift making. You'll also find music, instruments and hand-tuned wind chimes. The store is run by three sensitive, savvy women — Theresa Cook, Kalinda Wycoff and Christine Byrd — who know great buys when they see them. Their store also serves as a Floyd County information center of sorts. Their **"Here and Now" Art Gallery** features new exhibits monthly. New Mountain Mercantile rates as one of the outstanding handcraft stores in the entire Blue Ridge. They also have a branch store at the Virginia Explore Park and at Tanglewood Mall in Roanoke. You never know which Bluegrass artist will be performing out front to lure you in.

SPECIALTY STORES

A direct contrast to a simple country mountain way of life, **Chateau Morrisette**, (540) 593-2865, the sixth-largest winery in Virginia, is a delightful stop, not only to buy wine and baked goods at wholesale prices, but as a terrific gourmet place for lunch (see the Restaurants and Wineries chapters).

Wintergreen Farm Sheepskin Shoppe, (540) 745-4420, specializes in sheepskin products, of course, but also has fine American handcrafts, antiques and unique walking sticks. While there, visit the turn-of-the-century Farmstead Museum and Woodwright Blacksmith Shop. It's on U.S. 221, 2 miles south of Floyd.

Another uniquely specialized, interesting place is the **County Christmas House**, (540) 745-3565, on Va. 615. Formerly the Possum Hollow School House, it has everything to decorate your tree and home.

Bluegrass and old-time music lovers will want to see the largest distributor of such music in the world, **County Records or County Sales**, (540) 745-2001, on Main Street. Requests come in from the four corners for their old-time fiddle music and gospel albums.

OUTLETS

Better than an outlet store, with more fabric than you could ever find in any retail store, **School House Fabrics**, (540) 745-4561, on Locust Street, is a cloth addict's dream. An old three-story schoolhouse has been renovated and filled with everything from specialty fabrics to buttons and beads. What is amazing is how organized and well-grouped this massive mania of yard goods is. Each room is arranged according to fabric; for example, a downstairs room is devoted to bridal fabrics, lace, veils, beading and wedding goods. Out back, an extra building contains large reels of upholstery fabric, tapestry and some remnants.

Giles County

ANTIQUES

You can't miss **White Horse Antiques**, (540) 726-7021, on U.S. 460 between Pearisburg and Narrows. Look for the huge, white plaster horse in the window. You'll find a wide range of quality and prices: sets of Florentine dishes priced up to $100 and china plates for a dollar. Another interesting antique store is **Woodland**, (540) 921-1600, in tiny downtown Pearisburg. You can find some real gems among the rural offerings.

HANDCRAFTS

The New River Valley Arts and Crafts Guild operates a dynamic **Fine Arts Center Shop**, (540) 626-3309, in the Old Pembroke School on the main drag, U.S. 460. More than 50 categories of handcrafts are available from 60 working artists, with such original works as snake canes and Knobbits. In addition to a huge variety of first-class items for sale, the Guild has a floor loom in operation, on which beautiful rugs can be woven from old rags and discarded clothing. The service is open to the public for a small fee. There's also a year-round Christmas Corner.

Radford

ANTIQUES

Some dandy antique shops can be found in Radford: **Grandma's Memories**, (540) 639-0054, 237 First Street; **Collector's Corner**, (540) 639-9185, 327 First Street; and **Uncle Bill's Treasures**, (540) 731-1733, at 1103 Norwood Street.

SPECIALTY SHOPS

The combined **Norwood Art Gallery** and **Encore Gifts, Toys and Accessories Shop**, (540) 639-2015, 1115 Norwood Street, is the best place in the city to find unique gifts and original fine art. Merchandise ranges from the very unusual to the very trendy. Discover eclectic folk art, Toys That Touch the Senses and truly unique cards, gift items and packaging. After you're done shopping, you can dine on artfully prepared cuisine in a casual gallery setting at Gallery Cafe.

Pulaski County

Pulaski County and Main Street Pulaski offer the most tremendous shopping surprises of any place in the rural Blue Ridge. It's a Blue Ridge town, where time seems to have stood still just for the benefit of tourists. While Pulaski County's unusual shops have been established for some time, newcomers to Downtown Pulaski within the past three years will think they're dreaming when they see what has happened to a formerly neglected downtown area.

Roscoe Cox, a Pulaski native and retired executive, took up the town's languishing Main Street program several years ago and, within eight months, had 20 new stores and restaurants within two blocks of the town's newly rebuilt courthouse.

Some stores already there even before the revival are worth the trip in themselves. Theda and Rudolph Farmer of **Theda's Studio**, (540) 980-2777, have been in the portraiture business for more than 55 years, and a visit to their shop is like taking a trip through time, from the original tin-roofed ceilings to the arresting pictures of brides from the '50s and '60s. With an outside barber pole that still turns, **Sani-Mode Barber Shop**, (540) 980-6991, is like looking through the window into a Norman Rockwell painting. The prices of haircuts are a throw-back to that time, as are the lines of barber chairs from the '40s and '50s. This is a priceless

Insiders' Tips

— we repeat, priceless — experience that may not be on the Americana landscape for much longer.

R.P. Collectibles, (540) 994-0812, has a wide selection of antique clocks, Depression-era glass creamer sets and hundreds of knives. **Pulaski Antique Center**, (540) 980-5049, at 80 W. Main Street, has two full floors of quality antiques and post-1900 furniture, as well as a large selection of glassware and artwork. The shop also houses one of the South's largest selections of quality antique wicker.

New stores include specialty ones, such as **C&S Galleries**, (540) 674-0232, an authorized P. Buckley Moss dealer; **The Colony of Virginia Ltd.**, (540) 980-8932, specializing in items handcrafted in Virginia; and **New River Fine Arts Gallery**, run by the Fine Arts Center for the New River Valley, (540) 980-7363, which has been serving the arts and culture of the New River Valley for 15 years. In this spacious setting you'll find furniture, glassware, rugs, quilts, baskets and jewelry. Nationally known artists Annie Moon and Pam Tyrell are represented here. Also, don't miss **Upstairs, Downstairs**, (540) 980-4809, hand-painted furniture downstairs and a series of small boutiques upstairs. You'd find furniture like this for four times the cost in the metropolitan areas.

Nearby is The Count Pulaski Bed & Breakfast and Gardens. The Renaissance Restaurant, at 55 W. Main Street, is a nice place to stop for lunch; they serve a terrific selection of sandwiches, salads and entrees.

Main Street Pulaski's main thrust, however, is attracting first-class antique stores. It has succeeded wildly in this area. The list is long and still growing. By the time you ready this, who knows how many first-class, unusual stores Roscoe Cox will have attracted to Main Street Pulaski!

GENERAL STORES

Pulaski County offers some unusual specialty shopping in unique settings. **Draper Mercantile**, (540) 980-0786, on Va. 658, two minutes off I-81 at Exit 92, is a revitalized 1880s general store, doctor's office and fire station in what was old downtown Draper. Now it's a discount place to buy, among other things, the largest display of Ridgeway grandfather, wall and mantle clocks in Virginia. You also can buy, at a 40 to 60 percent discount, High Point, North Carolina, showroom furniture, gifts, crafts, floral arrangements, reproduction toys and Christmas ornaments. If you can't take it with you, the gracious owners, Lee and Katie LaFleur, will arrange to have it shipped to your home.

SPECIALTY STORES AND OUTLETS

Christmas store buffs, don't you dare miss the opportunity of a lifetime at the trio of **PJ's Carousel Collection Christmas Stores** in Newbern in Pulaski County, (540) 674-4300; Fort Chiswell, (540) 637-NOEL; and Wytheville, (540)

228-ELFS. The latter two are in Wythe County, and all are just off I-81. PJ's Carousel Village in historic Newbern is the original home of the famous full-size and miniature carousel horses, right next to the factory where they are manufactured. Factory seconds are available. The Carousel Village is 3,500 square feet of fun! Be sure to have some ice cream in the old-fashioned parlor. The stores down the road offer the world's only Christmas carousel (Wytheville) and a 150-year-old Christmas House (Fort Chiswell).

Alleghany Highlands Region

ANTIQUES

The Highlands are sprinkled with charming little shops in quaint downtowns and along out-of-the-way country roads in the counties of Alleghany, Highland and Bath. It's a junket you're bound to enjoy, whether you're hunting for top-quality antiques or just out enjoying the scenery.

Always unique, **Always Roxie's**, (540) 862-2999, 622 Main Street, Clifton Forge, Alleghany County, specializes in doll houses and miniatures. Their slogan is, "We can help make your mini-house a mini-home." The shop carries railroad items, crocks, jewelry and glassware.

Lovers of quilts and high quality, unusual quilted gifts and handcrafts should head for **Quilts Unlimited**, (540) 839-5955, a Homestead Resort shop on Cottage Row in Bath County. They handle both new and antique quilts, along with a fine selection of regional handcrafts.

In Highland County, plan a visit to **High Valley Antiques and Collectibles**, (540) 474-5611, which occupies a pre-Civil War era log home, and the **Woodlane Craft Shop**, (540) 499-2230, Va. 84, which offers antiques, crafts and junque.

GENERAL STORES

Over in McDowell, just off U.S. 250, you'll come across **Sugar Tree Country Store and Sugar House**, (540) 396-3469, a 19th-century country store featuring maple products, apple butter, pottery, baskets and some antiques. The store, in the scenic Bullpasture Valley, is a must-see during the annual Highland Maple Festival, when they have demonstrations of old-time methods of making maple syrup in iron kettles.

HANDCRAFTS

In Alleghany County visit the **Highlands Arts & Crafts Center**, (540) 862-4447, in downtown Clifton Forge, off I-64, for fine arts, handcrafts, antiques and collectibles. The Center is a run by a not-for-profit volunteer organization that encourages creativity and appreciation of the visual arts. Items for sale include pottery, wooden wares, jewelry, stained glass, needlework, quilts, fiber arts and watercolor and oil paintings.

In Bath County, shops in The Virginia Building at The Homestead offer country

---

If you're traveling and can't squeeze one more whimmy-diddle or whatchamacalit into your car, ask the shopkeepers if they'll ship your purchase to your home. If not, find a local shipper and do it yourself.

Insiders' Tips

crafts such as dolls, rugs, candles, baskets, tin and pottery.

Highland County's **Gallery of Mountain Secrets**, (540) 468-2020, on Main Street in Monterey, is a treasure of traditional arts and fine crafts. It's a very special store, down from the historic Highland Inn, that offers jewelry, pottery, wooden and quilted items and decorative accessories. Also on Main Street, **Highland County Crafts**, (540) 468-2127, gives a touch of country to all its gifts. It offers a Christmas corner and maple syrup and homemade preserves and pickles.

OUTLETS

It's worth a trip to the Alleghany Highlands just to shop at the **Bacova Guild Factory Outlet**, (540) 839-2105, on Main Street in Hot Springs, Bath County. You've seen the Bacova Guild's many silk-screened gifts, including mailboxes and doormats, in leading outdoor catalogs such as Orvis and L.L. Bean. The Bacova Guild's owners provided every family in Bath County with a free silk-screened mailbox — a county trademark undoubtedly unmatched in the United States and perhaps the world! The wildlife-motif items are made in Bacova, a charming village erected in the early 1920s as a lumber mill's company town. In 1965 the village was totally restored by philanthropist Malcolm Hirsh, whose brother, Philip, owns Meadow Lane Country Lodge in Warm Springs (featured in 1995 in a nationally-broadcast commercial for Tide detergent). A complete line of decorative, yet useful, gifts are at least 20 to 40 percent off regular prices. Summer shopping can yield an incredible Christmas gift bonanza!

SPECIALTY STORES

Across the Alleghany County border in Greenbrier County, West Virginia, shops at the Greenbrier Resort will remind you of New York City. They include a toy store and fabulous boutiques.

Bath County's Homestead Resort offers a great array of shops including **Ashleys**, (540) 839-3286, just off the main lobby, with products from Crabtree & Evelyn. Other Homestead shops are **The Captain's Cabin**, (540) 839-5447, **Bootery**, **Men's Shop**, **Tower Shop** with logoed items and linen, and a children's shops.

Highland County has the unique **Ginseng Mountain Farm**, (540) 474-5137, storefront off U.S 220. Hours of operation are erratic so call ahead for an appointment. You can get choice spring lamb cut to your specification, sheepskin products, stoneware, maple syrup and stove and fireplace bellows. The farm also has added a one-room bed and breakfast accommodation for visitors to this rugged land. Another great place is **The Personal Touch**, (540) 468-2145, Main Street, Monterey, which carries country fabric art, lampshades and stained glass.

Inside
Resorts

The Blue Ridge has an enviable concentration of resorts, the most famous of which are The Homestead and The Greenbrier, an embarrassment of riches within a half-hour's drive of each other. Charlottesville's Boar's Head Inn is legendary for its Old World decor, extensive sports facilities and special events such as its Thanksgiving Feast and Merrie Olde England Christmas. Mile-high Mountain Lake Resort was made famous by the movie *Dirty Dancing*, and Bernard's Landing on Smith Mountain Lake was the site of Bill Murray's zany hit, *What About Bob?* There are, of course, other resorts with great amenities that Hollywood has not found yet.

The listing that follows, from north to south and east to west, tells you a little about the resorts' histories, amenities and what sets each apart. Unless otherwise noted, major credit cards are accepted.

Shenandoah Valley Region

BRYCE RESORT

Basye   (540) 856-2121
Directions: The resort is on Va. 263 11 miles west of I-81 off Exit 273. From Washington, D.C., take I-66 W. to I-81 S. to the Mt. Jackson Exit, then take Va. 263 W. to Basye and Bryce Resort. Sky Bryce Airport is a five-minute walk from the resort.

Bryce Resort, in the Shenandoah Mountains that form the western lip of

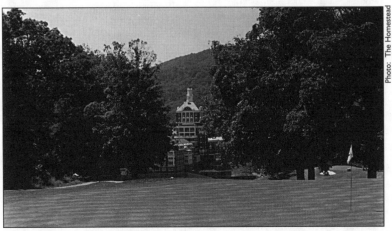

Photo: The Homestead

The Homestead in Hot Springs is a landmark resort.

the Shenandoah Valley, offers a wide range of family recreation and lodging in modern, privately owned studio condominiums, townhouses and chalets. All units have interesting decor, often reflecting the history of this colorful and friendly valley. Many are furnished with kitchenettes.

Bryce is especially attractive to golfers and outdoor enthusiasts. Popular as a winter skiing recreation getaway (see the Skiing chapter), it is also unique for its grass skiing (yes, we said "grass," in which participants glide down the resort's hills on short, tread-like skates during the summer months).

Bryce's 18-hole golf course is a par 71, 6,175-yard mountain layout. Facilities include a driving range, putting green, club and cart rentals, professional instruction, individual club storage and a fully stocked golf shop (see the golf section of our Recreation chapter).

While Mom and Dad are on the course, the children can enjoy Lake Laura, a 45-acre man-made private lake with its own sandy beach, offering swimming, boating, windsurfing and fishing. Beach admission is $3. Windsurfing is taught at a certified school, beginning on a dry-land simulator before you head for the water. The novice package costs $32.

From Memorial Day to Labor Day, the resort's T.J. Stables provides one-hour guided trail rides for $20 and pony rides for $5.

Mountain biking and in-line skating are growing sports at Bryce. "Diamond Back" mountain bikes can be rented at the ski shop for $25 day or $15 for three hours. Rollerblades are $20 and $13 for the same time periods.

Tennis is another favorite activity at Bryce Resort, which has lighted outdoor courts and a well-stocked pro shop. Court time is $10, light tokens $3 per hour.

Lodging prices vary according to accommodations. Condos on the ski slopes, each with a great fireplace, bedroom and bath, rent for $95 nightly (there's a three-night minimum during ski season); two-bedroom townhouses on the golf course rent for $115 nightly; and scattered chalets range from $250 to $700 for a two-night stay. The resort does not accept out-of-state checks.

MASSANUTTEN

Harrisonburg   (540) 289-9441
Directions: From I-81, take Exit 64, turn right on U.S. 33 E. and go 10 miles to Va. 644; the entrance is on the left.

Massanutten bills itself as "More than a Mountain, Your Place in the Fun . . ." with 5,300 acres of unspoiled beauty and unequaled recreation. The Massanutten experience can't be said any better than that! Massanutten is well-known for its skiing and winter recreation (see the Skiing chapter) and for its 18-hole championship golf course (see golf section of the Recreation chapter).

Guests also enjoy Massanutten's multimillion-dollar sports complex, Le Club, which has a gym, fitness center, racquetball courts and year-round swimming pools. Lighted outdoor tennis courts are available at no charge. Mountain bikes can be rented for $5 per hour.

Massanutten is family-oriented, with a host of programs geared to children, including tubing, canoeing, nature hikes, arts and crafts, miniature golf and pond fishing.

On-mountain dining is limited to a cafeteria-style restaurant in the sports complex, but nearby Harrisonburg, home of James Madison University, has a variety of restaurants.

Lodging ranges from $75 per night for a hotel room midweek to $225 per night for a two-bedroom condo on a weekend.

NATURAL BRIDGE OF VIRGINIA

Natural Bridge   *(540) 291-2121*
                        (800) 533-1410
Directions: Natural Bridge is 13 miles from the Blue Ridge Pkwy., minutes off I-81, 12 miles from I-64 and 39 miles north of Roanoke. Traveling up or down I-81, you can't miss it.

One of the seven wonders of the natural world, Natural Bridge Resort isn't posh in the same sense as some of the other great five-star resorts of the Blue Ridge, but it's definitely worth seeing and staying at overnight because of its unique character. Many make the trip just for the unique sunrise services, as well as for the nightly Dramas of Creation, a spectacular light and sound show. Both are held under the 23-story-high, 90-foot-long structure.

The story of Natural Bridge, a 36,000-ton limestone arch carved millions of years ago, is a historian's delight. Early on, the bridge was worshipped by the Monocan Indians. Thomas Jefferson was the first American to own the bridge, which he purchased from King George III in 1774. George Washington surveyed the bridge as a lad. In fact, you can still see the spot where he carved his initials. Colonists made bullets by dropping molten lead off the bridge into the cold creek water below. During the War of 1812, soldiers mined the nearby saltpeter cave to make explosives.

Additional attractions are the 34-story-high caverns (it is said they are haunted with ghostly voices still heard as late as 1988) and the Natural Bridge Wax Museum, which houses lifelike figures including a gallery of American presidents. A huge gift shop sells such tasty fare as homemade fudge and candy made to look like rocks, as well as fine gifts. For lunch or a snack, a deli featuring several fast-food stations is in the gift shop. For recreation, the tennis courts, indoor heated swimming pool and new 18-hole Mini-link Indoor Golf Course are popular features. Each attraction costs $8 per adult and $4 per child (ages 6 to 15); special combination rates are $7.50 per adult and $3.50 per child to visit the wax museum and caverns.

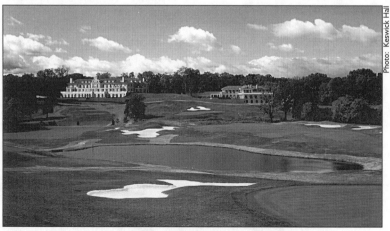

Photo: Keswick Hall

The award-winning Keswick Hall, just outside Charlottesville.

Accommodations feature 180 rooms in the newly refurbished Natural Bridge Inn and Conference Center and cozy Stonewall Inn. Room rates range from $29 to $69 weekday and $39 to $89 weekend, depending on the season. A three-room suite is $125 weekday and $150 weekend. Personal checks are accepted for advance deposits only.

East of the Blue Ridge Region

THE BOAR'S HEAD
INN & SPORTS CLUB
Charlottesville   (800) 476-1988
Directions: From I-64, take U.S. 250 W. 1½ miles to the Inn.

The Boar's Head, on a 53-acre country estate, has 174 guest rooms and suites, 12 meeting rooms, a grand ballroom, two dining rooms, three outdoor swimming pools, specialty shops and a modern Sports Club. Amenities include 20 tennis courts, massages, facials, aerobics, a complete fitness center and two platform tennis and four squash courts. The 18-hole championship Birdwood golf course is adjacent to the resort. Hiking, fishing, horseback riding and, or course, sightseeing, are available nearby.

Dining is available in the acclaimed Old Mill Room and at Racquets Restaurant in the Sports Club, which offers casual family dining focusing on heart-healthy entrees and light fare.

Highlights of the year are the traditional Thanksgiving feast, preceded by the Blessing of the Hounds of the Keswick Hunt at Grace Episcopal, and Christmas celebrations. At Christmas the Inn is draped in pine boughs, ribbons and sparkling lights; hot cider is served by the fireside. The season is busy with horse-drawn carriage rides, crafts and food demonstrations, puppet and magic shows, Virginia cloggers, wine tastings, concerts, including one on Christmas Eve, and lectures.

The Inn's architectural style recalls an earlier era, but its facilities offer all the modern amenities. The Boar's Head has one of America's 50 best tennis programs, and the hot-air balloon flights over the breathtaking countryside are not to be missed.

The history of the Inn, which takes its name from the Old English symbol for festive hospitality, is a colorful one. Three decades ago the Inn's founder, John B. Rogan, moved an 1830s mill to its present spot from near Thomas Jefferson's historic Monticello. The mill, with its massive hand-hewn beams, is the heart of the resort and home to The Old Mill Room, a premier restaurant and one of Virginia's highest rated. Regional delicacies and gracious service are the hallmarks here.

Public rooms are furnished with English antiques, and guest rooms feature custom-designed period reproductions. The manicured grounds are showcases for traditional Southern flowers and greenery.

Seasonal packages range from the traditional bed and breakfast to the whimsical bed, breakfast and ballooning. Golf and tennis packages are also available, as are the Historic Tour (Monticello and other historic sites) and the Wine Tour (tastings at local Virginia wineries).

KESWICK HALL
701 Country Club Dr.   (804) 979-3440
Keswick   (800) ASHLEY-1
Directions: From Charlottesville, go east on Bypass U.S. 250, east on Va. 22 and right onto Va. 744 until you reach a stop sign. Keswick is directly ahead. From Washington, D.C., take U.S. 29 S. to U.S. 250 and follow directions above. From Richmond, take I-64 W. to Shadwell/250 Exit.

For the ultimate in pampered living, Keswick lives up to its promise of "a fine estate drawing on the best traditions of

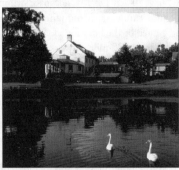
English County Life." Owner Sir Bernard Ashley, co-founder of the Laura Ashley company and founder of Ashley House Inc., has added a wonderful new chapter to the long and fascinating history of Keswick. Broad Oak, a pre-Civil War mansion, once stood here, replaced by Villa Crawford in 1912. Twice the location of the Virginian State Open Golf Tournament, it became a country club in the 1940s. Now it is the 600-acre Keswick Estate, a magnificent backdrop for Keswick Hall, a country house hotel; Keswick Club, an exclusive golf and leisure club; and attractive residences (see our chapter on Real Estate).

At Keswick Hall, Sir Bernard wants visitors to feel as if they were house guests in an old English house with a butler and a maid. Phyllis Napier, the Ashley House interior designer, has made each of the 48 rooms so distinctive that no two are alike. They are decorated with antiques from Ashley's collection and, of course, Laura Ashley fabrics in the familiar flowery prints and more sophisticated styles. All the suites have themes, and the inn emphasizes details such as pure cotton sheets, fluffy bathrobes and other comforts.

Public rooms include a library, a pretty chintz sitting room for English afternoon tea (with scones and jam), the inviting morning room with fireplace and piano and the snooker room for an after-dinner game. Informal meetings or functions are often held in these comfortable, naturally lighted rooms. The Keswick Board Room is perfect for private meetings.

Dining is a special aspect of the Keswick Hall experience. Dishes combine European classic recipes and the best of modern cooking methods, using fresh produce from the community and the estate's own herb garden. Complementing the fine food are wines from an extensive cellar — and the view of vine-covered terraces and lovely gardens. Dinner is $55 per person.

The Keswick Club, the centerpiece of which is an 18-hole Arnold Palmer-designed golf course, is a private club. However, guests at Keswick Hall are granted temporary house memberships which enable them to use the golf course, tennis courts and clubhouse facilities at an extra charge. Within the Pavilion Clubhouse is an indoor/outdoor pool, exercise room, spa and sauna. The Pavilion Pub, an Old English tavern with wooden floors and leather chairs, serves authentic ale, and light meals are served à la carte in the European-style bistro overlooking gardens and the course.

Lodging rates range from $195 for a room to $645 for a master suite, which includes a full country house breakfast and traditional afternoon tea.

WINTERGREEN

Wintergreen   *(800) 325-2200*
Directions: The resort is 43 miles southwest of Charlottesville, bordering the Blue Ridge Pkwy. From I-81 take U.S. 250 E. to Va. 151 S. to Va. 664. Follow signs to Wintergreen.

Wintergreen, an 11,000-acre resort along the spine of the Blue Ridge, enjoys a reputation as one of the most environmentally conscious resorts in the Blue Ridge, and has won awards for its conservation efforts.

Wintergreen is consistently listed among the Top 50 Favorite Family Resorts by *Better Homes and Gardens* and the Top 10 Family Mountain Resorts chosen by *Family Circle* magazine. *Tennis* magazine has named Wintergreen one of its Top 50 Tennis Resorts, and *Golf Digest* rated the resort's Stoney Creek course as one of the best new resort courses in the country in 1990. While Stoney Creek occupies the valley (giving guests the unique opportunity to play golf and ski on the same day), the resort's mountain top Devils Knob Course is the highest in the state (see the golf section of our Recreation chapter for details).

Tennis buffs have their pick of 20 composition clay and five all-weather hard surface courts. The court rate ranges from $12 to $28, and tennis clinics, workouts and ball machine rentals are available.

Swimmers can take advantage of an indoor pool at the Wintergarden Spa and five outdoor pools. Water enthusiasts also have 20-acre Lake Monocan for swimming and canoeing. Mountain bikes can be rented by the hour for $8 ($50 daily), and there is a 25-mile network of marked hiking/biking trails. Horseback riding and pony rides are offered seasonally (see the Recreation chapter). After all the activity, you might want to relax in a hot tub or have a massage at the Wintergarden Spa.

Special events such as the Spring Wildflower Symposium are featured throughout the year and include holiday celebrations such as an Appalachian Mountain Christmas, with horse-drawn carriage rides and candlelight dinners.

In summer a special children's program introduces youngsters to the beauty and wildlife of the Blue Ridge. Babysitting services are also available.

Six restaurants offer varied and delightful dining choices, from sandwiches in the Gristmill lobby of the recently renovated Mountain Inn to gourmet fare in the elegant Copper Mine. Seasonal restaurants are open according to golf and skiing schedules, and the resort has three lounges, one with live entertainment.

Wintergreen has 350 rental homes and condominiums, ranging from studio-size to seven-bedroom. Most have fireplaces and fully equipped kitchens, and many have spectacular views. Rates range from $100 to $550 depending on size and season. Various packages are available, including golf, tennis, family, sports and romantic getaways.

BERNARD'S LANDING

Moneta   *(800) 572-2048*
Directions: It is 45 minutes from either Roanoke or Lynchburg. From Roanoke, take U.S. 220 south to a left on Va. 697 at Wirtz. Follow this

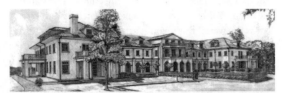
road to its intersection with Va. 122; turn left. Continue for approximately 7 miles, then turn right on Va. 616 at Central Fidelity Bank. Drive 7 miles, then turn left on Va. 940, which will dead end at Bernard's. From Lynchburg, take U.S. 460 W. to Va. 122 and drive about 25 miles to Va. 616. Turn left and follow above directions to Bernard's.

Bernard's Landing is a relatively new resort on relatively new Smith Mountain Lake. The largest lake in Virginia with 500 miles of shoreline, it has become a water playground getaway for people from all over the East Coast. This resort's majestic view and magnificent sunsets sinking into the crystal clear water have drawn artists from around the world.

Bernard's Landing was built in 1981 on what was once a prosperous farm worked by slaves of the Parker family. The family home, an original brick plantation house, still stands at the center of Bernard's activity. Appalachian Power filled the lake in 1966, submersing 22,000 acres and making many Franklin, Bedford and Pittsylvania county farmers instantly wealthy. Bernard's was built on the widest part of the lake and is one of few places where you can see the

magnificent view of the 7-mile-long Smith Mountain Lake.

Walt Disney Productions searched the entire United States for a lake resort with just the right combination to portray Lake Winnipesaukee, New Hampshire, an out-of-the-way vacation spot that still had luxurious amenities. In 1990 a staff of 100, including Bill Murray and Richard Dreyfuss, stayed nearly half a year for the filming of *What About Bob?* Many of the guests were so impressed with the pristine beauty of the lake that they stayed even longer. That's because Bernard's has become known as the place where people come to get away from it all. Although friendly, Franklin County residents grant you privacy, whether you're sailing, swimming or just drinking in the silence.

The well-planned waterfront community sits on its own peninsula and is designed to take advantage of its natural surroundings of mountains reflected by the sparkling lake. As you drive up, the resort impresses you with its huge expanse of lawn that separates the buildings. This could be a premier location for an international kite-flying competition. There are sandy beaches for swimming and sun bathing and an Olympic-size swimming pool. The plantation home serves as a clubhouse. A health club with exercise equipment, indoor handball courts and six tennis courts complement the recreational activities. Clearly, the draw is the water. But if you want more than a splendid view, there's plenty to keep you entertained.

Smith Mountain is an angler's paradise. Nationally known for its striped bass fishing, the lake boasts the state's record striper — weighing 45 pounds. If you're into fishing (see "Fishing" in our Recreation chapter), Bernard's operates a marina and rents fishing, pontoon and ski boats right at the dock. The Virginia Commission of Games and Inland Fisheries manages and maintains an adjoining 5,000 acres for hunting enthusiasts.

The resort's restaurant, The Landing, with premier chef Howard Wilcox, serves gourmet meals. The Landing packs many a picnic lunch for boaters and consistently earns *Roanoker* magazine's Best Restaurant on the Lake award. Probably every resident at the lake has enjoyed Bernard's sumptuous Sunday brunch, truly worth a tasting trip. The savory omelets are the most requested item. Prices are reasonable for great sandwiches at the dockside restaurant or evening entrees.

Bernard's rental facilities run from one- to three-level townhouses to single-level homes or one- to three-bedroom condos. They feature fireplaces, decks, skylights and

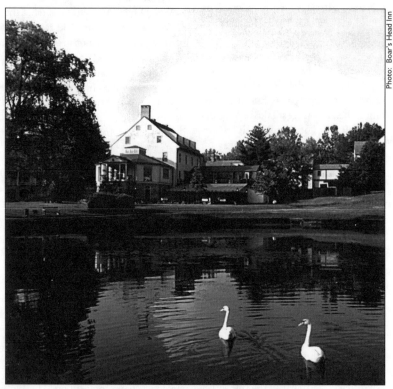

Photo: Boar's Head Inn

The Boar's Head Inn and Sports Club, Charlottesville.

cathedral ceilings. Nightly rentals in peak season range from $105 for a one-bedroom condo to $195 for a three-bedroom townhouse.

Alleghany Highlands Region

THE HOMESTEAD RESORT

Hot Springs   (800) 838-1766
Directions: From I-81, take Mt. Crawford/Va. 257 Exit west to Va. 42, going south to Millboro Springs, then take Va. 39 west to Warm Springs and U.S. 220 south to Hot Springs. Ground service is available from Roanoke Regional Airport. Ingalls Field, Hot Springs, is nearby, serving private and corporate aircraft.

The Homestead, one of the South's major resorts, is grandly situated on 15,000 acres in the Allegheny Mountains. It has been one of the highest-rated resorts for more than 30 years, yet it's as homey as its name suggests and is famous for its afternoon teas in its long, wide lobby. Washington and Jefferson strolled these grounds, and Lord and Lady Astor honeymooned here. The most unusual "guests" of all began their visit December 29, 1941, three weeks after the attack on Pearl Harbor, when 363 Japanese diplomats, along with many Japanese citizens in the United States, were placed at The Homestead for a three-month internment.

The Homestead has been pampering guests since the late 1700s, when the aristocracy of Virginia went to the mountains, with their refreshing springs, instead of enduring the lowland heat with the common folk. In those days, it was fashionable in high-society to move from one mountain spring to another, virtually en masse. Originally valued for medicinal purposes by Native Americans, the springs around The Homestead became centers of social activity.

Hot Springs, where The Homestead has stood for more than a century, was one of the most prominent springs in Virginia. The lineage of The Homestead as a resort and its tradition of "taking the waters" can be traced back to 1766. The spa of today was built in 1892, the dream of M.E. Ingalls, great-great-grandfather of the owner who sold it recently to Resorts International of Dallas, Texas. Designed with the grandeur and technological expertise of today, the spa offers treatments that are still among the most popular services here. The two covered pools and the sheltered drinking spring have been preserved in their natural condition. Eleanor Roosevelt's special chair is still at one of them.

Legions of visitors swear by the springs' curative properties. The magnificent, ornate indoor pool is fed continuously by waters of the Octagon Pool, which can be viewed in front of the spa. The most popular spot is where the natural mineral waters come rushing out under the see-through canopy. The spa has two outdoor pools as well.

The Homestead is undergoing approximately $12.5 million worth of improvements, including new furnishings and plumbing in guest rooms, refurnished hallways in the East Wing and redecoration of the Great Hall and dining room. The spa and playground have been redone; renovations are expected to be completed by 1997.

Today, golfers are often the ones who swear by the Homestead's magical abilities to renew youth and vigor. And no wonder! Golf is king at this resort. Championship play is available on three 18-hole courses, one of which has been the site of the U.S. Amateur and boasts the oldest first tee in continuous use in the United States. Golf Digest and Golf magazine rank the Cascades Course among the top in the nation. John D. Rockefeller used to spread his wealth here by tossing shiny dimes into the pool of water in back of the first tee for the caddies to fight over. President William Taft nearly created a scandal by playing the "frivolous" game of golf on the Fourth of July holiday here at the turn of the century. Golf carts are included in the rates, which range from $76 to $101 for the champion course.

The Homestead has a new sports center and golf practice facility.

Tennis is also superb at The Homestead, with 19 courts, including four all-weather ones. Singles are $10 per person and doubles are $7.50 per person, per hour.

Fishing is another favorite sport (permits cost $20), as is skeet, trap and sporting clays at The Shooting Club, where a round of 25 birds costs $22. Hiking and horseback riding are other popular activities; a carriage ride along scenic trails in a fringe-topped surrey is a pleasant option. Indoor entertainment includes bowling and movies.

Winter brings a whole new round of sports with skiing (see the Skiing chapter), and ice-skating. Half-day skating sessions cost $5.50 weekends and holidays. Some winter weekends are priced for the budget-minded pocketbook. Bring the kids!

The Homestead is a classic. Six hundred spacious guest rooms fill the sweeping Colonial-style building topped by a modern high-rise clock tower. Inside are white Corinthian columns, high-ceiling rooms and turn-of-the-century crystal chandeliers.

Daily room rates in high season, November through April, are $258 to $308 for double occupancy; in value seasons, $218 to $268. Children younger than 12 may share their parents' room at no charge. Prices include breakfast and dinner in the main dining room or in the casual atmosphere of Sam Snead's Tavern in the Village.

THE GREENBRIER

White Sulphur Springs, W.Va. (800) 624-6070
Directions: Take White Sulphur Springs Exit off I-64. Turn right onto W.Va. 60 and travel 2 miles; the entrance is on the left. The Amtrak Station is across the street. Accessible by air from Greenbrier Valley Airport and Roanoke Regional Airport, the resort is two hours away by limousine.

"Monumental" is the first word that comes to mind about this five-star National Historic Landmark set in 6,500 acres of breathtaking scenery. Both its history and its current style, as well as its star-studded guest list, have enchanted people for two centuries. The Greenbrier has hosted world summits and celebrities in the midst of the sleepy little town of White Sulphur Springs. One never knows when TV star Bill Cosby or former British Prime Minister Margaret Thatcher will be seen on the grounds. In 1981, when the U.S. government wanted the ultimate in rest and recreation for its former Iranian hostages, it chose the Greenbrier.

Its history has been nothing short of incredible, beginning in the 18th century when aristocratic Southerners came to drink the mineral waters, stroll and chat while avoiding the summer sun. Twice during wartime, the U.S. government took over and used the resort as a hospital, first in 1861, when the Confederacy also claimed it as its military headquarters. It came perilously close to total destruction during the 1864 occupation by Union troops, when it was ordered burned. Only a plea from a U.S. senator saved it. Later Gen. Robert E. Lee used it as his summer home. During World War II, former guest Gen. George Marshall (for whom the museum in nearby Lexington, Virginia, is

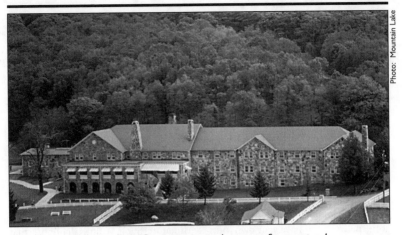

Photo: Mountain Lake

Mountain Lake Resort is situated on one of two natural freshwater lakes in Virginia.

named) turned it into a 2,200-bed hospital named Ashford General. According to locals, many a wounded soldier, upon awakening, thought he had died and gone to Heaven.

After the war, again a resort, The Greenbrier was refurbished and redecorated. Its interior designer used more than 30 miles of carpeting, 45,000 yards of fabric, 40,000 gallons of paint, 15,000 rolls of wallpaper and 34,567 individual decorative and furniture items on the job. The outstanding results stand today.

In 1992 the Pentagon confirmed that a secret underground bunker large enough to house the president, his cabinet and Congress, was constructed here during the nuclear attack threat of the Cold War. Locals have known of its existence for years, but it's a fact the Greenbrier wouldn't discuss. However, resort officials have requested that the bunker be declassified.

Staff outnumber the guests, with 1,600 employees and a 1,200-guest capacity. Accommodations and facilities include 639 guest rooms, 69 cottages, 33 suites, 30 meeting rooms, three championship golf courses, 20 tennis courts and a $7 million spa. To ensure you are adequately fed, there are 110 chefs (no kidding — 110!) to serve you six-course dinners in The Greenbrier's acclaimed combination of classical, continental and American cuisine, in five settings. The list of culinary awards is seemingly endless. The Greenbrier is acclaimed for its own cooking school, La Varenne.

Next door is the world-famous Greenbrier Clinic, a diagnostic center where CEOs can have a checkup in the morning and play golf in the afternoon on a course designed by Jack Nicklaus.

Golf also gets a lot of attention at this resort. Sam Snead, the Greenbrier's golf pro emeritus, played his best game ever here, setting a PGA record of 59 in the third round. You might see him motoring around the course in his golf cart, which is specially fitted with a platform for his dog. Bob Hope, Bing Crosby, Arnold Palmer and the Prince of Wales have played here. In 1979 the course served as the site of the International Ryder Cup matches and the 1994 Solheim Cup. Golf is complimentary for guests during December, January and February; fees range from $45 in the off season to $90 in peak season. The golf cart is extra at $34.

For the tennis set, 15 outdoor Har-Tru courts and five indoor Dynaturf courts await play. Doubles are $42 per hour indoors. Other recreational possibilities are croquet, indoor and outdoor swimming, bowling, billiards, trout fishing, hiking, horseback riding, carriage rides, mountain biking, falconry, white-water rafting, cross-country skiing, trap and skeet shooting and shopping in a large gallery of wonderful stores. For a touch of heaven, give yourself a gift of one (or more) of the 18 treatments at the new spa and have your own nutritionist and exercise trainer design an individual program for you. A five-day spa package costs $2,350.

You won't miss a meal at The Greenbrier. Nobody does. The Greenbrier's food is so excellent that First Lady Hillary Clinton spirited away The Greenbrier's head chef to work at the White House.

Rates are based on a Modified American Plan, which includes breakfast and dinner in the main dining room. Nowhere else is The Greenbrier's Southern heritage more apparent than at the breakfast table, with fresh brook trout, hominy grits, Virginia ham and bacon, cornbread and biscuits. Dinner of six courses is truly an event. A string ensemble provides music, and dinner is served amid candlelight and chandeliers. The vichyssoise is a favorite of Greenbrier regulars, as is its famous peaches and cream for dessert. In 1989 The Greenbrier delivered 10,000 of its famous handmade chocolate truffles for former president George Bush's inaugural dinner.

The Greenbrier's multitude of accommodations is available in a variety of packages, including golf, tennis and family. Its tariff schedule ranges from $145 to $197 per person nightly November through April on the Modified American plan to $183 to $260 per person April to October.

You don't have to stay overnight to enjoy the Greenbrier. Dessert and beverage for two can be had for about $25. Have a snack and then tour the Presidents' Cottage Museum or visit the Miniature Shop, a little dollhouse that sells only miniatures. Then, save your dollars for the total experience!

New River Valley Region

MOUNTAIN LAKE RESORT

Mountain Lake   *(800) 346-3334*
Directions: Take U.S. 460 Bypass around Blacksburg to Va. 700, following this road for 7 winding, scenic country miles to Mountain Lake.

If you saw the great, nostalgic sandstone lodge in the hit movie *Dirty Dancing*, you saw Mountain Lake Resort. The majestic beauty of this grand old hotel was forever captured in 1986 after filmmakers, searching for a gentle, romantic c. '60s resort, saw an ad for Mountain Lake in a magazine. The rest is history. Everyone wants to know where Patrick Swayze slept when he stayed there.

But there's far more history than that to Mountain Lake, one of only two natural freshwater lakes in Virginia and one of the highest natural lakes in the East. It was formed when a rock slide dammed the north end of the valley, creating a 100-foot-deep lake fed by underground streams that rarely allow the water temperature to rise above 72 degrees.

The first report of a pleasure resort here was in 1857, and the first hotel was wooden. In the early '30s, William Lewis Moody of Galveston, Texas, purchased the property and built the present huge hotel from native stone. His elder daughter, Mary, who died in 1986, loved to sit under the great stone fireplace in the lobby, which is still inscribed with "House of Moody." Mary ensured her beloved Mountain Lake, where she stayed each summer, would keep its 2,600 acres of natural paradise in perpetuity by establishing a foundation in her name.

Mountain Lake's motto is "We'll Put You On Top of the World." And they do. When you sit in a rocking chair on the great stone front porch overlooking the lake, you can't help but feel refreshed and renewed. Summer offers the opportunity to relax in cool mountain air, and in the autumn, few fall foliage vistas can compare to Mountain Lake's.

Open May 1 to October 31 only, the resort offers a variety of boating, fishing (guests must furnish own equipment), hiking, tennis, swimming and lawn games. A health club is equipped with a whirlpool, exercise equipment and sauna. And the Recreation Barn offers games, snacks and several shops featuring Appalachian arts and gifts. Mountain Lake celebrates the fall season with an Oktoberfest on the last two Saturdays of September and every Friday and Saturday in October.

The food is always superb in the dining room, where guests lucky enough to get window tables will see a panorama of bluebirds, canaries and redbirds scolding spoiled squirrels awaiting guests' handouts. Deer are common visitors to the grounds, and other wildlife is prevalent. Neat attire is requested for evening meals, which are a gourmet's delight and unbelievably priced for such fare in a beautiful setting. Brunch is $14.95 and dinner is $19.95 per person. Many Virginia Tech parents make the 17-mile trip just for the meal, which can be booked with a reservation.

Accommodations include the 50-room hotel, whose room amenities may include fireplace and whirlpool; the 16-room Chestnut Lodge; and 15 wooden cottages with fireplace. Prices for couples range from $105 nightly to $195 in the lodge, with a small additional charge for each child. Most guests stay on the Modified American Plan, which includes lodging, breakfast, dinner and use of all facilities and equipment. Personal checks are accepted. The air is rare, and so is the experience!

Southwest Virginia Region

DOE RUN LODGE
RESORT AND CONFERENCE CENTER

Mile 189 Blue Ridge Pkwy   (540) 398-2212
Hillsville   (800) 325-6189

Just across the border of Floyd County, in Patrick County, Doe Run Lodge Resort and Conference Center and its High Country Restaurant are nestled in the most beautiful part of the Blue Ridge Parkway. With Groundhog Mountain as the midpoint on this road of pastoral beauty, your senses will be overwhelmed by what this year-round resort has to offer.

Doe Run Lodge Resort and Conference Center was built to fit the beauty of this environment. The chalets are constructed of wood beams and stone; floor to ceiling windows allow magnificent views. Each large suite has a fireplace, two bedrooms, two full baths and a living/dining area. The chalets and villas are furnished and have complete kitchens. Millpond Hideaway, designed for executives and honeymooners, has a whirlpool tub, luxury shower and steam cabinet, full-suite stereo and TV, fireplace and enclosed garage.

The historic Log Cabin dates back to 1865 and was moved to the Lodge. The exterior remains primitive, but the interior features a queen size bed, a whirlpool tub, a shower, natural stone fireplace and TV/VCR. The Executive Suite is a modern chalet with whirlpool tub, luxury shower and steam cabinet, and full-suite stereo and TV. The area also boasts personal homes and building sites available for sale.

High Country Restaurant offers regional fare such as country ham steak, fresh rainbow trout from their own stocked pond, as well as seafood and beef dishes. The restaurant will pack picnic lunches too.

Rates range from $125 to $175 per night.

Inside
Bed and Breakfast and Country Inns

Isn't it time you got away from it all? Slip into the tranquility of country life at an old stagecoach inn on the Valley Turnpike in Woodstock, linger for a while at the Inn at Narrow Passage or get closer to heaven at the Bent Mountain Lodge that sits high in the Blue Ridge. No matter what your interest, you can find the perfect place to relax.

Each of these grand old bed and breakfast inns and country inns has its own distinct charm, with histories as varied as the decor. How many of us dream of spending the night in a real mansion? Experience just that at Lynchburg's Mansion Inn. You can stay on the former site of an ancient Native American village at Silver Thatch Inn in Charlottesville. Or you may be swept away by the beauty of bubbling springs at Meadow Lane in Warm Springs, featured this year on a national Tide detergent TV commercial.

A significant number of the inns are in restored, historic properties. Historic and other attractions of exceptional interest, plus skiing, fishing, boating, swimming and horseback riding are all within reach of a bed and breakfast inn. Many provide dinners, weddings, receptions and other social and meeting functions.

You'll find that Blue Ridge innkeepers are among the most cordial hosts in the world, genuinely concerned about your well-being and comfort. Virginia is internationally known for Southern hospitality, and these antique country manors can convey to you a sense of tranquility hard to find anywhere else.

As in our Other Accommodations chapter, we provide a dollar key to assist you in determining the cost of a stay for two at the inns we've listed in this chapter. Most inns have similar price ranges of between $50 and $120 dollars per night, and most require a deposit of one night's lodging to confirm reservations. Rates may change at different seasons, so bear this in mind when calling for reservations.

$45 to 65	$
$66 to $85	$$
$86 to $105	$$$
$106 and higher	$$$$

Reservation Services

The following services are available to assist you in selecting a bed and breakfast or country inn and making reservations.

This state-wide association has just issued a CD-ROM showing 182 of Virginia's finest bed and breakfast inns. It includes pictures, a calendar of events, listed monthly by region and other general Virginia tourism information. The cost is $15.95 for the CD-ROM or $10.95 for the diskette version.

• **Bed & Breakfast Association of Virginia**, P.O. Box 791, Orange 22960; (703) 721-3951

• **Blue Ridge Bed & Breakfast**, Route 2, Box 3895, Berryville 22611; (703) 955-1246

• **Guest House Bed & Breakfast**, Charlottesville; (804) 979-7264

• **Princely Bed & Breakfast Inc.**, Alexandria; (703) 683-2159

• **Shenandoah Valley Bed & Breakfast Reservations**, P.O. Box 634, Woodstock 22664; (703) 459-8241

• **Shenandoah Valley Lodging Services**, Route 3, Box 119F, Luray 22835; (703) 743-2936

Shenandoah Valley Region

Boyce

THE RIVER HOUSE
U.S. 50 E., off I-81
Exit 313A   *(504) 837-1476*
$$-$$$$

Cornelia and Donald Niemann will make your stay on this historic property near the Shenandoah River a memorable one. The site, known in 1780 as Ferry Farm, part of the huge Carter Hall estate, was surveyed by a young George Washington for Lord Fairfax. It served as a field hospital in the Civil War and, in the 1940s, was a popular restaurant and tavern.

Renovations and expansions have created an imposing Virginia fieldstone residence with five air-conditioned guests rooms, each with a private bath and working fireplace. Each room is elegantly appointed, spacious and has a unique personality. Snacks and an early continental breakfast in one of the two kitchenettes may precede a hearty brunch in the dining room. Rooms are accessible to the

handicapped, equipment is available for small children, and corporate rates are available. Each room has a telephone, and a fax and copier are available.

The surrounding 15 acres of open woodland and river frontage, just an hour from Washington, D.C., give the inn a distinctively rural ambiance. Numerous historic sites, horseback riding, biking, strolling, golf, tennis, antique and other shopping and award-winning dining are all within easy travel distance.

The Niemanns hold special theme weekends, one of the most popular of which is "Enter Laughing — A Weekend in the Country," with role-playing and other hilarity wrapped around a peaceful retreat. Three-day Country Houseparties are tailored for groups — families, couples, friends — and can include wine and cheese gatherings, candlelight dinners, picnics, planned activities and a gourmet brunch.

Front Royal

KILLAHEVLIN
1401 N. Royal Ave.   *(540) 636-7335*
$$$-$$$$

Irish immigrant and limestone baron William Carson built his home on the highest spot in Front Royal, calling it "Killyhevlin" for the place in Northern Ireland he cherished as a child. The house was designed by the architectural firm that created Washington's grand old Executive Office Building.

During the Civil War, it is said that two of Mosby's men were hanged here, and Union troops often camped in this strategic spot.

Owners Susan and John Lang were captivated by the brick Edwardian mansion and instructed their interior designers to make sure the taste of Ireland re-

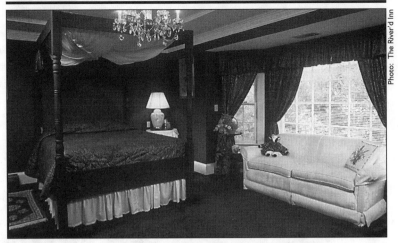

One of the elegant rooms at the River'd Inn in Woodstock.

mained foremost in the house's decor. Each of the three rooms has a queen-size bed, working fireplace, private bath with tub and shower and wonderful views. The two suites have enormous bathrooms with whirlpool tubs.

Breakfast is a sumptuous repast of fresh fruits and breads and a variety of entrees elegantly served.

Front Royal is not only the gateway to the Skyline Drive, but a lively place with several wineries and many local festivals.

Woodstock

COUNTRY FARE

402 Main St.   *(540) 459-4828*
$

Historic Lee Highway (U.S. 11) leads to this small-town bed and breakfast inn. A half-acre of glorious magnolia, boxwoods and Japanese cherry trees encircle the home. Proprietor Bette Hallgren extends old-fashioned hospitality in a home that exudes charm and history. Country Fare was built in the late 18th century; a section was added in 1840. From 1861 to 1864, the building served as a hospital. The house has been completely restored.

The three guest rooms are furnished with antiques and country collectibles. Each has been hand-stenciled in original designs. The master bedroom has a private shower, another room has a queen-size bed and a Boston rocker, and a cozy double-bedded room has accents of brass.

A continental breakfast of home-baked muffins and breads and surprises from Grandmother's cookbook is served before the wood-burning stove in the dining room on cold mornings or on the brick patio in summer.

After breakfast, take a walk into the village of Woodstock to explore the town's history. The courthouse, designed by Thomas Jefferson in 1792, is the oldest building of its kind still in use west of the Blue Ridge Mountains. Nearby natural attractions include Shenandoah National Park, Skyline Drive, Luray Caverns and various vineyards. New Market Battlefield, Belle Grove Plantation and Wayside Theater are a short distance away. The Shenandoah Music Festival and the Shenandoah County Fair are held nearby each summer.

Photo: The River'd Inn

THE INN AT NARROW PASSAGE

1-81 and U.S. 11 S.   *(703) 459-8000*
$-$$$

This log inn overlooking the Shenandoah River has been welcoming and protecting travelers since the 1740s, when it was a haven for settlers against Indian attacks along the narrow passage, where only one wagon could pass and travel was dangerous. It also served as Stonewall Jackson's headquarters during the Valley Campaign of 1862. Ed and Ellen Markel have taken great care in restoring this landmark to its 18th-century look and maintaining the warm ambiance of the original inn.

The inn is furnished in antiques and Colonial reproductions. Each bedroom has comfortable amenities; some have wood-burning fireplaces. The inn is centrally heated and air-conditioned. Breakfast is served in the Colonial dining room, often before a cheery fire; relax by the

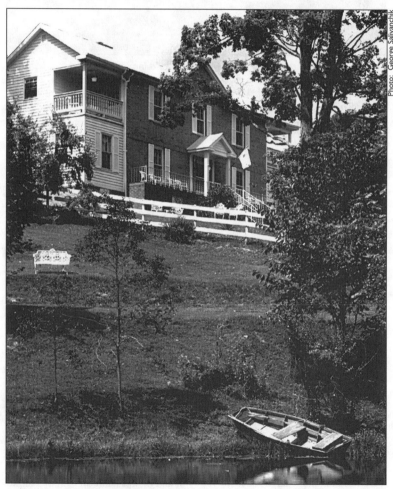

Photo: George Salivanchik

The Inn at Union Run sits on 12 acres outside of Lexington.

massive limestone fireplace in the living room or enjoy the views of the sloping lawns and river from the porch.

Hiking and fishing are options at the inn. Nearby you'll find historic battlefields, wineries, caverns and skiing at Bryce Resort. The inn is 2 miles from I-81, off Exit 283, just south of Woodstock. A conference room is available for executive retreats.

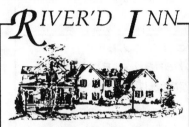

RIVER'D INN

A secluded Victorian Inn nestled at the base of the Massanutten Mountains on the Shenandoah River.

Woodstock, Virginia 22664
1-800-637-4561   (540) 459-5369

RIVER'D INN

Va. 663, off U.S. 11   **(540) 459-5369**
$$$$

Cross over a low-water bridge on the north fork of the Shenandoah River and, if the river rises, the locals say you are "rivered in." This Victorian inn, at the base of Massanutten Mountain, sits on one of the famous seven bends of the Shendandoah. Hosts Alan and Diana Edwards oversee the 25 acres of secluded natural areas offering picnicking, hiking and relaxing. A wraparound veranda and swimming pool are other leisure options.

Country auctions, antique and craft shops, horseback riding, fishing and other river-oriented activities beckon. Nearby attractions include the New Market Battlefields and Civil War Museum, Massanutten and Bryce ski resorts, Skyline Drive, caverns, Wayside Theatre and numerous other historic and cultural sites.

The inn offers quiet dining in three country-elegant dining rooms, each with a distinctive fireplace and intimate seating. Meals are elegant, candlelit affairs with fresh-cut flowers, linen, china and gourmet cuisine. Highlights of a typical brunch might be chilled peach champagne soup with fresh strawberries, eggs Benedict, local pan-fried trout and pecan tartlett with fresh whipped cream. Dinners feature such gourmet mainstays as lobster tail, filet mignon and chicken cordon bleu.

The inn is centrally heated and air-conditioned and rooms are furnished in fine antiques.

Luray

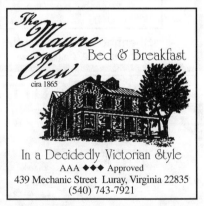

The Mayne View Bed & Breakfast
cira 1865

In a Decidedly Victorian Style
AAA ◆◆◆ Approved
439 Mechanic Street Luray, Virginia 22835
(540) 743-7921

THE MAYNE VIEW

Mechanic St.   **(540) 743-7921**
$$$

This bed and breakfast inn in the heart of Virginia's lush Shenandoah Valley offers fine accommodations and breathtaking mountain views from its position between the Shenandoah National Park and the Washington and Jefferson National Forest. Guest rooms are well-appointed with feather beds, fireplaces and private baths. Fine cuisine is another attraction here.

In Virginia's Shenandoah Valley

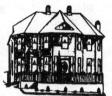
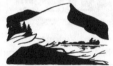
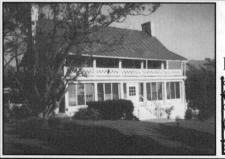
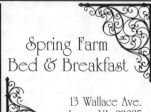

In Virginia's Shenandoah Valley

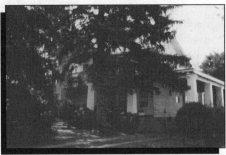
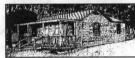
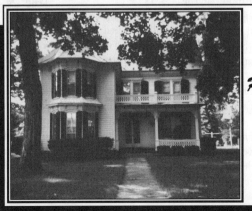
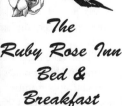

Just minutes from hiking, championship golf and other outdoor activities, The Mayne View is also convenient to tourist attractions, including Luray Caverns and New Market Battlefield.

The Shenandoah sunrise is a great backdrop for the morning meal, which includes gourmet coffees, teas and homemade muffins, pastries and jams. If you want to sleep in, a bountiful breakfast buffet and cooked-to-order breakfasts are also available. For the ultimate indulgence, make plans ahead for breakfast in bed.

SPRING FARM INN

Wallace Ave., off U.S. 211   *(540) 743-4701*
$$-$$$$

This 200-year-old historic brick Colonial sits on 10 acres of grounds with mountain panoramas visible from nearly every vantage point. A gazebo, hammocks and a patio bring guests outdoors to enjoy the secluded, natural setting, which is part of a bird sanctuary. A veranda running the full length of the house commands views of the Blue Ridge Mountains, while a porch on the other side of the house frames a view of Massanutten Mountain.

Guests may choose from three large bedrooms with a shared bath, a suite with a private bath and a glass-enclosed sitting area (the better to see those gorgeous mountains!) or the cottage, which also has a private bath. Innkeeper Thelma Mayes provides a full breakfast each morning and refreshments every hour of the day.

This serene retreat is near numerous natural and historic sites and a lot of recreational opportunities. It is 2.5 miles from Luray Caverns, 8 miles from the entrance to Skyline Drive, and fine restaurants within a short drive. The inn is 90 miles from Washington, D.C.

Gift certificates are available, and the inn plans memorable wedding packages.

WOODRUFF HOUSE

330 Mechanic St.   *(540) 743-1494*
$$$-$$$$

This highly rated inn is described by the Woodruffs as an "1882 fairytale Victorian," and it delivers on that promise with its antiques, Oriental rugs and hallmarked silver catching the firelight in cozy Victorian parlors. Each of the three guest rooms has a private bath and fireplace. An elegant evening high-tea buffet dinner, morning gourmet coffee service in your room and a fireside candlelit breakfast are included in the room price. Innkeeper Lucas Woodruff is a chef, so fantastic food is *de riguer*.

In the garden, which is lit by candles after dusk, is a heated Jacuzzi that sets the tone for a romantic, relaxing evening. By day, the active can avail themselves of bicycles and canoes or visit nearby attractions such as Luray Caverns, New Market Battlefield, Massanutten Resort or the Skyline Drive.

Stanley

JORDAN HOLLOW FARM INN

Stanley   *(540) 778-2209*
$$$$ *(540) 778-2285*

Jordan Hollow Farm Inn is a beautifully restored Colonial horse farm that has been converted into a country inn. The farm has 45 acres nestled in a secluded hollow surrounded by the Shenandoah National Park and the George Washington National Forest.

The buildings, except for Rowe's Lodge, are the original farm buildings, renovated to provide cozy but modern facilities. An overall family farm environment is nurtured here, a blend of roll-

Inns to *Bed & Breakfasts*

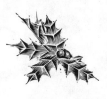
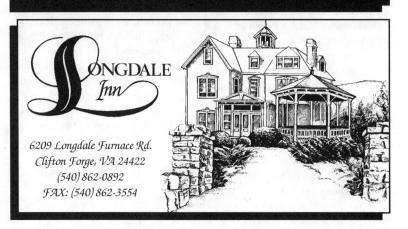

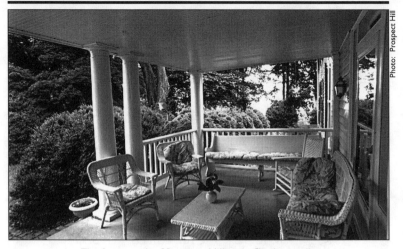

Photo: Prospect Hill

The front porch of Prospect Hill near Charlottesville.

ing hills, lush meadows and fragrant woods.

The sun deck surrounding Rowe's Lodge is a good place to oversee the farm's activities. The inn has 21 guest rooms, decorated with country antiques and artifacts. Each has a private bath and some have fireplaces and Jacuzzis. The Colonial farmhouse has four dining rooms.

The food, described as "country cosmopolitan," is outstanding home-style cooking with a French flair and a touch of African and Mideastern seasonings. The selection includes quail, chicken, veal, steak, fish and pasta, complemented by home-baked bread, a garden salad and fresh vegetables.

For indoor entertainment, visit the library, cable TV lounge and pub, named The Watering Trough, that was originally a stable. Live entertainment is provided on Friday and Saturday nights, and you may find yourself challenged to a game of pool or chess. A stable on the property can accommodate riding for the beginner or expert, as well as pony rides for children younger than 8.

Other nearby activities include swimming, hiking, canoeing, fishing, skiing, museums, antiques and craft shops. The farm is a short drive from Lake Arrowhead, Luray Caverns, Shenandoah National Park and George Washington National Forest. Limited boarding facilities are available for pets or horses. You need to let them know if you are bringing children when making reservations.

MILTON HOUSE BED & BREAKFAST
Va. 340 Busi.   *(540) 778-3451*
$$$-$$$$

John and Karin Tipton, innkeepers, pamper their guests with Southern hospitality in their beautifully refurbished 1915 Southern Colonial home ordered from Sears' *Big Book Catalog.* The inn, 7 miles south of Luray, is filled with antiques, Karin's hand-made quilts, floral arrangements and dried flower wreaths. A collection of Steiff bears and rabbits, along with June McKenna limited edition Santa Clauses, are charming distractions.

The inn is rich in detail: long sweeping porches cooled by stately fir trees, leaded-glass windows that create a kaleidoscope of sunbeams in the morning, detailed stenciling and other architectural attractions.

Rates include a leisurely candlelight dinner, a soak in the outdoor garden Jacuzzi, early morning coffee and a sumptuous breakfast of Belgian waffles with fresh fruit or stuffed French toast with orange-apricot sauce.

All rooms have private baths, and a suite with a double shower is available. The property also includes a log cabin, built in 1991, with two deluxe accommodations that include living/seating areas, queen-size beds, private baths, gas log fireplaces and decks with mountain views (one unit has a kitchen). The inn also offers a mountain retreat nestled at the foot of Massanutten Mountain with panoramic views of the Blue Ridge Mountains. The Shenandoah River and a 15-acre lake are five minutes away. The retreat has two bedrooms, a living room with a stone fireplace, cathedral ceilings, a fully equipped kitchen, bath, screened porch and stone barbecue.

Smoking is permitted in designated areas. Weekly rates are available.

THE RUBY ROSE INN
BED AND BREAKFAST
Stanley   (540) 778-4680
$$-$$$$

This lovely Victorian home, c. 1890, is the ideal setting for a peaceful retreat — just ask members of the British Parliament, who are the inn's most famous guests. Comfortably furnished and newly remodeled, The Ruby Rose has a private cottage with fireplace and Jacuzzi, the Mayhew Suite and spacious guest rooms with private baths.

Guests awaken to a full breakfast, and beverages and homemade goodies are always available. The inn is surrounded by mountains, tall oaks and colorful flower beds and sits in the Valley between Shenandoah National Park and George Washington National Forest, scenic areas for hiking and biking. Other "neighborhood" activities include horseback riding, golfing, fishing, canoeing, rafting, antiques shopping and tracing historic Civil War battles and skirmishes by markers, which dot the area. The famous New Market Battlefield, just a few miles away, hosts a spring re-enactment.

Package plans include a professionally guided nature and birding hike with a picnic lunch. Inquire about estate sales, trail maps, box lunches and tee times. In the Cottage, you can get breakfast in bed and personal touches, such as flowers or a homemade cake, for special occasions.

Discounts are available for multiple nights and other specials from November through March. Pets are not allowed. Guests must refrain from smoking inside buildings, but a flagstone patio is available for guests who wish to smoke.

Weyers Cave

THE INN AT KEEZLETOWN RD.
Va. 276   (540) 234-0644
$$

This elegant 100-year-old Victorian in the quaint village of Weyers Cave has spectacular views of the Blue Ridge Mountains. The four large guest rooms are furnished with antiques and comfortable beds and have quiet sitting areas. Each has a private bath, air conditioning and cable TV.

The innkeepers, Sandy and Alan Inabinet, provide a full country breakfast that includes fresh eggs from the inn's own chickens. Dinner reservations may also be made. The grounds have gardens and a goldfish pond, and guests may walk on the adjacent trail through the town's park or sit and rock on the inn's porch. Historic sites are within easy driving distance, as are the airport and several colleges. Orchards, vineyards, hiking trails, antique shops, caverns, ski resorts and other attractions are nearby.

Children 14 years old and older are welcome. Smoking is limited to the garden and porch. Pets are not permitted. The inn is a mile east of I-81.

Harrisonburg

JOSHUA WILTON HOUSE, INN AND RESTAURANT

412 S. Main St.   *(540) 434-4464*
$$$

Roberta and Craig Moore welcome guests to their elegantly restored Victorian home, which lies in the heart of the Shenandoah Valley. Restoration efforts have preserved much of the original architecture.

The Moores will spoil you with a complimentary glass of wine or beer, and their gourmet breakfast, including homemade pastries, fresh fruits and a delicious pot of coffee, is enough to summon anyone out of bed in the morning.

The inn's bedrooms are furnished with period antiques to give them the charm of the 1880s. You can choose from three dining rooms, a sun room or an outdoor terrace and dine on meals famous throughout the Shenandoah Valley. All five bedrooms have private baths and reading areas.

The Wilton House is within walking distance of James Madison University and downtown Harrisonburg. There is also a variety of athletic activities, such as golfing, biking, hiking, swimming and skiing, accessible from the inn. This old

mansion is an oasis of quiet charm and gracious living surrounded by the Blue Ridge Mountains.

Penn Laird

HEARTH N' HOLLY INN

Penn Laird   *(540) 434-6766*
$$

Doris and Dennis Brown's pleasant bed and breakfast is 5 miles from I-81 Exit 247A, 10 minutes from Massanutten Four Seasons Resort and James Madison University. Situated on 15 acres, the Colonial and Victorian inn has three guest rooms with queen-size brass beds, private baths and fireplaces.

There are two seatings, at 8 AM and 9 AM, for a full country breakfast. Dinners are also available on request, and the innkeepers love pulling out all the stops to host weddings and other special events.

The new picnic pavillion has a hot tub and a queen-size hammock for maxiumum relaxation.

Diversions within easy reach are the theater, arts and sports events at the university; golf, skiing and a host of other activities at Massanutten Resort; Skyline Drive and the Blue Ridge Parkway; Civil War battlefields; Endless, Grand and Luray caverns. Be warned: It will be hard to leave the inn, with its sunroom, picnic pavilion, hot tub, queen-size hammock and wooded walking trails.

Staunton

ASHTON COUNTRY HOUSE

1205 Middlebrook Ave.   *(540) 885-6819*
$$-$$$ *(800) 296-7819*

With 24 beautiful acres surrounding this country retreat, it's hard to believe the center of town is a mere mile away. A c. 1860 Greek Revival manor house,

$\mathcal{I}$nns to $\mathcal{B}$ed & $\mathcal{B}$reakfasts

Joshua Wilton House

Harrisonburg's most elegant lodging dining facility in a beautifully restored Victorian home. Within walking distance of James Madison University and historic Downtown Harrisonburg. Eat our fine cuisine in the Restaurant or dine casually in The Cafe.

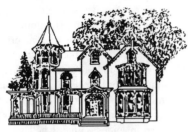

412 S. Main Street
Harrisonburg, VA 22801
(540) 434-4464

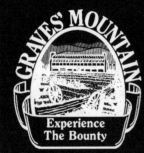

Experience
The Bounty

Our Blue Ridge Mountain country inn specializes in home-cooked food and gracious hospitality. Enjoy hiking, fishing, swimming and good old-fashioned fun.

Rt. 670 Syria, VA 22743 (540) 923-4231

Frederick House

A Small Hotel and Tearoom

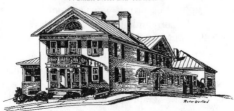

FREDERICK AND NEW STREETS
P.O. BOX 1387, STAUNTON, VIRGINIA 24402-1387
540-885-4220   800-334-5575

Ashton has been owned since 1991 by Sheila Kennedy and her husband, Stanley Polanski, a professional jazz pianist. The 40-foot center hall hints at the manor-house stylings you'll find throughout, including the rosewood grand piano.

No detail is overlooked in their guests' comfort, including flannel sheets in the winter and cool cotton chambray in the summer — plus four plump pillows. Ah, luxury! Lovely English country-style furnishings, immaculate housekeeping and gracious common rooms enhance your stay. Four double guest rooms and one suite are available, each with a private bath or shower (or both). Four of the rooms have a fireplace and one features a balcony.

A generous breakfast includes fruit, scones, scrambled eggs, bacon and potatoes prepared with a professional touch by Sheila, a graduate of the New York Restaurant School, and accompanied on the grand piano by Stan.

Three porches overlook the expansive grounds, populated by several dogs, numerous cats and a pair of genteel goats.

Children older than 15 are accepted. Wheelchair access and a specially equipped bathroom are available.

BELLE GRAE INN

515 W. Frederick St.   *(540) 886-5151*
$-$$$$

This authentically restored 17-room inn built in 1870 will please you with its luxurious rooms and appetizing menu. It is named for two of the surrounding mountains, Betsy Belle and Mary Grae. The Scotch-Irish settlers in the area, reminded of their homeland, named the mountains for Scottish landmarks. Belle Grae sits atop a hill in historic Staunton. Wicker rockers invite relaxation on the veranda; white gingerbread decorates the porch of the main, original building.

One of the first things a guest sees is four stained-glass panels in the double entrance door and a crystal oval in which the Inn's name is engraved. Period reproductions and antiques, which are for sale, are found throughout the dining rooms, bistro, lounge and other lovely rooms. The bedrooms are each furnished a little differently, but all fit the period. You can sit in front of your cozy fireplace (most rooms have them) and sip complimentary sherry from long-stemmed glasses. All rooms have private baths with such amenities as English herb soaps and bath oils. Joined by pathways and boradwalks are five restored 1870s to 1890s vintage houses available to families or for executive retreats.

The popular chef at this fine establishment prepares meals using fresh breads and fruit, and the best meats and vegetables. A full American breakfast is included in the room price. Or, if you prefer to relax, a continental breakfast and newspaper will be delivered to your room.

Activities in the area include walking tours through gorgeous historic Staunton, shopping at a gigantic antique warehouse or chess and backgammon in the quiet of the inn's sitting room.

FREDERICK HOUSE

Frederick and New Sts.   *(540) 885-4220*
$-$$$ *(800) 334-5575*

Three stately old townhouses were rescued from demolition and transformed into Frederick House. These Greek Revival buildings have been restored and the rooms inside graciously appointed with antiques and paintings by Virginia artists. The oversize beds add an extra touch of comfort. Each of the eight rooms and six suites has its own private bath, cable TV, telephone, radio, air conditioning and private entrance. A full, delicious

Inns to Bed & Breakfasts

The River House
Bed & Breakfast on the Shenandoah

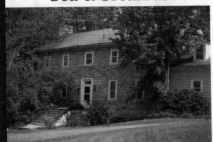

- 5 rooms, each with a private bath, fireplace & a/c
- Full breakfast/brunch in the Dining Room
- Corporate rates available for business travelers
- Telephones in all rooms, fax, & copier available
- special comedy and murder mystery weekends scheduled during the winter months

**Boyce, VA
(540) 837-1476**

The INN at Narrow Passage
WOODSTOCK

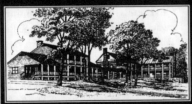

Historic Lodging on the Shenandoah River

Relax in this historic log inn with 5 acres on the Shenandoah River near fishing, hiking, antiquing, vineyards, caverns and fine restaurants. 90 minutes from D.C.

EXECUTIVE CONFERENCE FACILITIES

Rt. 11 S. (I-81, Exit 283) Woodstock, VA 22664 • (540) 459-8000

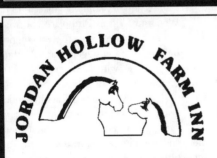

The 150 acre restored horse farm has cozy lodging, an excellent restaurant, horseback riding and walking trails. It's located in Virginia's lovely Shenandoah Valley only 2 hours west of Washington. D.C. and 8 miles south of the Luray Caverns and Skyline Drive.

**540-778-2209 or 540-778-2285
Route 2, Box 375, Stanley, Virginia 22851**

home-cooked breakfast is served each morning in Chumley's Tea Room.

One activity we recommend is a relaxing stroll through the town to photograph Staunton's gorgeous architecture and to visit the town's antique shops. Woodrow Wilson's birthplace is only two blocks away, and Mary Baldwin College is next door. Cycling, hiking and touring are perfect activities in the surrounding Blue Ridge and Allegheny mountains. Hosts Joe and Evy Harman will point out places of interest and provide a bit of history as well.

Fine dining is available at McCormick's Restaurant, adjacent to the Frederick House, and at six other restaurants within lazy walking distance.

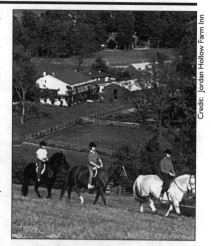

Credit: Jordan Hollow Farm Inn

Riders enjoy a leisurely outing on the hills surrounding Jordan Hollow Farm in Page County.

KENWOOD

235 E. Beverley St. (540) 886-0524
$$

Kenwood, a beautifully restored turn-of-the-century brick Colonial Revival home, is in the historic district, next door to the Woodrow Wilson Museum and Birthplace and within walking distance of Staunton's finest restaurants and shops. Filled with period furniture and antiques, the inn offers comfortable accommodations in a relaxed atmosphere. A full Shenandoah Valley breakfast is included with your stay.

Guests have their choice of three upstairs bedrooms with queen-size beds and private baths.

Your hosts, Liz and Ed Kennedy, can suggest many ways to spend your days in the area, many within a short walk or drive of the inn. Take the Staunton walking tour, visit Mary Baldwin College and Stuart Hall and see the exhibits at the Museum of American Frontier Culture and the Statler Brothers' Museum. Stroll along picturesque East Beverley to see the antique shops or have a gourmet meal at one of several restaurants. Wintergreen Resort, Harrisonburg, Lexington and Charlottesville are about 30 minutes away, and Skyline Drive and Blue Ridge Parkway are only 15 minutes away.

THE SAMPSON EAGON INN

238 E. Beverley St. (540) 886-8200
$$-$$$ (800) 597-9722

This elegant inn, which has won preservation awards, is in the historic Gospel Hill section of Staunton, adjacent to the Woodrow Wilson Birthplace and Mary Baldwin College. The property's original owner, Sampson Eagon, was a Methodist preacher who held services on the grounds here during the 1790s.

Don't expect any preaching today, however: The inn is tailor-made for privacy, with three distinctive guest rooms and two suites, each furnished with beautiful period pieces, a queen-size canopied bed, cozy sitting area and modern bath. Private TVs with VCRs are also standard in the rooms, and the inn even has a fax machine, just in case you can't get away from the office completely.

The day begins with a full gourmet breakfast in the formal dining room (although the accent is on casual). Entrees include such entrees as pecan Belgian waffles, Grand Marnier souffle pancakes and an array of egg dishes.

The inn was selected in 1993 by *Country Inns Magazine* as one of America's Best Inn Buys, and *Gourmet* magazine writes that proprietors Frank and Laura Mattingly "take the second 'B' in B&B seriously." This is indeed the place for a memorable retreat.

THORNROSE HOUSE AT GYPSY HILL
531 Thornrose Ave.   (540) 885-7026
$-$$

Otis and Suzanne Huston are the innkeepers at this beautiful bed and breakfast inn in Staunton's Gypsy Hill area. The moment you step into the grand entranceway, you begin to discover the charm of this Georgian Revival brick home and its five comfortable guest rooms, each with private bath.

You'll awaken to the aroma of a heart-healthy breakfast, after which you'll want to venture out and see the sites that make Staunton so special. Nearby attractions include the P. Buckley Moss Museum, Monticello, Grand Caverns and the Museum of American Frontier Culture. Across the street is the 300-acre Gypsy Hill Park, where you can play golf, tennis (rackets and balls provided) or swim.

Thornrose House has lovely gardens gracing its acre of grounds. The wraparound veranda with rocking chairs is perfect for a afternoon refreshments. The sitting room has a fireplace and grand piano. Children older than 4 are accepted.

Steeles Tavern

STEELES TAVERN MANOR
Steeles Tavern   (540) 377-6444
$$-$$$$ (800) 743-8666

Hospitality in this small town on Lee Highway (U.S. 11) dates back to 1781, when David Steele provided lodging to travelers between Staunton and Lexington. The home that Steele's descendants built in 1916 underwent extensive restoration in 1994. In 1995 innkeepers Eileen and Bill Hoernlein opened its doors as a highly rated inn, completing the circle.

The inn has five guest rooms, each with a private bath, and some with whirlpool baths or VCRs. Each room is named for a flower — dahlia, buttercup, wisteria, hyacinth and rose — and has a king- or queen-size bed and a sitting area. The house and guest rooms are tastefuly decorated in antique furniture, quilts and lace.

The Hoernleins bring out their fine china, light the candles, and put on classical music, creating a special atmosphere for their sumptuous country breakfast. If you're an early riser, Eileen will have a thermos of hot coffee waiting on your doorstep. Afternoon tea is served between 4 and 5 PM. Guests can also arrange to have Saturday night dinner at the manor. Children younger than 14, pets and smoking are not permitted in the inn.

The area is excellent for antiquing and craft shopping, for golf on several nearby courses, and for sightseeing in Lexington, Staunton or the Skyline Drive. By the way, Cyrus McCormick built his revolutionary reaper in Steeles Tavern, and James Gibbs perfected his Wilcox Gibbs sewing machine just outside of town.

THE SUGAR TREE

Steele's Tavern   (540) 377-2197
$$$-$$$$

Sarah and Hal Davis' getaway is set on 28 wooded acres 2,800 feet up in the Blue Ridge Mountains (take Exit 205 off I-81). In spring, the woods are a riot of trillium, rhododendron, laurel and dogwood blossoms, and fall presents a palette of yellow, rust and scarlet. From the broad porch of this mortise-and-peg timber and stone lodge, you can see 40 miles across the mountaintops and watch wildlife from 100 feet or less.

Sugar Tree opened to national acclaim in 1983, then slipped into a hiatus which was broken by the Davises in 1994. Everything has been refurbished. Eleven spacious rooms and suites occupy three buildings, including the main lodge's Sugar Tree Country Room with a king-size bed, vaulted ceiling and oversized whirlpool bath with a mountain view. Each room has a woodburning fireplace and private bath; some have whirlpool baths, ceiling fans and VCRs.

Dinners are served nightly — romantic, candlelit affairs featuring stuffed quail or beef tenderloin medallions with mushroom sauce — and sumptuous breakfasts are served in a glass-walled dining room overlooking a field of wildflowers. Lexington, Staunton, and the Blue Ridge Parkway are nearby.

Swoope

LAMBSGATE

Va. 254 and Va. 833   (540) 337-6929
$

This restored 1816 farmhouse 6 miles west of Staunton is a comfortable lodging with a bountiful Southern breakfast and spectacular mountain views. Dan and Elizabeth Fannon invite you to relax in their home on the Middle River, surrounded by seven acres, a working sheep farm. You can hike or bike the back roads or watch the day-to-day activities of life on a farm. Children especially enjoy the animals and the garden behind the house that grows everything from spices to grapes. Poles are provided for fishing on the nearby river.

Wooden floors, solid furniture and warm quilts hand-made by Mrs. Fannon are homey touches, as are the sheepskin rugs at your bedside. The house's three guest rooms share a bath.

A mouthwatering breakfast stars Dan's bran muffins and homemade peach and strawberry preserves. Breakfast orders are taken the evening before; the daily newspaper and greet guests at the day's first light.

Lambsgate is open all year, offering three double guest rooms, with a maximum of six sharing a bath.

Waynesboro

THE IRIS INN

191 Chinquapin Dr.   (540) 943-1991
$$-$$$

The charm and grace of Southern living in a totally modern facility surrounded by woods — that's the Iris Inn. The brick-and-cedar inn was built in 1991 and is ideal for a weekend retreat, business accommodation or tranquil spot for the tourist. Its focus is on comfort, with seven spacious guest rooms decorated in nature and wildlife motifs, each with private bath.

The main building has six guest rooms, each furnished with 18th-century reproductions, family pieces and antiques and each having specific themes, such as Deer Room, Wildflower Room, Pine Room, Bird Room and Duck Pond. The bright and airy rooms

Inns to Bed & Breakfasts

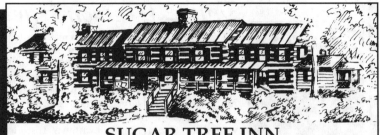

Did you know there are over 600 Bed & Breakfasts in the Commonwealth of Virginia and still continuing to escalate?

Inns to Bed & Breakfasts

The Inn At Union Run

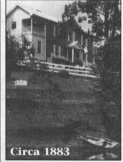

Circa 1883

Offering country quiet on our creek fronted mountainside. 8 gracious accommodations filled with antiques. Relax on the pastoral grounds and hear conservations steeped in Civil War history. Enjoy the nouvelle, American cuisine served in our candlelight restaurant and select from our award winning wine list. 5 minutes from downtown, Historic Lexington. Please Come!

1-800-528-6466 or (540) 463-9715
Union Run Rd. Rt. 674 • Lexington, VA

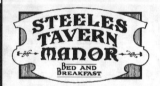

STEELES TAVERN MANOR
BED AND BREAKFAST

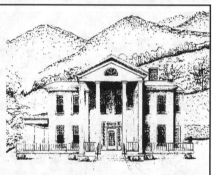

". . . quiet country elegance in a 1916 Manor House. 15 minutes from Historic Lexington"

Rt. 11   Steeles Tavern, VA   1-800-743-8666

❦ *Brierley Hill* ❦

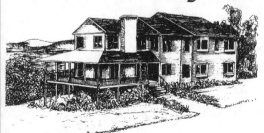

A
Bed & Breakfast
Country Inn in
historic
Lexington, VA.

A Charming,
restful retreat.
Come Relax &
Enjoy

1-800-422-4925   (540) 464-8421   Borden Rd., Lexington, VA. 24450

all have king- or queen-size beds (some have a daybed for a third person). One room is equipped for the handicapped. A seventh guest room, the Hawk's Nest, is an efficiency unit, complete with kitchenette and sitting area, ideal for longer stays and a favorite of honeymooners.

The Great Room, in addition to being the breakfast room, provides a gathering place around the high stone fireplace where guests may relax and enjoy the woodland views. Beverages are available at the check-in, and the "bottomless" cookie jar is on the sideboard. A balcony library overlooks this beautiful room, providing panoramic views of the Shenandoah Valley. Wraparound porches on both floors and a three-story lookout tower — a hot tub is on its first floor! — are popular with guests.

The full breakfast includes home-baked breads, juice and fruit, fresh-brewed coffee and an entree that changes daily. Nearby attractions are Waynesboro's Virginia Metalcrafters and P. Buckley Moss Museum, the historic Monticello and Ash Lawn-Highland near Charlottesville, Skyline Drive, Blue Ridge Parkway and the Appalachian Trail.

Rockbridge and Lexington

BRIERLEY HILL

Borden Rd., Lexington	*(800) 422-4925*
$$-$$$$	*(540) 464-8421*

Guests at this 2-year-old bed and breakfast inn rave about the wonderful food and beautiful accommodations, not to mention the breathtaking views from the large veranda. Situated on eight acres of hillside farmland, the inn is quiet and romantic, and the hospitality is second to none. Owners Barry and Carole Speton enjoy the finer things in life and want to share them with their guests. Barry is a former lawyer and is interested in antique books, prints and furniture. Carole is the former director of the Canadian Figure Skating Association who enjoys gardening, quilting and cooking.

The inn is decorated throughout with Laura Ashley wall coverings, fabrics and linens. Each of the five guest rooms has an elegant bed (four are canopy beds and one is an antique brass bed), a private bathroom and sitting area. The Deluxe King Room has an additional day bed, fireplace and TV. A new two-room suite has a fireplace, Jacuzzi and private patio looking out to spectacular views. The inn is fully air-conditioned, and fireplaces in the dining and living rooms warm the winter chill.

Guests feast on a full country breakfast of Grand Marnier French toast, buckwheat banana pancakes, French scrambled eggs with cream cheese and herbs, eggs Benedict and Belgian waffles with strawberries and sour cream, along with juice, fresh fruit and ham, bacon or sausage. Afternoon tea includes homemade cakes, breads, scones and cookies. Advance notice is required for dinner — and it is worth it! Dinner features fresh herbs and vegetables from the garden, as well as entrees such as boneless salmon steak with red wine and mushroom sauce, ribeye roast with herbs and red wine sauce and spicy stuffed chicken breast with sun-dried tomatoes.

You can relax in the serenity at Brierley Hill by lounging on the veranda or strolling down a country road. If you're up for a little more adventure, you can go sightseeing in historic Lexington or take advantage of special packages for theater, horseback riding, winter getaways and specials for midweek stays. Children older than 14 years are welcome. Smoking is restricted to the veranda or garden. No pets are allowed.

THE KEEP BED AND BREAKFAST
116 Lee Ave., Lexington
$$-$$$ (540) 463-3560

This bed and breakfast inn in a gorgeous Victorian home sits on a quiet corner in the heart of Lexington's historic residential district. Owners Bea and John Stuart offer guests two suites and a double-bed room, each with a private bath. Don't expect a lot of frou-frou here; the decor is elegant and understated. The Stuarts put on a lavish breakfast, complete with linens on the table, and also serve dinner upon request. At tea time, the owners are always happy to share tea, coffee or sherry with their guests. "We like to spoil nice people," says Bea Stuart.

Summertime travelers to Lexington will be grateful for the central air conditioning at The Keep, which is a short walk from museums and shops in downtown Lexington. The inn does not allow children younger than 12 but does welcome small, well-behaved pets on a request basis. Rates are $75 a night for the double room and $100 for the suite.

THE INN AT UNION RUN
Va. 674, Lexington   (540) 463-9715
$$

A friendly, down-to-earth couple, Roger and Jeanette Serens have won rave reviews for the service and enticing cuisine they offer. The inn is situated on roughly 12 acres about 4 miles from town and is bordered by a bird sanctuary. Union Run Creek, named for the Union Army that camped on the grounds in June of 1863, winds through the property. The Federal-style home was built in 1883.

The main house has a small dining area, living room and den for guests downstairs and three guest rooms with private porches upstairs. Two of those rooms are equipped with Jacuzzis. An adjacent carriage house has four guest rooms, each with a private bath. American and Victorian antiques fill the rooms in both the carriage house and the main building. Other interesting collectibles include an array of Toby mugs dating from 1755, a walnut desk that belonged to Winston Churchill, Meissen porcelain figurines and Henry Wadsworth Longfellow's clock.

The Serens serve tea in the afternoon, if requested, and wine or beer upon arrival. A full gourmet breakfast features such specialties as French toast made with English muffins and topped with fresh strawberries, whipped cream and powdered sugar, gingerbread pancakes, specialty souffles and an eggs Benedict-type of dish with spinach and artichokes instead of Canadian bacon. They also offer gourmet meals to guests and to the public in a romantic dining room. Discriminating gourmands from around the Shenandoah return repeatedly for the cuisine (see our Restaurants chapter).

The Serens offer special packages for guests who want to combine their stay with fox hunting, horseback riding or a trip to see a play or concert at the outdoor Lime Kiln Theater nearby.

SEVEN HILLS INN
408 S. Main St.
Lexington   (540) 463-4715
$$-$$$

This inn's seven guest rooms are named after the seven historic estates in Rockbridge County that are connected to the Grigsby family who settled here in the 1700s. The estates themselves are magnificent, and the Seven Hills Inn reflects this grandeur. It's a southern Colonial-style home that was actually built by a Washington & Lee fraternity in 1928. It passed through several hands before being purchased by its current owners, Ben and Carol Grigsby. Ben's mother, Jane Daniel, is the executive innkeeper.

All the guest rooms are furnished with either the family's antiques or with 18th- or early 19th-century hand-crafted reproductions. A gorgeous, handmade needlepoint rug from Portugal graces the living room, and decorative items purchased during the family's trips to the Orient are displayed throughout the house.

All the rooms have private baths except for Liberty Hill and Cherry Hill, which share an enormous connecting bathroom. Those rooms are often used as a suite by families. Speaking of families, the inn welcomes well-behaved children. Rates are from $75 to $95, depending upon the size of the room. Rates are based on double occupancy; a third person costs an extra $15. Included in the cost are a deluxe continental breakfast and afternoon tea, upon request. Guests can watch television, read or play games in the Chapter Room in the basement where the fraternity used to hold its meetings.

LLEWELLYN LODGE AT LEXINGTON

603 S. Main St., Lexington   (540) 463-3235
$-$$$ (800) 882-1145

This charming 55-year-old brick Colonial home is in the heart of Lexington, within walking distance of all the city's historic sights. Ellen and John Roberts are your hosts at this lovely home. She's a gourmet cook who has been a part of the airline, travel, hotel and restaurant industries. John is a Lexingtonian who will be happy to share his knowledge of the surrounding area.

The friendly atmosphere is noticeable from the start as you are met at the front door with refreshments. The comfortable living room, which has a large

fireplace, is a perfect setting for good conversation. The Lodge has a separate television and telephone room and is air-conditioned. Each of the bedrooms is distinct and designed to meet the needs of a variety of guests. Each room has extra-firm bedding, a ceiling fan and private bathroom. Highlights include a pencil-post bed, wicker furniture, an oak spindle bed, brass beds and four-poster beds. A first-floor room can accommodate handicapped persons who do not require a wheelchair.

A gourmet breakfast awaits you each morning: fantastic omelets, Belgian waffles, French toast, Virginia maple syrup, homemade muffins and breads, bacon, sausage, ham, juice, coffee and teas. After breakfast, take on the great outdoors, such as on the Chessie Trail, bicycle riding, canoeing on the Maury River, tubing at Goshen Pass and golf and tennis at Lexington Golf and Country Club. You might even find that John is willing to share his "secret" fishing spots with you. In the summer, you can visit the drive-in movie theater or the Lime Kiln Arts Center, featuring regional historical dramas and concerts.

Smoking in the guest rooms or dining room is not permitted, nor are pets of any kind. The Lodge is designed with adults in mind, although children age 10 and older are welcome.

FASSIFERN

Va. 39, Lexington   (540) 463-1013
$$-$$$

Visitors to the Virginia Horse Center pass right by Fassifern. It's a place of striking beauty: tall weeping willows surround a small pond, and bright flowers abound when the weather is warm.

Fassifern is situated on three acres, just across the road from the Art Farm, a gallery with summer workshops that teach the traditional methods of Chinese painting. On the other side of the Art Farm is the Horse Center.

This bed and breakfast inn's main building is a beautiful old home, built in 1867. There's also the Dependency, which used to be an ice house and servants' living quarters and now houses two guest rooms.

Owners Ann Carol and Arthur Perry live on the property in their own separate quarters. Guests need not feel they must tiptoe around someone's private home, because this house is set up for guests and their needs. The guest living room is elegant but cozy, furnished with an old pump organ and piano, a stuffed leather chair and sofa and lots of magazines and books. Or you may choose to relax in one of the other two private sitting areas.

The beautifully decorated dining room is the setting for a hearty continental breakfast that includes freshly squeezed orange juice, homemade granola, fresh fruit, croissants and other breads, country ham spread and hot chocolate, coffee and tea.

Each of the five guest rooms is air-conditioned and has a private bath. The Austrian Room is furnished with gorgeous European antiques, while the Country Room is more casual, with golden oak furniture and bright reddish print wallpaper. The three other rooms are also beautifully furnished and appear to be very comfortable.

Rates range from $79 to $88, which include breakfast. Children ages 8 and older are welcome. The owners recommend calling as far in advance as possible to make reservations.

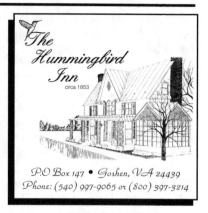

The Hummingbird Inn
circa 1853

P.O Box 147 • Goshen, VA 24439
Phone: (540) 997-9065 or (800) 397-3214

THE HUMMINGBIRD INN

Wood Ln., off Va. Alt. 39   (540) 997-9065
Goshen   (800) 397-3214
$-$$

This unique Victorian villa has operated on and off as an inn since it was built in 1853. Its owners, Jeremy and Diana Robinson, have done a beautiful job redesigning the interior. Its five guest rooms, furnished with antiques, are colorful and spacious and each has a private bath (two have double Jacuzzis). Full breakfasts include country bacon or sausage, homemade bread and foods unique to the area. The house features wraparound verandas on the first and second floors, original pine plank floors and a rustic den, solarium and music room.

During Goshen's boom days in the late 1800s and early 1900s, the inn was directly across from the town's railroad station, and the steps from the tracks to the inn's private road are still in place. Trains still roll through several times a week, but never at night to disturb guests' sleep.

In the 1930s the inn played host to Eleanor Roosevelt (one of the rooms is named after her) and Ephraim Zimbalist Sr., among other notables.

A wide trout stream defines one of the property lines, and only five minutes away is the gorgeous Goshen Pass, a popular spot for kayaking, picnicking and sunbathing in warm weather. This place is not to be missed when the rhododendron are in bloom!

Guests can also enjoy a relaxing float in inner tubes along Mill Creek, which flows behind the inn. Just 20 minutes away is historic Lexington, with its fine restaurants and shops, the Virginia Horse Center, George Marshall Museum, Stonewall Jackson House and other historic sites.

The Robinsons offer a prix fixe four-course dinner for $27.50, including a carafe of wine. Among their varied specialties are chicken with wild mushrooms, salmon filet with dill sauce and rabbit in herbs and cognac. Twenty-four hour advance notice is required since all food, including French baguettes, is prepared to order. Rates are between $70 to $95 breakfast only or $130 to $155 including dinner.

LAVENDER HILL FARM

Va. 631, Lexington   *(540) 464-5877*
$-$$ *(800) 446-4240*

Cindy and Colin Smith have restored a 200-year-old farmhouse on about 20 acres a few miles outside Lexington. The house sits on the banks of Kerrs Creek and has three light, airy guest rooms with private baths. One of the queen-size rooms can be rented as a suite; it connects to a second room with a double bed.

Horseback trips led by Virginia Mountain Outfitters are a unique aspect of a stay here. Trail rides and riding workshops are geared to all levels of riding experience. The inn was designed with animal lovers in mind. Sheep, cows and friendly Nubian goats roam over the land that surrounds the farmhouse, and a border collie and cat stay close by.

Colin Smith is a gourmet chef who loves to cook with fresh herbs grown on the farm. In fact, he has written a book on cooking with herbs. Four-course dinners cost $24.50 per person and are optional. Reservations are required. Available anytime are picnic lunches, perfect to take along to the theater or to Goshen Pass. The four-course picnic meals cost $20 per person.

The Horse Lovers Holiday package costs from $245 to $259 per person, based on double occupancy, and includes a two-night stay, breakfast, dinner and picnic lunches both days, along with the use of horses, tours and all instruction.

Guests can get special theater packages during the summer months, when the local Lime Kiln Theater puts on its outdoor plays and Sunday night concerts. The Smiths will purchase tickets and pack a gourmet picnic dinner to take along to Lime Kiln, where the bucolic grounds are conducive to sipping wine and feasting.

The Smiths don't allow pets or smoking inside the house. But, quips Cindy, they do welcome children accompanied by "well-behaved adults."

Roanoke and Salem

THE MARY BLADON HOUSE

381 Washington Ave. S.W.
Roanoke   *(540) 344-5361*
$-$$

This 1890s Victorian home is nestled in the heart of Roanoke's Old Southwest neighborhood. Bill and Sheri Bestpitch want The Mary Bladon House to be your home away from home as you explore the beautiful Roanoke Valley. The Rococo Revival, Renaissance Revival and Eastlake-style furnishings, antique English china, original brass light fixtures and even the Victorian playing cards on the writing table in the parlor help recapture the charm of "a time when elegant comfort was a way of life," say the Bestpitches. Guests will feel the spirit of the Victorian age while relaxing in the rocker in their room or on the swing on the wraparound front porch.

The guest rooms are decorated with crafts and period antiques. Families traveling with children are welcome in the Garden Room. Modern amenities, such as air conditioning and a 24-hour telephone answering service, are provided.

Breakfast includes the cook's choice of eggs, pancakes, waffles or French toast served with bacon, ham or sausage, along with home fries, hot and cold cereals, juice, coffee and tea. With advance notice, the cook can accommodate special dietary requests.

Afterwards, spend the day in downtown Roanoke. Visit the restored Farmers' Market and Center in the Square, an arts and entertainment mecca. The home is also only five minutes from the Blue Ridge Parkway. You'll also find easy access to Natural Bridge, Dixie Caverns, Mabry Mill, Smith Mountain Lake, Peaks of Otter and more. Afternoon tea is served from 4 to 6 PM, and with advance reservations you can savor a terrific dinner in the dining room.

The inn cannot accommodate pets. Smoking is permitted on the verandas only. Long-term and business rates are also available.

THE INN AT BURWELL PLACE
601 W. Main St., Salem   (540) 387-0250
$$-$$$$

Michel Spence Robertson is the innkeeper of this turn-of-the-century mansion at the southern end of the Shenandoah Valley. The magnificent front porch allows for a panoramic view of the Blue Ridge Mountains and the

Roanoke Valley. Each of the five bedrooms is decorated with queen-size beds, period furniture and antiques, and each has a private bath. A large suite with fireplace and whirlpool is perfect for families with children or for couples desiring privacy and romance.

After a large country breakfast of eggs, French toast or pancakes, fresh fruit, home fries, muffins and more, visit the sights of Salem. The historic downtown area is full of antique shops. Roanoke College and Salem's Farmers' Market are within walking distance, and a short drive will take you to Dixie Caverns, the Blue Ridge Parkway, Mabry Mill, Peaks of Otter, Natural Bridge and historic downtown Roanoke. Return after a day's exploring to afternoon tea on the porch.

Pets are not permitted, and smoking is not allowed inside the inn.

WALNUTHILL
436 Walnut Ave. S.E.
Roanoke   (540) 427-3312
$

Before coming to Roanoke, innkeeper Alexandra Condron commuted between her homes in Montreal and Florida. During her drives along I-81, she fell in love with Virginia, and while staying in Roanoke saw a huge three-story yellow brick house for sale. She knew this was where she wanted to settle and open her bed and breakfast inn.

The house, built in 1916, was obviously meant to last, as it was reinforced with steel beams. The front door has windows of leaded glass with beveled panes. The formal living room and foyer are decorated with a blend of American antiques and modern and continental styles. The family room features a sectional sofa, TV, stereo with classical music and a collection of books. The guest rooms are bright

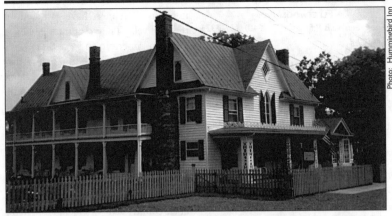

Photo: Hummingbird Inn

The Hummingbird Inn in Goshen, only a 20-minute drive from Historic Lexington.

and airy, with queen-size beds and an eclectic mix of furnishings, such as a contemporary bed with lighted-mirror headboard, a Louis XIV reproduction desk and chair, Victorian lace curtains and a large Persian rug. Another room is furnished with a replica of a French bedroom suite, with a triple dresser, antique tilt-top table, two stuffed rocking chairs and Oriental rugs. The third room is very private and features white wicker furniture, a daybed and queen-size bed, sitting area with TV and Aubusson rugs. Each guest room has a private bath. One of the bathrooms is a converted sun porch with a wall of windows and a hot tub. Occasionally, Condron will open her apartment to guests when the other rooms are full.

The dining room is decorated simply but with elegance. A long table covered with a Belgian lace tablecloth. The china matches an antique cobalt German chandelier Condron picked up at an auction. A full gourmet breakfast is served on antique Rosentahl and Meissen serving dishes. Choose from secret-recipe pancakes, Virginia ham, bacon or sausage, homemade biscuits with sausage gravy or eggs. Also a favorite is Walnuthill's special homemade fig syrup.

After breakfast the large veranda is a great place to relax, especially in one of the two hammocks. Or head for adventure in historic downtown Roanoke. Children are welcome, as are well-behaved pets. No smoking is allowed. Rates range from $49 to $59.

East of the Blue Ridge Region

Loudoun County

CORNERSTONE BED AND BREAKFAST
Paeonian Springs   (540) 882-3722
$$$

Molly and Dick Cunningham preside over this historic gem in the Catoctin Mountains, just five minutes from Leesburg's historical district. Two guest rooms with private baths are comfortably furnished with antiques, in the tradition of Victorian railstop guest homes. On the grounds are exquisite gardens and a pool.

Guest awake to a sumptuous full breakfast. Nearby attractions include historic Harpers Ferry, vineyards, and hunt country events.

FLEETWOOD FARM

Evergreen Mills Rd.   (540) 327-4325
Leesburg   (800) 808-5988
$$$$

Carol and Bill Chamberlin have only two guest rooms, but that means they lavish more attention on their guests. Their 1745 Historical Landmark home and sheep farm south of Leesburg is a highly rated accommodation. Guest rooms have air-conditioning, fireplaces and private baths (one has a Jacuzzi) and are decorated in antiques. Carol adds touches such as soft robes, wine, homemade shortbreads and fresh flowers.

Croquet, horseshoes and cookout facilities are set up outside, and guests can help with the gardening or fruit-picking if they like.

Breakfast is a feast featuring whatever fruits and vegetables are in season on the farm. That could mean apple butter pancakes, orange French toast with maple-orange syrup, blueberry pancakes or Eggs Fleetwood, a secret recipe. Bacon, sausage and scrapple accompany every meal, and there's always honey from the farm hives to put on fresh muffins.

Arrangements can be made to ride at a nearby stable, or you can take the farm canoe out on the reservoir a mile away. Whatever you do, you'll want to hurry back to Fleetwood.

Fauquier County

1763 INN AND RESTAURANT

U.S. 50, Upperville   (540) 592-3848
$$$$ (800) 669-1763

Uta and Don Kirchner have turned a complex of six old farm buildings on 50 acres into a heavenly getaway steeped in history and comfort. The cozy restaurant in the main farmhouse overlooks a pond with swans and is decorated in items the Kirchners have gathered on their travels. The restaurant menu is German-American and a credit to Uta's homeland. Sixteen bedrooms are dispersed among the main house, log cabin cottages and a stone barn atop a hill. Each room is distinctively decorated, one with a two-person hot tub, fireplace and buffalo head, another with a museum-size portrait of FDR which once hung in the Mexican Embassy.

Other amenities are a swimming pool, tennis courts and a fishing pond. Nearby horse country activities include spectator events such as horse shows, steeplechases, and foxhunts, as well as hiking and shopping in Middleburg.

THE ASHBY INN

U.S. 50, Paris   (540) 592-3900
$$$-$$$$

Yes, Virginia, there is a Paris in the Piedmont. Adding to the charm of this Fauquier County village is The Ashby Inn and Restaurant, which occupies a home dating back to the 1820s and serves some of the best food west of the Washington Beltway. Six guest rooms in the main building are decorated with studied, elegant simplicity to let the magnificent view of the mountains reign. Of these, the Fan Room, with its two skylights, fan window and private balcony, is among the most coveted. Four delightful rooms occupy Paris' former one-room schoolhouse, each with its own private porch facing the Blue Ridge. Quilts, blanket chests, and rag rugs impart a country feel to all rooms, but you won't find creaky floors or clanking pipes. Everything at The Ashby Inn is absolutely first class.

Hosts Roma and John Sherman are busy during dinner hours at the restaurant, but you may get to know them over breakfast, a feast reserved for guests. Roma is an avid horsewoman who also takes humanitarian trips to Bosnia, and John is a former House Ways and Means Committee staffer who still writes the occasional speech for Washington and New York clients.

Sperryville and Washington

BELLE MEADE BED & BREAKFAST
353 F.T. Valley Rd.
Sperryville   *(540) 987-9748*
$$-$$$$

Understated luxury and comfortable elegance describe what you can expect from

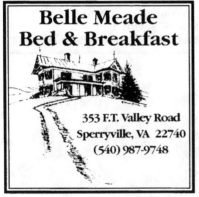

Belle Meade Bed & Breakfast

353 F.T. Valley Road
Sperryville, VA 22740
(540) 987-9748

this turn-of-the-century Victorian inn. Renovated in 1994, the inn has three guest rooms, each with scenic views and a private bath.

A hearty breakfast starts a busy day here. The 137 acres are gorgeous in any season — fall foliage and winter cross-country skiing are especially enticing — and hiking and birding are popular pastimes. The inn has a 60-foot swimming pool and hot tub.

Attractions in the area include Old Rag Mountain, a popular hiking destination. Skyline Drive and Luray Caverns are nearby, as are many fine restaurants and wineries. On weekends, parents can leave their children at the inn's summer day camp while they explore the area.

BLEU ROCK INN
U.S. 211, Washington   *(540) 987-3190*
$$$-$$$$

This cozy country inn is situated on 80 acres in Rappahannock County. It overlooks lush meadows, a pond and tall shade trees, with a vista of the mountains beyond. Several acres are carefully tended vineyards which supply wines for the inn, a renovated farmhouse with five guest rooms, each with a private bath. After a glass of wine in the lounge, you can dine fireside in one of three dining rooms. An open-air terrace overlooks the vineyards of Cabernet Sauvignon, Chardonnay and Seyval grapes.

You can stroll through pastures where horses graze, or try your hand at catching bass, catfish and blue gills from the pond. Rappahannock County offers ample opportunities for skiing, bicycling, canoeing, golfing, hiking and caving. Historical sites and wineries are not far from the inn.

Bernard and Jean Campagne are the owners and operators of Bleu Rock Farm and Inn. Jean has been honored with the Medals of Merite Agricole de France, Academie Culinaire de France, Cordon Bleu and Maitre Cuisinier de France. But you won't need his credentials to tell you that the food here is delicious. Breakfast, which is only served to overnight guests, is spectacular. It begins with fresh orange juice and coffee served with hot biscuits, croissants and muffins. Next is a fruit plate from from the inn's orchards. Then main course could be an omelet of ham, shiitake mushrooms and cheddar cheese, or Santa Fe French toast served with maple syrup and creme fraiche. Both are

$\mathcal{I}$nns $_{to}$ $\mathcal{B}$ed & $\mathcal{B}$reakfasts

Heritage House, Inc.
BED & BREAKFAST

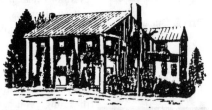

Main Street • P.O. Box 427 • Washington, Virginia • 22747
Telephone: (540) 675-3207

BLEU ROCK INN

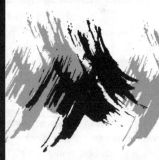

Fine French-American
Cuisine & Lodging
Complete with a
Blue Ridge
Vista

U.S. Rt. 211, Rt. 1, Box 555, Washington, Virginia 22747, (540) 987-3190

THE FOSTER HARRIS HOUSE
Bed & Breakfast

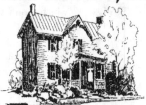

P.O. Box 333, 189 Main Street
Located in Historic Washington, VA • 1-800-666-0155

accompanied by a spicy homemade pork sausage and sauteed apples. This breakfast will really knock your socks off, and the dinners are equally superb.

Pets are not allowed, but children older than 10 years are welcome if supervised by an adult when they are outdoors near the pond or horses. The inn is closed Monday and Tuesday.

FOSTER-HARRIS HOUSE

Washington	(540) 675-3757
$$$-$$$$	(800) 666-0153

Phyllis Marriott's turn-of-the century frame home on the Main Street of this popular little tourist town offers four air-conditioned guest rooms, each with a private bath and a wonderful view of the mountains or the grounds' perennial gardens.

The Mountain View Room has a whirlpool tub big enough for two and a wood-burning stove for winter evenings. The Garden Room, which has the village's first indoor bathroom (now modernized), overlooks the inn's side spring garden.

Phyllis, a former Washington, D.C., caterer and delicatessen owner, prepares a full breakfast every morning and serves afternoon refreshments in the parlor, on the porch or beneath a grand old plum tree.

Smoking and pets are not allowed.

Area attractions include orchards, vineyards, fairs, antique shops and local theater. Hiking, biking and horseback riding are available too.

THE GAY STREET INN

Washington	(540) 675-3288
$$$-$$$$	

At the end of a quiet, dead-end street sits this 150-year-old stucco home, a re-

Gay Street Inn
Bed & Breakfast

Located in a quiet corner
of historic Washington, VA
(540) 675-3288

stored farmhouse with three spacious guest rooms, its resident dog and cat and lovely gardens out back. All rooms have views of the mountains, private baths and Colonial wallpaper from the Shelbourne Museum Collection. One room has a canopy bed and a working fireplace.

Innkeepers Donna and Robin Kevis prepare a marvelous morning feast, which sometimes includes frittata, smoked turkey sausage, homefries and homemade corn muffins.

The Gay Street Inn is charming, homey and convenient to Washington's shops and restaurants. The Shenandoah National Forest is nearby, as are caverns and other natural attractions.

HERITAGE HOUSE

Main St., Washington	(540) 675-3207
$$$$	

Jean and Frank Scott's elegant inn dates back to 1837 and is said to have been used by Confederate general Jubal Early as a command center during the Civil War. It's in the heart of "little" Washington, a minute's stroll from shops, historic landmarks and the famous Inn at Little Washington. The great outdoors are at your back door here, including Shenandoah National

Park and Skyline Drive. Not far away are the Rapidan, Rose and Thornton rivers and other well-known trout streams.

The four gracious guest rooms have air-conditioning and private baths. Each has its own theme. For instance, the suite has a sitting room/sun porch with a view of the Blue Ridge. The Lace Room has blue-flocked wall coverings, crystal lamps and antiques, while the Amish Room is decorated with a simple antique double bed, rag dolls and an original Thomas Palmerton landscape. Charles Dickens' *Old Curiosity Shop* and the city of London create the theme of the British Room, featuring David Winter cottages and castles.

At 9 AM, the Scotts serve a sit-down gourmet breakfast of hot entrees, fruit, home-baked fruit breads, juice and a variety of coffees and teas. Freshly baked treats and hot beverages are available to guests all day.

THE INN AT LITTLE WASHINGTON
Middle and Main Sts.   *(540) 675-3800*
$$$$

If you want to be pampered beyond your wildest dreams and eat food more delicious than you thought possible, then The Inn at Little Washington should certainly be No. 1 on your list. Surrounded by a quiet Rappahannock county town, the Inn is the one of the top-rated inns in the United States. Praise has come from far and wide, including *USA Today*, *People* magazine, *The New York Times* and the *San Francisco Chronicle*.

Reinhardt Lynch and Patrick O'Connell are the owners. Lynch takes care of the day-to-day operations at the Inn, little stuff such as making sure the 3,000 requests for Saturday night dinner are narrowed down to 65. O'Connell causes all the commotion with his culinary masterpieces.

The prix fixe dinners include cocktails, wine, five to six courses and after-dinner drinks. Diners select from 11 entrees and 15 desserts.

The Inn's 12 guest rooms are furnished with antiques, overstuffed reading chairs and canopied beds and elegantly decorated with faux bois woodwork and draped fabrics. The scent of freshly cut flowers mingles with that of potpourri. Old-fashioned silhouettes hang on the wall. Colorful pillows form a mountain of comfort on the bed, but don't succumb before soaking in a tub of pine-scented bubbles in the marble-and-brass bathroom. Swathed in a plush white robe, you can watch the fountain from your balcony and pinch yourself to see if you're still awake. The Inn is very popular, so advance registration is a must.

THE MIDDLETON INN
176 Main St., Washington   *(540) 675-2020*
$$$$

The Middleton Inn is a grand Federal home in a rural setting with mountain views. The house, which has an impressive center hall and high ceilings throughout, was built in 1850 by Middleton Miller, who designed and manufactured the uniform worn by Confederate soldiers. The house has eight working fireplaces, including one in every bedroom, and each of the four guest rooms has a private marble bath.

Sharing a five-acre knoll with the house are three other original buildings: the summer kitchen, the smokehouse and the slave quarters. The latter is now a two-story guest cottage with a working fireplace and Jacuzzi.

The inn combines the best of town and country, with cattle grazing in an adjoining pasture and shops just two blocks away. Washington and the surrounding area is rich in antique and craft shops, natural wonders such as the Skyline Drive and small-town festivals that pull visitors into the spirit of the place.

Culpeper County

FOUNTAIN HALL BED & BREAKFAST
609 S. East St., Culpeper   (540) 825-8200
$-$$$$ (800) 29VISIT

George Washington, the first county surveyor of Culpeper, referred to the town as "a high and pleasant situation." It still is, and Fountain Hall enjoys an enviable location in this charming village, once part of a large tract owned by Virginia's Royal Governor, Sir Alexander Spotswood. Hosts Steve and Kathi Walker have decorated their five large sunlit guest rooms with antiques but provided the modern conveniences of a telephone and private bath in each. Some have whirlpool tubs and outdoor porches.

Games are set up on the lawn, and formal gardens are perfect for strolling. The streets of Culpeper beckons history and antique buffs.

Breakfast in the sunny morning room is a leisurely affair of fresh croissants topped with country preserves, cereals and juices.

Madison County

GRAVES' MOUNTAIN LODGE
Syria   (540) 923-4231
$-$$

Graves' Mountain Lodge is a family-owned resort on the edge of Shenandoah National Park. It's a family-oriented place, with family-style meals and a variety of activities: swimming, tennis, softball, volleyball, horseback riding, hunting, fishing and hiking. The recreation center has books, magazines, games, a piano and a television for rainy days. The gift shop sells mountain crafts, Native American and folk carvings and jewelry.

Stop in at the old-time country store, Syria Mercantile Company, where you can buy groceries, dry goods and other necessities.

The lodge has 10 accommodation styles. The Ridgecrest Motel has 22 rooms and two conference rooms; Hilltop Motel has 16 rooms, some with televisions; and the Old Farm House has seven rooms with half-baths and a portico to the shower house. Nine cottages are in the vicinity of the lodge.

To get to the lodge from U.S. 29 S., turn right and go 7 miles south of Culpeper on Va. 609, then right on Va. 231 and left on Va. 670.

THE INN AT MEANDER PLANTATION
U.S. 15, Locust Dale   (540) 672-4912
$$$-$$$$ (800) 385-4936

In the heart of Jefferson's Virginia, the Inn at Meander Plantation offers the charm and elegance of Colonial living. The stately mansion, built in 1766 by Joshua Fry, is the centerpiece of an 80-acre estate. Converted to a bed and breakfast inn in 1993, the house contains five sun-drenched bedrooms, each with private bath. Four-poster queen-size beds are piled high with plump pillows atop down comforters.

Throughout the house are private nooks for reading, and guests often gather in the parlor that was often visited by Thomas Jefferson and Gen. Lafayette. A baby grand piano awaits impromptu concerts.

A full plantation-style gourmet breakfast is served daily in the formal dining room or under the arched breezeway. Full dinners and picnic lunches can be arranged.

Inns to Bed & Breakfasts

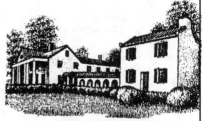
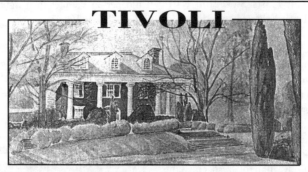
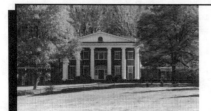

Outdoors, white rockers line both levels of the expansive back porches, providing peaceful respites for sipping afternoon tea. The boxwood gardens are dotted with secluded benches and a hammock. Croquet, volleyball, badminton and horseshoes are set up on the lawns, and the woods are made for strolling. Overnight boarding for horses is available at the stables.

The innkeepers are Suzanne Thomas and Suzie and Bob Blanchard. Suzanne, a former newspaper publisher, finds time now for freelance writing. Susie continues her career as a food writer, and Bob has a training and consulting company.

The inn is located in a bend of the Robinson River, 9 miles south of Culpeper and 8 miles north of Orange. The best of the countryside is close at hand, including wineries, antique shops and historical sites.

Greene County — Stanardsville

EDGEWOOD FARM BED & BREAKFAST
Va. 667   (804) 985-3782
$$ (800) 985-3782

A 130-acre farm with rushing streams and deep woods surrounds this beautifully restored house, which was built in 1790 and expanded in the 1860s. Each of the three period-decorated bedrooms has a fireplace and private bath (with special touches such as pleasantly scented goat's milk soap, lotion and shampoo made in nearby Charlottesville).

Hosts Norman and Eleanor Schwartz, greet guests with refreshments and smiles, and that's just the beginning of the pampering. When you open your door to the aroma coffee and fresh muffins wafting up to your room, you'll find a silver service of hot coffee and fresh flowers and the morning paper. Breakfast is a generous array of home-baked muffins, coffee cakes and other breads, and fresh fruit. Picnic lunches are available by special arrangement.

On the grounds is a plant nursery that specializes in herbs and perennials. Within a 30-mile radius of the farm are historical and natural attractions such as Skyline Drive, Monticello, Montpelier, Ash Lawn-Highlands and the University of Virginia. Vineyards and antique and craft shops are also close by.

Orange County

ROCKLANDS
17439 Rocklands Dr.
Gordonsville   (540) 832-7176
$$$-$$$$

The Classic-Revival mansion, which is surrounded by 1,800 acres of woods and fields, is registered as a Historic Landmark by both Virginia and the U.S. Department of Interior. The setting offers breathtaking views from the front veranda, which overlooks a pond, woods and the Blue Ridge Mountains.

The present dwelling was build in 1905 on the site of an antebellum home. The Neale family has operated the estate since 1926. Formal gardens, bridle trails, croquet and volleyball courts, a swimming pool and miles of private hiking trails await outdoors, or you can relax in the library. The inn has 11 guest rooms, five in the manor house and the others in adjacent structures. A full Virginia-style breakfast is served each morning.

The inn is an executive retreat, offering a conference center and other amenities for productive meetings.

Gourmet dining is a hallmark of Rocklands, a country inn, which serves meals to the public as well as to guests. Menus are varied, focusing on fresh ingredients and local and international flavors, complemented by wines from the inn's wine cellar.

Nearby attractions include Charlottesville's historic and cultural offerings, Skyline Drive, Montpelier, Civil War sites and museums, wineries, antique shops and more.

TIVOLI

9171 Tivoli Dr.	(540) 832-2225
Gordonsville	(800) 840-2225
$$-$$$$	

Tivoli is a three-story 24-room Victorian mansion atop a hill. Framed by 14 massive Corinthian columns, the house commands views of the Blue Ridge Mountains in the distance and its own 235-acre working cattle farm. Four carefully restored bedrooms — two with private baths, two with shared baths, and each with a working fireplace — are available for guests. Owners Phil and Susie Audibert pride themselves on their "don't leave hungry" breakfasts, featuring big, brown fresh eggs.

With its ballroom (complete with a Steinway grand piano), 12-foot-high ceilings, state-of-the-art kitchen and antique-filled living and dining rooms, Tivoli also offers ample space for wedding receptions, private parties, small conferences and seminars. Wineries, Civil War battlefields, Monticello, Montpelier, gourmet restaurants, amateur theatre and Shenandoah National Park are all within easy driving distance. Guests are also encouraged to walk the farm's rolling pastures and miles of wooded trails.

WILLOW GROVE INN

14079 Plantation Way	(540) 672-5982
Orange	(800) WG9-1778
$$$-$$$$	

If you want to live and breathe history, consider this antebellum mansion with for-

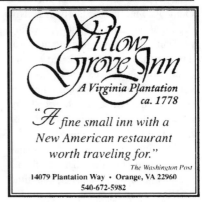

mal gardens and sloping lawns. Willow Grove Inn, listed on the National Register of Historic Places, was built by the same craftsmen chosen by Thomas Jefferson for work on the University of Virginia.

The mansion, the exterior of which is a prime example of Jefferson's Classical Revival style, fell under siege during the Civil War. You can still see trenches near the manor house, and a cannonball was recently removed from its eaves.

Tucked into 37 secluded acres, the mansion retains its original Colonial atmosphere. Fine American and English antiques decorate the manor house, and English boxwood, magnolias and willows grace the lawns.

But don't let this intimidate you. Owner Angela Mulloy has figured out how to help her guests unwind. A newspaper and pot of fresh coffee will be at your door in the morning, along with freshly baked muffins if you want something before the hearty breakfast.

The inn also serves dinner in distinctive dining rooms offering varying atmospheres: Clark's Tavern is dark, cozy and casual, while the Dolley Madison Room is formal and resplendent in delicate china and crystal.

Antique furnishings, wide pine flooring and original fireplace mantles preserve the traditional character of each of the inn's three rooms and two suites. You'll also find fresh flowers, down pillows and comforters, and coconut milk baths in your private bathroom.

SLEEPY HOLLOW FARM

Va. 231, Gordonsville   *(540) 832-5555*
$-$$$

This cozy 18th-century house is filled with nooks and crannies and bedrooms that feel like private hideaways. Flower and herb gardens surround the house, and the broader surroundings are woods and rolling fields where cattle graze. Beverley Allison and her daughter, Dorsey Allison-Comer, run the inn, which has been the Allison family home for decades.

The atmosphere here is casual and comfortable, with dog and cats serving as the palace guards. In their rooms, guests find a welcome basket stocked with Virginia peanuts, fruit and homemade chocolate chip cookies. If this isn't enough to snack on, a freshly baked cake is always available in the sitting area. The formal dining room is very pretty and overlooks the herb garden and distant rolling hills.

Three rooms have private baths, and the three suites share a private bath each. One room has a working fireplace and whirlpool. A beautiful pond on the grounds can be used for swimming or fishing, and ducks and their offspring glide around the pond each spring. Speaking of babies, Sleepy Hollow is one of the few bed and breakfast inns in the area catering to children. A baby crib and playpen are available, and the suites are popular with families.

Rates include a sumptuous full country breakfast and afternoon tea, if requested. Private dinners are also offered by prior arrangement, and the owners like to hold wine tastings when several guests stay more than more night.

Skyline Drive, Monticello and Montpelier are nearby.

Charlottesville Area

CLIFTON — THE COUNTRY INN

1296 Clifton Inn Dr.   *(804) 971-1800*
$$$$

Clifton wins rave reviews around the country for its elegance, comfort and

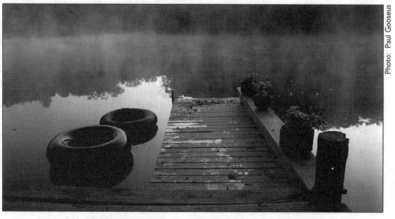

Lake Leana, Clifton Country Inn's 20-acre private lake.

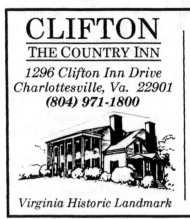
gourmet dining. *Country Inns* magazine calls it one of the top 12 inns in the nation. And Judith Martin, Miss Manners herself, listed Clifton as one of her four favorite hotels in the world in her book, *Miss Manners Guide to the Turn of the Millennium*. Clifton is an imposing 18th-century manor house with pillared veranda and a clear view to Monticello when the trees are not in leaf.

Clifton was built by Thomas Mann Randolph, husband of Thomas Jefferson's daughter, Martha, on land that once adjoined the Shadwell Plantation, Jefferson's birthplace. It is believed to have been built as an office for Randolph, but it became his home in his later years. Clifton offers overnight guests a slower pace, where the only important decisions are whether to play a few wickets of croquet, read a book by the fire, float around the lake on an inner tube or practice a Chopin prelude on the grand piano.

Innkeepers Craig and Donna Hartman set the mood at Clifton with their obvious and genuine affection for people. Tea is served at 4 PM, complete with gourmet teas, fresh fruits and freshly baked treats.

Every room has its own fireplace, freshly laid with wood and ready for the strike of a match. Guests are also warmed by down comforters on antique beds. All the rooms and suites have private baths, as individual and unusual as the rooms themselves. One of the most popular rooms, the Martha Jefferson, has walls, bed hangings and a rug the color of rich vanilla ice cream. The carriage house is a spectacular guest suite featuring a stair railing and other architectural artifacts from the dismantled Meriwether Lewis home. This seems especially fitting because Martha and Thomas Randolph's affection for Lewis was such that they named their fourth son after him.

Outside, flower beds surround a manicured croquet court. Down the lawn from the enclosed veranda is a spacious gazebo, and a little farther is a tennis court and a swimming pool with waterfall and heated spa. All this is surrounded by 40 acres of dense forest through which a short walk brings you to a dock on the private lake. This is the perfect point from which to begin a swim or a lazy float in an oversized inner tube.

Full breakfasts include fresh fruit, sausage or bacon, a lavish entree, juice and coffee or tea. Clifton also operates a restaurant that serves gourmet dinners to the public nightly. Exquisite meals consist of five or six courses and are prepared by Craig Hartman and assistant Jennifer Wilson-Devaney, both award-winning chefs and graduates of the Culinary Institute of America.

Light refreshments — freshly baked cookies and a self-serve refrigerator stocked with wine, sodas, beer and water — are always available for guests. The Clifton staff will prepare luncheons and private dinners to order.

Clifton is just off U.S. 250 E. 5 miles from Charlottesville and 4 miles from Monticello.

THE 1817 ANTIQUE INN

1211 W. Main St.
Charlottesville   *(804) 979-7353*
$$$-$$$$ *(800) 730-7443*

If you suspect this inn in a historic townhouse might be too stiff and formal for your fancy, consider: the friendly black lab sitting quietly in the hallway, so happy for a scratch behind the ears; or owner Candace DeLoach Wilson, who encourages her guests to sit back and relax in the living room and munch on the M&Ms she keeps in a big bowl.

Eclectic decor makes this place unique in tradition-bound Charlottesville. For instance, the living room is decorated with items as disparate as Biedermeier chairs, American Empire chests, Venetian tables and a big zebra skin rug. The total effect is exciting but comfortable.

This is precisely the aim of Candace, who grew up in Savannah, graduated from college in South Carolina and then moved to New York, where she worked as an interior designer for 10 years. She met her husband, Jon, a fellow South-erner, in New York and the two married and moved to Charlottesville for his industrial engineering position in 1992.

In the spring of 1993, Candace opened DeLoach Antiques in a townhouse that adjoins the inn. All the antiques and furnishings in the inn are for sale, at reasonable prices for the Charlottesville area.

Both buildings were built in 1817 by one of Thomas Jefferson's master craftsmen, James Dinsmore of Northern Ireland. Dinsmore was the principal carpenter at Monticello and several original dormitories at the University of Virginia. With another master builder, Dinsmore was Jefferson's principal carpenter for the Rotunda, which is only a few blocks from The 1817 Inn.

Breakfast includes hearty muffins, granola, yogurt, piles of fresh fruit, juice and coffee. The Tea Room Cafe is a delightful addition to The 1817. Here, you can order gourmet lunches Monday through Friday; prices are very reasonable. Homemade soups, salads, sandwiches and desserts are served in the solarium and on the back porch.

All the bedrooms evoke a romantic mood, whether it be the spacious Mattie Carrington room, with French antiques and a glass chandelier, or the exotic Lewis and Clark room, with an African cowhide rug, fur pillows and English hunt pictures. The Sleeping Porch is also enchanting, furnished with two double beds draped with mosquito netting canopies and made up entirely in cream linens.

Our favorite is Mrs. Olive's Room in the back, with its many white-shuttered windows hung with silk balloon valances and loveseat, chair and tufted ottoman that make for a comfortable place to read and write letters.

The inn's convenient location makes it a popular destination for parents of UVA students. Within easy walking distance is The Corner, a block or two of restaurants, clothing stores and other shops across from campus. Some of Charlottesville's most appealing restaurants are along Elliewood Avenue in this neighborhood.

THE INN AT SUGAR HOLLOW FARM

White Hall   (804) 823-7086
$$-$$$$

Dick and Hayden Cabell are the innkeepers at this 70-acre wooded farm in the Moorman River Valley, at the edge of the Shenandoah National Park. The site served as a trading post originally, and its history goes back to the days of Thomas Jefferson.

The new inn is custom-built and has five distinctive bedrooms with cozy corners for reading and relaxing, as well as several comfortable common areas. Each bedroom has a connecting private bath, and two rooms have whirlpool baths. Wood-burning fireplaces warm you in four of the bedrooms, and one guest room meets the needs of the physically handicapped.

The oak-beamed country-style family and dining rooms open to a broad, blue-stone terrace offering a grand view across the gardens and fields to Pasture Fence Mountain and the Blue Ridge. A library and sun room are other relaxing options.

Breakfast features egg specialties, homemade granola, fresh fruit from the inn's gardens and freshly baked muffins or pastries. Freshly prepared refreshments are always on hand.

Exploring the outdoors tops the list of activities here; the nearby national forest offers hiking and biking trails. Equestrian events at Foxfield and Montpelier and Charlottesville's numerous historic attractions are nearby, and Wintergreen Ski Resort is within an hour's drive.

INN AT THE CROSSROADS

North Garden   (804) 979-6452
$-$$

Surrounded by beautiful countryside 9 miles south of Charlottesville, the Inn at the Crossroads commands spectacular vistas of the foothills of the Blue Ridge and is near many of the regions's finest natural attractions, including Crabtree Falls, Devil's Knob Mountain, the James River and Sherando Lake National Recreation Area.

The aptly named inn and one-time tavern, built in 1820, sits at the crossing of two Colonial roads, a north-south route linking Charlottesville with Lynchburg and an east-west pike connecting the James River with the Shenandoah Valley. Five comfortable bedrooms with shared baths await guests, as do two common rooms replete with books, antiques and curios.

A full breakfast is included in the reasonable room price.

INN AT MONTICELLO

Va. 20 S., Charlottesville   (804) 979-3593
$$$-$$$$

Carol and Larry Engel invite guests to "spend the day at Thomas Jefferson's beloved Monticello. Spend the night with us." This country manor house was built in the mid-1800s in the valley of Jefferson's Monticello Mountain. On the grounds of the house are dogwoods, boxwoods and azaleas and beautiful Willow Lake. Croquet is set up on the manicured lawn, and a lazy hammock beckons.

Inside are five elegant bedrooms, each furnished with period antiques and reproductions. The beds are made up with crisp cotton linens and down comforters. Some

Inns to *Bed & Breakfasts*

The Inn at Monticello

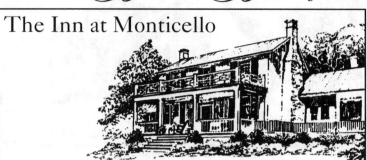

"A Cozy Charmer" — Country Inns Magazine, June '92
Route 19, Box 112 Charlottesville, Va. 22902 804-979-3593

Ginger Hill

Bed & Breakfast

Ginger Hill is a secluded country cottage, located on 14.5 acres, convenient to Charlottesville and Richmond, Virginia. Many historic and recreational areas are within a short driving distance.

Rt. 5, Box 33E, County Road 800, Louisa, Virginia 23093
(540) 967-3260

The Inn at
Sugar Hollow Farm

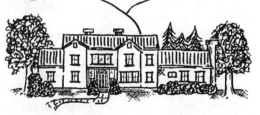

P. O. Box 5705 Charlotesville, VA 22905 • (804) 823-7086

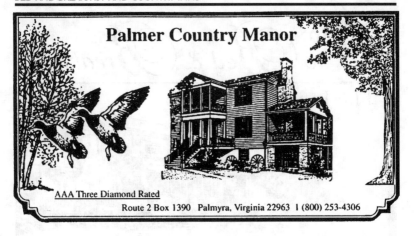

Palmer Country Manor

<u>AAA Three Diamond Rated</u>

Route 2 Box 1390 Palmyra, Virginia 22963 1 (800) 253-4306

rooms have special features, such as a working fireplace, four-poster canopy bed or private porch. Every room is air-conditioned and has a private bath.

Let the aroma of freshly brewed hazelnut coffee lure you from your warm bed. The ever-changing menu includes such delicious entrees as crab quiche and orange yogurt pancakes.

The inn is convenient to Monticello (the home of Thomas Jefferson), Michie Tavern, Ash Lawn-Highland (the home of James Monroe), Montpelier (the home of James and Dolley Madison) and many vineyards.

GINGER HILL BED & BREAKFAST
Va. 800, Louisa   *(540) 967-3260*
$$

Ginger Hill, a country cottage on 14½ secluded, wooded acres not far from Charlottesville, is surrounded by natural diversions: a fishing pond with a canoe, two beaver ponds and a variety of birds and animals to watch. The inn is also a good base for daytrips to historic, recreational and cultural sites.

The home was built in 1992 with generous features — 10-foot ceilings, a fireplace and porches — found in older

homes but the modern amenities of air-conditioning, bathrooms and ample parking for cars, trailers and boats. The inn has two sunny guest rooms, each with a private bath and sitting area.

Innkeepers Ron and Ginger Ellis provide a full Southern breakfast in the formal dining room, on the porch or even at the picnic table by the pond. Afternoon and evening refreshments are available, and a light supper can be arranged at an additional cost.

The inn can accommodate pets with prior notice. Special occasion packages are available, as are corporate rates and special activities such as a fishing trip or cruise on Lake Anna or a tour of Civil War sites.

To get to the inn from Charlottesville, take Exit 143 off I-64, go east on Va. 208 and then right on Va. 800 to the second drive on the left.

PALMER COUNTRY MANOR
Va. 640, Palmyra   *(800) 253-4306*
$$$-$$$$

This estate of 180 acres was once part of a 2,500-acre plantation known as Solitude. Palmer Country Manor was built by Richard McCary, a mason who also built

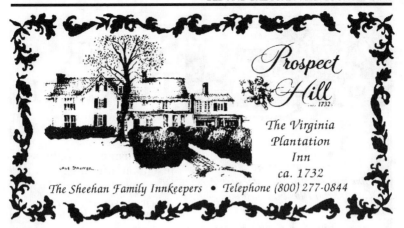

Prospect Hill

The Virginia
Plantation
Inn
ca. 1732

The Sheehan Family Innkeepers • *Telephone (800) 277-0844*

the Palmyra Stone Jail and Carysbrook Plantation. McCary prospered, and within 20 years he and his wife owned 583 acres. However, in 1858 he was arrested for murder, put in the jail he built and found it necessary to sell the entire plantation.

Owners Kathy and Greg Palmer opened the estate as a bed and breakfast in 1989, with the furnishings and ambiance of an 1834 plantation house. You can stay in two rooms in the historic plantation house, with its library, parlor and screened porch, or in one of the 10 suites in private cottages. Each air-conditioned cottage has a fireplace, king- or queen-size bed, color television, full bath and large private deck. Each can accommodate as many as four people. Guests are served a complimentary breakfast every morning, and a lavish dinner is available every night.

Adventurous types may want to raft the white water on the James River or hike, picnic, fish or relax in the nearby woods. Romantics can opt for a champagne balloon ride at sunset.

PROSPECT HILL INN

| Trevilians | (540) 967-0844 |
| $-$$ | (800) 277-0844 |

A graceful English tree garden shades the manor house, and a boxwood hedge lines the entrance way to this 1732 mansion. A few steps away are the slave quarters, the overseer's house, slave kitchen, smoke house and carriage house. A large open lawn rolls on for a quarter mile. This is Prospect Hill, a plantation that is more than two centuries old. Michael and Laura Sheehan are the innkeepers today, but the tradition of hospitality began long before their time.

After the Civil War, the son of the plantation owner returned to find Prospect Hill overgrown and run down. In order to make ends meet, he was forced to take in guests

Many inns and bed and breakfasts offer greatly reduced rates in the off season. You'll not only save money, but you can fully enjoy amenities such as fireplaces, hot cider and snow-covered meadows.

Insiders' Tips

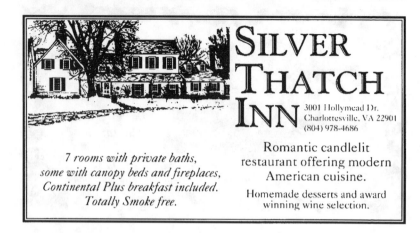

from the city. In 1880 he built an addition to Prospect Hill and remodeled the old slave quarters for guest bedrooms. This renovation created an interior as beautiful as the extraordinary magnolias, tulip poplars and giant beeches in the yard. The slave quarters have beamed ceilings and warm, crackling fireplaces. The rooms in the manor house are adorned with antique furnishings and lovely quilts, and all have fireplaces. A private veranda offers a view over the hillside. The inn has 13 guest rooms, each with a modern bathroom, some with Jacuzzis. There are also three private dwellings on the grounds.

A full country breakfast is served to you in bed or at a table in your room. Dinner is served as well; a bell will ring to summon you to one of three candlelit dining rooms for your five-course feast. Dishes are traditional French with Provençal and American accents. Tea time is a ritual at Prospect Hill, and you can also sip a glass of Virginia wine before dinner.

On the grounds or nearby you can go hiking, picnicking, fishing, biking or swimming. Sunset champagne balloon rides are easily arranged. The inn is in the Green Springs Historic District of Louisa County, near Skyline Drive, Blue Ridge Parkway, Monticello, Ash Lawn, University of Virginia, Montpelier, the Barboursville Vineyards or Oakencroft Vineyard and Winery.

SILVER THATCH INN

3001 Hollymead Dr.
Charlottesville (804) 978-4686
$$$$

Built in 1780 by Hessian soldiers, the Silver Thatch Inn's central house brings to mind the architecture of Colonial Williamsburg. It is an immaculately restored white clapboard building surrounded by dogwoods, magnolias and pines.

The Hessian Room of the inn is named for Hessian soldiers captured in New York during the Revolutionary War and marched south to Charlottesville. They built a two-story log cabin on the site of a former Native American settlement, where the Silver Thatch Inn now stands. In the 19th century, the inn served as a boys' school, then a tobacco plantation and after the Civil War, a melon farm. A wing was added in 1937, and a cottage was built in 1984 to complement the main building.

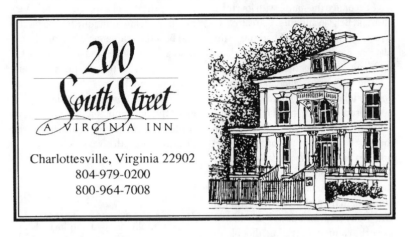

200
South Street
A VIRGINIA INN

Charlottesville, Virginia 22902
804-979-0200
800-964-7008

Owners Vince and Rita Scoffone have decorated the inn with early American folk art, quilts, reproduction furniture and antiques. The seven guest rooms are named for Virginia-born presidents. The Thomas Jefferson Room has a pencil-post, queen-size canopy bed and fireplace. All rooms have private baths and several have fireplaces. Guests will find fresh, homemade cookies waiting for them in their rooms.

The Silver Thatch Inn has a restaurant with three dining rooms, a sun room and a bar where guests can have a complimentary glass of wine or beer before dinner.

Dinner is served Tuesday through Saturday. The menu changes frequently but always includes a vegetarian special and entrees such as grilled filet mignon to satisfy conventional tastes. Two of the more exotic items on one winter menu included roasted quail Sonoran (served with a Southwestern sauce of tomatoes, onions, olives, bacon and garlic) and lamb chops Fez (grilled with Merguez sausage, Moroccan tomato sauce and couscous). Among the desserts were a hazelnut/brown sugar tart with Frangelica cream, and flourless chocolate cake with pecans.

Silver Thatch is a short drive from the University of Virginia, Monticello, James Madison's Montpelier and Ash Lawn-Highland. Skyline Drive and the Blue Ridge Parkway are a half-hour's drive away. Guests have access to an outdoor swimming pool and tennis courts near the inn.

200 SOUTH STREET

South St., Charlottesville   (804) 979-0200
$$$

200 South Street is actually two restored houses in downtown Charlottesville. The restoration was completed in 1986, and every detail of the inn was meticulously recreated or renewed, including the classical veranda and a two-story walnut serpentine hand rail. The larger of the two buildings was built in 1856 for Thomas Jefferson Wertenbaker, son of Thomas Jefferson's first librarian and close friend, and remained a residence until the 20th century. In the following years, the building was believed to have housed a finishing school for girls, a brothel and then a boarding house before it was transformed into the inn.

Innkeepers Brendon and Jenny Clancy

have decorated the rooms with lovely English and Belgian antiques. You can choose a room with a whirlpool bathtub, a fireplace, a canopy bed or a private living room suite. Every room has a private bath.

The inn's main gallery houses an ongoing exhibition of Virginia artists and part of the private collection of Holsinger photos of historic Charlottesville. A complimentary continental-style breakfast, afternoon tea and wine are available to guests.

200 South Street is only blocks from the finest restaurants, shops and entertainment in the area and 5 miles from the University and Monticello. It's hard to leave the comforts of the inn, though; the library, sitting room, upstairs study, veranda and garden terrace beckon.

Nelson County

LOOKING GLASS HOUSE

Va. 151, Afton   (703) 456-6844
$$-$$$ (800) 769-6844

This 1848 farm house near the Blue Ridge Parkway is an English country-style inn that takes its name from a Lewis Carroll tale. The inn is within a half-hour's drive of Charlottesville, Monticello and Wintergreen Resort.

Innkeeper Mary Haviland has decorated her four guest rooms (each with private bath) with antiques gathered during her travels in England. Vintage linens are used on all guest beds. Two wicker-furnished porches offer views of the countryside, while the library and formal drawing room are comfortable settings for reading, parlor games, and television. Refreshments are served to guests each afternoon.

Breakfast in the formal dining room starts with freshly baked muffins or breads and juice, followed by a second course of seasonal fruits and then the main course, which could be heart-shaped waffles,

puffed pancakes or a special egg dish. Victorian silver, linen, antique serving pieces, and beautiful china make the meal even more special. Coffee and tea are available to early risers on the antique hutch outside the rooms.

Fresh-cut flowers from the garden grace the inn's interior, and guests may stroll through the rose garden or the plantings along the two stream banks.

THE MARK ADDY

Va. 151 S. and Va. 613 W.
Nellysford   (804) 361-1101
$$$-$$$$ (800) 278-2154

Beautifully restored and lovingly appointed, the Mark Addy offers the richness and romance of a bygone era. The inn is a former estate house, Upland, that was begun as a four-room farmhouse in 1884 and expanded to its current size by 1910.

Guest rooms are decorated in individual

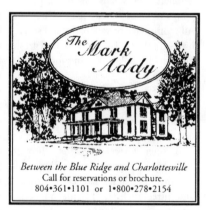

The Mark Addy

Between the Blue Ridge and Charlottesville
Call for reservations or brochure.
804•361•1101 or 1•800•278•2154

themes: Oriental, English, Victorian or the military-style Colonel's Room. Each has a private bathroom with either a double whirlpool bath, double shower or an antique claw-foot tub with shower. Five porches and a hammock are available for lounging. Public rooms include a dining room, parlor, sitting room with cable TV, VCR, games and phones and a library.

Each room has a decanter of liqueur, and breakfast is a hearty meal. Innkeepers John Maddox and Saverio Anselmo take pride in their cuisine de grandmére.

Nearby attractions include Skyline Drive, Monticello, wineries, Wintergreen Resort and all the shops, museums, restaurants and social activities of the university city of Charlottesville. For those who are happiest when browsing through curiosity shops, Tuckahoe Antique Mall and Jordan's are just a few miles away. For the more adventurous of spirit, canoeing, hiking and rafting are minutes away.

THE MEANDER INN
AT PENNY LANE FARM
Va. 612 and Va. 613
Nellysford   *(804) 361-1121*
$$-$$$$

The Rockfish Valley of Nelson County is the setting for this country farmhouse on 50 acres of horse-grazed pasture and woods. Rick and Kathy Cornelius are the innkeepers of the Meander Inn, an 80-year-old Victorian home on the Rockfish River. The five guest rooms are decorated with Victorian or country antiques and four-poster beds. If you rise early enough, you can help fetch the morning eggs from the hen house and give the horses their breakfast grain. Or you can just wake in time to savor a tasty country breakfast.

Leisurely afternoons can be spent taking tea on the porch or watching the guinea hens play in the brush. As the inn's name suggests, you can meander along Skyline Drive and behold the spectacular scenery. Among the activities within easy reach are skiing, canoeing, horseback riding, tennis, golf, fishing, hiking, swimming and biking.

After a day's activity, it's fun to enjoy a glass of Virginia wine and sit around the wood stove listening to the antique player piano or soak in the outdoor hot tub by starlight.

TRILLIUM HOUSE
Wintergreen, Nellsyford   *(804) 325-9126*
$$-$$$

What an enviable setting! Betty and Ed Dinwiddie's Trillium House is in the middle of the posh Wintergreen Four Seasons Resort, overlooking the 17th fairway of the Devil's Knob Golf Course. Guests have the use of the resort's 11,000 acres, with its tennis, golf, swimming and skiing facilities and several excellent restaurants. However, you may not want to dine anyplace but the Trillium House, where sumptuous breakfasts are served to guests and dinners Friday and Saturday by appointment.

The inn was built in traditional style in 1983 and has 10 individually decorated, sound-proofed rooms and two suites, all with private baths and controlled temperature.

The cedar inn has a Great Room with a 22-foot-high ceiling, a large family library, TV area, garden room and a spacious dining room.

If you can tear yourself away from the resort, the glories of Charlottesville, with its historic sites and excellent shopping, as well as the Skyline Drive and Blue Ridge Parkway, await.

Amherst, Monroe and Lynchburg

DULWICH MANOR
Va. 60, Amherst   *(804) 946-7207*
$-$$$

You will know your journey is over when you turn onto the winding country lane and see the inviting porch of this estate, set on five secluded acres in Amherst County. Flemish bond brickwork and fluted columns decorate the outside of this late 1880s English-style manor house. Nestled in the countryside and surrounded by the Blue Ridge Mountains, Dulwich Manor abounds with beauty and country appeal.

Hosts Bob and Judy Reilly have created a serene getaway. Period antiques decorate the rooms, and the living room and study each have a large fireplace to set a cozy, relaxed mood. The six bedrooms are reminiscent of an English country home — beds are canopied brass or antiques — and you can choose a room with a fireplace or window seat for relaxing afternoons or evenings. The Scarborough Room also offers a whirlpool tub and a canopied queen-size bed.

Each day begins with a full country breakfast, including fresh fruits and juices, inn-baked muffins and breads, country sausage, herb teas and hot coffee. Take a stroll after breakfast and see the natural beauty of the Washington and Jefferson national forests. The Blue Ridge Parkway is nearby for hiking, picnicking or photographing the view. Natural Bridge and Caverns, Peaks of Otter and Crabtree Falls are all scenic spots for a lunch. This area of the country is also full of history: Washington, Jefferson and Patrick Henry were all born near here. The Appomattox Courthouse, Monticello, Ash Lawn and Poplar Forest are all within a short distance of Dulwich.

FAIRVIEW BED AND BREAKFAST

Va. 778, Amherst   (804) 277-8500
$-$$

"I used to feel somewhat apologetic because there's not more activity in our area, but I discovered that most people come here because it's quiet and beautiful and restful,"

says innkeeper Judy Noon. "When you look out the window, all you see is mountains. 'Fair View' is an understatement. Even the stars seem brighter than they do ohter places, so our guests tell us."

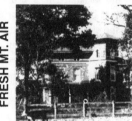

Fairview Bed & Breakfast

FABULOUS VIEWS FRESH MT. AIR

FINE BREAKFASTS FAMILY RATES

804-277-8500 FAX 804-277-8311
LOWESVILLE RD. AMHERST, VA 24521

Tootsie, an enthusiastic laborador, takes her welcoming duties quite seriously, and it's okay if you bring your pet too as long as you clear it with Judy and husband Jim.

Fairview was built by a Yankee doctor two years after the Civil War, as is indicated by the inscription on a dining room window pane: "This house was built in 1867. Fairview July 22 in 87." Local legend says the doctor fell in love with a local girl. The home he built for her is most unusual, in that its Italianate style is more common in New York's Hudson River area. "It's a toned-down Italianate," says Judy. "They can be very grand, with fountains, terraza and marble floors — but this is just a big, comfortable farmhouse."

The three guest rooms, each with a private bath, are furnished with antiques "which are meant to be used," says Judy. A fourth room, the Duck Room, is available for children or a third person. The house is fully air-conditioned.

Judy started a modest teddy bear collection some years ago, which has grown to a delightful hodgepodge of more than 50 bears, thanks to donations from her guests.

Judy customizes breakfast to the dietary needs of her guests, but she loves to whip up a hearty country eye-opener featuring her specialty, grits quiche, and fried green tomatoes.

"We're an old-fashioned kind of bed and breakfast in the European style, not the glitzy, hot tub sort," says Judy.

ST. MOOR HOUSE
BED & BREAKFAST
High Peak Mountain Rd.
Monroe   (804) 929-8228
$

Warm Virginia and British hospitality greet you at this lovely house, which sits among large trees facing majestic High Peak Mountain in Amherst County. The nature lover can stroll along acres of fields and woods and see the pastures, horses, cows and clear pond. The sight is even more breathtaking when the peach and apple orchards on the adjacent land are in full bloom. Or you can sit on an outside deck and enjoy the birds and landscapes.

The home's interior is every bit as lovely as the vistas outside. The old chestnut post-and-beam architecture makes St. Moor House unique. A cathedral ceiling, handmade brick fireplace and plenty of gorgeous antiques and Orientals make the atmosphere inside warm and inviting. The building is centrally air-conditioned, and private or semiprivate baths are available.

The aroma of a delectable breakfast will wake you each morning. Nearby are the natural wonders of the Blue Ridge Parkway, Natural Bridge and the James River. Advance registration is required. Children are welcome, but pets are not allowed.

LANGHORNE MANOR
313 Washington St.
Lynchburg   (804) 846-4667
$$-$$$

You can share in the comforts and heritage of this 27-room classical mansion, built c. 1850 for the Langhorne family. It stands today in the heart of Lynchburg's historic Diamond Hill neighborhood. Antebellum architecture, mahogany and walnut furnishings and crystal and brass chandeliers decorate the interior of Langhorne Manor. The three bedrooms and two suites are full of massive antique furniture and Langhorne family heirlooms. Each has a private bath, most with clawfoot tubs, and all are air-conditioned.

A homemade breakfast is served in the oak-paneled dining room. The staff will also prepare dinners, late night snacks and picnic lunches. The gallery displays changing exhibitions of sculpture and other works by Virginia artists.

Proprietors Jaime and Jaynee Acevedo are proud of the history in this home, on the National Register since 1979, and others in the quiet neighborhood. Mountains, orchards and antique shops surround the inn, which is also not far from Poplar Forest, Fort Early, Natural Bridge and Crabtree Falls.

Reservations are accepted with the receipt of one night's fee. Smoking is not permitted on the upper floors, and pets are not allowed. Call to discuss children before bringing them along.

LYNCHBURG MANSION INN
BED AND BREAKFAST
405 Madison St., Lynchburg   (804) 528-5400
$$-$$$$ (800) 352-1199

Built in 1914 for James R. Gilliam Sr., this 9,000-square-foot Spanish Georgian Mansion sits on a half-acre in the Garland Hill Historic District. A six-foot-high

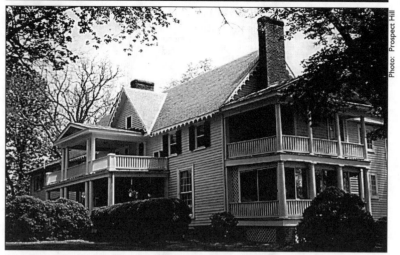

Photo: Prospect Hill

Prospect Hill is a historic plantation inn 15 miles east of Charlottesville.

iron fence surrounds the main house and carriage house. Three separate entrance gates are anchored in massive piers, and upon arrival guests drive under the columned porte-cochere to the six-columned entry portico. The front door opens onto the 50-foot grand hall with restored cherry columns and wainscoting. Just inches from the back door is a hot tub. The cherry and oak staircase has 219 spindles.

Garden level and first-floor accommodations are also available, and the bedrooms here are the ultimate in luxury. Family suites are also available. Some rooms have fireplaces, and all beds are king- or queen-size. Every room has a full, private bathroom, plenty of storage space, air conditioning, color television and telephone. Decor varies from the Victorian-style Gilliam Room, with mahogany four-poster bed with steps, a rose-patterned comforter, plump pillows and billowing lace, to the light and airy Country French Room that's done in crisp Laura Ashley prints, with a bleached four-poster bed and armoire.

The morning newspaper is delivered to

your door along with a freshly brewed pot of coffee and a pitcher of juice, and a full breakfast is served in the dining room, with fine china, crystal and silver. You can plan your outings at an information center in the back hall. After a day of sightseeing and shopping, you can retire to the elegant living room and sink into an overstuffed fireside chair.

Smoking is permitted only on the veranda. The request is for well-behaved children and no pets.

THE MADISON HOUSE
BED & BREAKFAST

413 Madison St.
Lynchburg   (800) 828-MHBB
$$-$$$$ (804) 528-1503

The Madison House, c. 1880, was built by Robert C. Burkholder for wealthy tobacconist George Fleming. This example of Italianate and Eastlake Victorian architecture, notable for its elaborate New Orleans-style cast-iron porch, sits in the historic Garland Hill District of Lynchburg.

Irene and Dale Smith have maintained the original floor plan, which has remained untouched for more than a century. Distinctive features include crystal chandeliers, an intricate peacock stained-glass window and numerous fireplaces and original woodwork. The Madison House library has books from as far back as the late 1700s, as well as many Civil War books and artifacts; the Smiths will provide a free packet of Civil War material pertaining to Lynchburg and Appomattox.

Each bedroom includes a mixture of antiques and modern conveniences, such as telephones and televisions. Your comfort is considered in such details as soft robes provided in your room, 100 percent cotton linens and bath towels and air conditioning. The Gold Room has a bay window, a king-size canopy bed, sitting area and antique vanity. The Madison Suite has a private sitting room with TV and writing desk and a bed chamber with a queen-size canopy bed. The Rose Room has a queen-size brass bed with dresser and armoire and a fireplace, and the Veranda Room has a screened-in sitting porch with Victorian-style white wicker. Each room has a private bath, two featuring original fixtures from the turn of the century.

A leisurely breakfast in the dining room consists of freshly perked coffee, fresh fruit, homemade coffee cakes, oven-baked omelets and English drop pudding. Eggs Benedict may also be served. Return to the Madison House for afternoon English tea each day. Irene prepares the homemade delicacies herself and displays the food on antique and Wedgewood plates.

After breakfast, you can visit some of the historical sights in and around Lynchburg, such as Poplar Forest, the Old Court House Museum and Appomattox Court House. The Blue Ridge Parkway, Skyline Drive and underground caverns are also close by. Check with the Smiths about walking-tour brochures and points of interest.

Smoking and pets are prohibited. Bringing children is discouraged, although some exceptions may be made. Reservations are strongly recommended.

WINRIDGE BED & BREAKFAST
Corner of Va. 675 and 795
Madison Heights (804) 384-7220
$-$$

Winridge Bed and Breakfast, 14 miles off the Blue Ridge Parkway, offers a panoramic view of the Blue Ridge Mountains and the simple elegance of country living. The Colonial Southern home sits on a 14-acre country estate built in 1910 by Wallace A. Taylor, president of the American National Life Insurance Company of Richmond. LoisAnn and Ed Pfister are the hosts now, and the landmark has been restored to its original grandeur. Four massive columns adorning the entry portico, and grand windows allow views of the surrounding countryside from anywhere in the home.

The inn has three guest rooms. The Habecker Room has a queen-size, four-poster bed and private bath with ceramic-tiled shower. The Walker Room has a queen-size cannonball bed, and the Brubaker Room has two twin beds. The Walker and Brubaker Rooms share a hallway bath with footed tub and brass and porcelain shower.

Breakfast is served every morning in the lovely old dining room. The estate offers plenty of entertainment: Explore the meadows, swing under the big shade trees or relax on the porches. The library and living room are full of books, magazines and games. If you prefer to venture off of the grounds, the Blue Ridge Parkway, National Historical Park at Appomattox Courthouse, Poplar Forest (Thomas Jefferson's summer home) and several colleges are all within a short drive. Nearby natural sites include Crabtree Falls, the Peaks of Otter and Natural Bridge and Caverns.

Smoking is permitted only outside. Children are welcome and are invited to play with the Pfister children.

Chatham

HOUSE OF LAIRD

$$$-$$$$ **(804) 432-2523**

Built in 1880, this Greek Revival house has been totally restored and professionally decorated with antiques, quality reproductions, Oriental rugs, imported draperies, wall coverings and moldings.

The House of Laird's romantic Library Suite is a favorite with guests. It has two working fireplaces and an Irish-estate canopy bed draped with 40 yards of fabric; other niceties include roses, chocolates, cable TV, a private bath with heated towels and gourmet breakfast in front of the fire. The Empire Room has a 100-year-old canopy Empire bed, working fireplace and luxurious decorator touches such as a Chinese Oriental rug, Belgium-imported draperies and hand-screened French wallpaper in the bath.

The Lairds' famous hospitality is evident in their gourmet breakfasts of traditional Southern foods served on antique china, silver and damask table linens.

Three blocks from the Colonial-era village of Chatham, named after the Earl of Chatham, who sided with the American revolutionaries, the house sits in a garden surrounded by 200-year-old oaks. This setting is a short distance from historical houses and battlefields, vineyards, seasonal festivals, antique auctions, fine dining, scenic mountain drives, horseback riding, hiking, fishing and boating.

The House of Laird offers weekday business discounts and hosts small weddings and meet-the-author literary weekends.

Rocky Mount and Wirtz

THE CLAIBORNE HOUSE
BED AND BREAKFAST

119 Claiborne Ave.
Rocky Mount   (540) 483-4616
$-$$$$

English-style gardens surround the 1895 Victorian Claiborne House, an elegant turn-of-the-century home in Franklin County. This tranquil getaway is nestled between the Blue Ridge Parkway and Smith Mountain Lake. The best place enjoy the scenery is from 130-foot wraparound porch furnished with white wicker furniture.

Victorian-era furnishings add charm to the interior. Each room has a king-, queen- or twin-size bed and private bath. Breakfast is a gourmet meal that may include fresh berries or other home-grown fruits in season or homemade bread. Specialties are eggs Benedict, blueberry crepes, spinach souffles and sourdough pecan waffles. Guests awaken to fresh coffee placed outside their doors.

You can spend our day reading a book from the lending library, or watch the house cat, Rascal, spend his day by the goldfish pond. Margaret and Jim Young are your hosts and can help you plan a day in the area. Smith Mountain Lake offers year-round activities — fishing, golf, tennis and biking — on its 500 miles of shoreline. Booker T. Washington National Monument is just moments away. Ferrum College and its Blue Ridge Farm Museum, Mabry Mill, Peaks of Otter, Mill Mountain Zoo and Roanoke's historic Farmer's Market are all within a short drive.

Well-behaved children are welcome. Sorry, no pets are allowed. Smoking is restricted to the outside only, and advance reservations are requested.

THE MANOR AT TAYLOR'S STORE
U.S. 122, Wirtz   *(540) 721-3951*
$$-$$$$

In 1799 Skelton Taylor first established Taylor's Store as a general merchandise trading post at this site in Franklin County. It served the community and travelers alike for many years. Later, the building functioned as an ordinary and a U.S. Post Office. The original manor house was built in the early 1800s as the focus of a prosperous tobacco plantation. The present-day home, once featured in *Southern Living*, has emerged as a lovely blend of the periods in which it has been restored. Lee and Mary Tucker are your hosts at this 120-acre estate.

The manor itself features several common areas, a formal parlor with a grand piano, a sunroom full of plants and a great room with a large fireplace. You may also enjoy the billiard room, guest kitchen or the fully equipped exercise room. The home is furnished with period antiques. Each guest room has a unique decor and ambiance. You can stay in the Castle, Plantation, Victorian, Colonial or English Garden suites. The Toy Room is decorated with antique toys, quilts and an extra-high queen-size canopied bed with steps. The Christmas Cottage is ideal for families with children; it has three bedrooms, two baths, a fully equipped kitchen, den with stone fireplace and a large deck with gorgeous views of the six ponds and wilderness area. Each guest room has a private bath, and some have a private balcony or kitchen.

After a fresh gourmet breakfast — Mary specializes in heart-healthy cooking and published a cookbook in 1995 — you can go hiking, picnicking, canoeing and fishing in one of its spring-fed ponds on the estate. There are also swimming docks, a gazebo and even a resident flock of geese! You can soak in the hot tub or lounge on the sun decks. Nearby are Smith Mountain Lake, Booker T. Washington National Monument, the Blue Ridge Parkway and all of Roanoke's sights.

Smoking is not allowed in the Manor house, and pets are not allowed in the house or the cottage. Children are welcome in the cottage. Advance reservations are important.

Blacksburg

BRUSH MOUNTAIN INN B&B
3030 Mount Tabor Rd.   *(540) 951-7530*
$-$$$

A Virginia Tech administrator and Bronze Star Vietnam War veteran Mode Johnson welcomes you to his "cottage-inn-the-woods" that specializes in personalized service. This 20-acre site is at the foot of Brush (or Brushy) Mountain. From your roomside deck, you can watch the native wildlife, inhabitants of Jefferson National Forest.

The cottage, built of laminated cedar and pine logs from Montana, features a timber-framed great room with a 20-foot stone fireplace, knotty pine walls, a wood stove, large whirlpool and an outdoor balcony off each bedroom. Normally, only two guest rooms are available, but special arrangements may be made to accommodate more guests. The Sunrise Room faces east, and the Forest Room is a suite on the first floor. TV, telephone and refrigerator are available for guests' use. Munchies, bottled water and magazines are little extras that make lounging around the woodstove even more comfortable.

A game room has darts and puzzles, while outdoor activities include trails and horseshoes. The surrounding forest has hiking paths (Mode keeps a stock of blaze-orange apparel for guests to use during fall hunting season). The Audie Murphy Monument is 6 miles away.

This inn is a great getaway for families. While many bed and breakfast inns will not allow children, here kids of all ages and pets are all welcome (with notice). Unique treats can be planned for honeymoon, anniversary, birthday or other special weekends. Smoking is restricted to decks and balconies.

L'ARCHE

301 Wall St.   *(540) 951-1808*
$$-$$$

An elegant 1907 Federal Revival-style home takes you away from it all — right in the heart of downtown Blacksburg. This renovated landmark, just a block from Virginia Tech, was opened by Vera Good in 1993. Six comfortable guest rooms are decorated with fluffy comforters and handmade quilts. Each features a private bath, queen-size bed and fresh flowers. One room is accessible to the physically challenged. The Country Room will accommodate a family with two children.

Guests may read, chat and relax in the drawing room, and the two cavernous dining rooms overlook the gardens. Share a table for two on the wide porch or sit under the Jeffersonian gazebo, which is sometimes the setting for weddings. Recreation is close at hand: white water rafting on the New River, boating at Claytor Lake State Park or picnicking by Cascades Waterfall. You'll find horseback riding, horse shows and carriage rides at Dori-Del Equine Center.

Nearby Virginia Tech and Radford University provide cultural and athletic events.

Breakfast at L'Arche is an event! The inn serves fresh fruit, home-baked breads, muffins and cakes, homemade granola and spiced teas. The morning repast may also include French toast, fluffy omelets or pancakes and waffles. Special dietary needs can be accommodated. Dinner may be served upon request.

Reservations are strongly encouraged. A two-night minimum stay is necessary on football weekends, commencement, parents' weekend or other special events. Smoking is permitted outside on the grounds. Gift certificates are available.

THE SYCAMORE TREE

P.O. Box 10937   *(540) 381-1597*
Blacksburg 24061   *(800) 381-1598*
$$-$$$$

The Sycamore Tree offers guests a peaceful country setting. Charles and Gilda Caines welcome you to share their custom-built home on 126 acres at the foot of Hightop Mountain. The Caineses settled in Virginia after living in Alabama, Kansas and New Jersey during Charlie's career.

The inn has six light, airy rooms decorated with antiques and old home pieces from the famous Hotel Roanoke. One room has a skylight, and each room has a connecting private bath, central heat and air conditioning. One room is specially designed for use by physically challenged guests. Guests can relax in the parlor, look out on the mountain skyline and watch the wildlife. The family room has a fireplace.

The Sycamore Tree entices you with nature, but for a little city life you can travel to nearby downtown Blacksburg, 6 miles away, or historic downtown Roanoke, 25 miles away. Cultural activities include theater and summer festivals, and academic and athletic events take place at nearby Virginia Tech, Radford University and Roanoke College. Outdoors enthusiasts can hike on the Appalachian Trail or take the 2-mile walk to the Cascade Waterfalls. And the Caineses start your day off with breakfast.

Advance reservations are required. Football games, parents' weekends, graduation and large family groups require a minimum two-night stay. Pets, smoking and alcoholic beverages are not allowed. Children older than 12 are welcome.

TWIN PORCHES

318 Clay St.   (540) 552-0930
$$

Kelly and Susan Mattingly bought an old, rundown boarding house in 1991 and transformed it into the inviting Twin Porches bed and breakfast inn. The Mattinglys had been students at Virginia Tech years before and decided to move back to the Blacksburg area after living in Northern Virginia. Susan loved this "diamond in the rough" because of its special little features, such as gingerbread trim, the ornately carved front door and porches on both levels. Just before they opened in 1992, Twin Porches won a civic beautification award as part of Blacksburg's 10th anniversary awards ceremony.

Comfortable guest rooms are decorated with antiques and quality reproductions. Rooms have queen- and full-size beds, and private baths in two rooms are equipped with original clawfoot tubs. The kitchen was converted into a lovely formal dining room, where a full breakfast is served each morning. The parlor offers a stereo and cable television.

For the sports lover, Lane Stadium is just 500 yards away. Virginia Tech is a terrific source of entertainment and diversion year round. Downtown Blacksburg is within walking distance for shopping and fine dining. Huckleberry Trail, a walking and cycling path built on the bed of the Huckleberry rail line, is just a block away.

Special weekday and corporate rates are available. Smoking is not permitted.

Christiansburg

THE OAKS

311 E. Main St.   (540) 381-1500
$$$$

Massive oak trees, believed to be 300 years old, surround this estate in Christiansburg, one of the most highly rated inns in the state. It earned four crowns from the American Bed and Breakfast Association, the top rating in its category. A green lawn stretches for what seems like miles and the home itself stands like a fairytale castle. Major W.L. Pierce built the buttercup-yellow Queen Anne Victorian for his family. Construction was complete in 1893. The home remained in the Pierce family for almost 90 years.

Margaret and Tom Ray converted The Oaks into a country inn. The luxurious manor is well-suited for both leisure and business travelers. Guest rooms have queen- or king-size canopy beds with Posturepedic mattresses, fireplaces and window nooks. The private baths in each room are stocked with plush towels, fluffy terry robes and toiletries. The garden gazebo houses a Hydrojet hot tub. A small, separate cottage has a sauna, efficiency kitchen and bathroom with shower.

In 1994 the inn was listed in the National Register of Historic Places, and has been named one of America's Most Romantic Inns. It also recently was selected for the PBS TV series *Inn Country USA*.

Each morning, guests wake to freshly ground coffee and a newspaper. The breakfast menu is varied and features such specialties as curried eggs, shirred eggs in spinach nests, rum-raisin French toast or whole wheat buttermilk pancakes in praline syrup. Sausage, bacon, ginger-braised chicken breasts and oven-fresh breads are all favorites. A bounty of fresh fruits and juices are available in season.

Take some time after breakfast to lounge on the wraparound porch with Kennedy rockers and wicker chairs. Investigate the books and games in the parlor or study. Or have a nice chat in the sunroom. Cable television and a VCR are also provided. Nearby, you can hike on the Appalachian Trail and boat or fish on Claytor Lake. The historic Newbern Museum, *Long Way Home* outdoor drama, Mill Mountain Theatre, Center in the Square, Smithfield Plantation and Chateau Morrisette Winery are all only a short drive away. The Oaks' Victorian Christmas each December is a special event.

Gift certificates are available. Advance payment and a two-night minimum are required for special-event weekends at local universities.

Pulaski

THE COUNT PULASKI
BED & BREAKFAST AND GARDENS

821 N. Jefferson Ave.   (800) 980-1163
$-$$

The move to 821 N. Jefferson was Florence Byrd Stevenson's 63rd — and last! She, along with her husband William H. Struhs, established the first bed and breakfast inn in Pulaski in this house that is more than eight decades old. The four-story brick home has three stairways and three upper guest rooms. The American Room has a canopied four-poster bed that is so high off the floor you have to climb into it using a stepstool. A crested plate

on the door to the Polish Room represents the royalty of the Polish count for whom Pulaski is named. Twin beds come together to make a king-size bed. Hand-decorated wooden pieces around the writing desk show fairy stories. James Michener's *Poland* lies on the desk, a gift given to Stevenson as a child. The French room is decorated with lithographs of Parisienne scenes. The seats of its two rosewood chairs were done in needlepoint by Stevenson's mother.

All the rooms have private baths. The rest of the house is decorated with furnishings from her life in Europe and Asia, along with family antiques. A 1912 Steinway baby grand sits in the living room and a Vietnamese temple bell sits on the mantle, along with a Byrd clock, which has been in the family for more than 100 years. Ceiling fans, air conditioning and fireplaces add comfort throughout the house. Start the day with a full breakfast in the dining room or on the porch. Then explore Pulaski's revitalized Main Street, famous for its antique shops; nearby are museums and national and state parks. Later, you could try a lunch or dinner cruise aboard the *Pioneer Maid* at Claytor Lake.

Reservations are suggested. Young children and pets can't be accommodated. The Count Pulaski is a smoke-free establishment.

Floyd County

BENT MOUNTAIN LODGE

Off U.S. 221 (Bent Mountain Rd.)
Copper Hill   (540) 929-4979
$-$$$$

The views are heavenly — in beauty and proximity — from this lodge overlooking the Blue Ridge Parkway from 3,200 feet up. Mornings are made for sit-

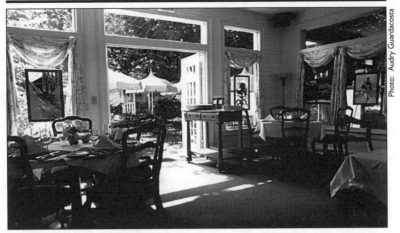

One of the three dining rooms in the Joshua Wilton House in Harrisonburg.

ting in a big rocking chair on your deck and gazing at the mountains and rolling countryside, a scene that innkeepers David Wood and Michael Maiolo get to see every day! Wood has been a teacher, a textbook salesman, director of food services for the Texas Rangers baseball club and a real estate agent who writes literature for young people. Maiolo is a former high school English teacher with a passion for Faulkner.

There are no planned activities, just areas for you to explore. The beauty of nature is emphasized a great deal. The owners have cut back the trees so the wildflowers — black-eyed Susans, daisies, fire pinks, sundrops and many more — can grow in abundance. Nature trails wind through the woods.

The lodge is decorated with country elegance and has five guest rooms and one two-room suite, each with a private bath with Jacuzzi and plush carpet. Quilts cover some beds, and some of the rooms have high ceilings. The large dining room is oak-paneled and constructed with hand-hewn timbers; bookshelves run

from the floor to nearly the 20-foot-high ceiling. A glass wall of French doors opens onto the 3,000-square-foot deck. A huge fireplace rounds out the room. The entire lodge is air-conditioned.

The lodge serves its guests three meals a day. The specialty is a country dinner with pot roast, chicken or country ham and fresh vegetables, bought from local farms, when available. Virginia wines are also featured. The restaurant is only open to non-guests from 5:30 to 9 PM Friday and Saturday and noon to 3 PM Sunday, but they will serve breakfast or lunch to a group of 10 or more.

Many weddings and conferences have been held here. Bent Mountain Lodge is also a great place for small weekday business meetings. These are generally held in the lounge, which has a fireplace and a bar from the former Floyd Mercantile store. Whatever the reason for your stay, Wood and Maiolo want you to feel at home. For that reason, they place few restrictions on their guests. Children and pets are welcome, smoking is OK and there is no minimum stay. So, relax and enjoy the view. The

Lodge is closed from January 2 through April 15 each year.

Alleghany Highlands Region

Clifton Forge and Covington

LONGDALE INN
BED & BREAKFAST
Longdale Furnace Rd.
Clifton Forge   (540) 862-0892
$-$$$$

Stone gates welcome you to Longdale Inn, formerly known as Firmstone Manor. Driving up the arched drive lined with flowering plum trees offers you a view of Longdale Inn's dusty-rose mansion and the Allegheny Mountains. A myriad of flowers and exotic shrubbery enhance the charm of this 1873 Victorian inn set near the southern tip of Virginia's beautiful and historic Shenandoah Valley.

Kate and Bob Cormier greet guests in the magnificent entrance hall, which takes you back in time to when Ulysses S. Grant was president and Virginia's first hot-blast iron furnace was established at Longdale. You can explore Longdale Inn's 23 rooms, each superbly restored and decorated with many original items from the Firmstone-Johnson mansion, owners and ironmasters of the Longdale Iron Works. Architectural details abound, and floor-to-ceiling windows bring let in mountain breezes and soothing sounds of the surrounding Allegheny Mountains.

The inn has 10 bedrooms and suites, furnished in Victorian, European or Southwestern decor. One suite furnished in white wicker with muted peach and gray tones is especially popular with honeymooners. A country breakfast, served in the dining room or in the privacy of your suite, includes freshly brewed Allegheny Star coffee, fruit, juices and cereals, followed by the chef's entree. You can request a picnic lunch for your outing; afternoon refreshments are also served. Relaxing activities here include croquet on the side lawn beneath century-old shade trees or strolling the 12 acres of grounds rich with wildflowers and songbirds that surround Longdale Inn.

Shopping and recreation sites are plentiful in the area. One mile west of the Inn, Longdale National Recreation Area has a variety of trails and a mountain lake for swimming. Outdoor enthusiasts and photographers will want to see the North Mountain Trail. Nearby National Forest roads and trails are ideal for cross-country skiing and mountain biking. You can soak in the fabled mineral waters of the Hot and Warm Springs or the Sweet Chalybeate Springs, or go to Douthat State Park and Lake Moomaw for swimming, boating, fishing and hiking. Highland has many antique shops and auctions, and Lexington offers the Virginia Horse Center and outdoor theater, concerts and several museums. Several challenging golf courses are nearby.

Longdale Inn also hosts gatherings, such as family reunions, meeting, seminars, retreats and weddings.

MILTON HALL
BED & BREAKFAST INN

207 Thorney Ln., Covington   (540) 965-0196
$$-$$$$

The Hon. Laura Marie Theresa Fitzwilliam, Viscountess Milton, built this manor in 1874. Lord Milton was ill and Lady Milton hoped the peace and tranquility of the countryside and beautiful mountain scenery would help return him to health. Today, Milton Hall still stands on 44 acres just west of Covington, in the community of Callaghan. Surrounded by the Allegheny Mountains, the house, with its gables, buttressed porch towers and Gothic trimmings, is a contrast to its rustic surroundings. The inside of the house is not as ornate, and, while it is spacious, is more of a large country home than a mansion.

A roomy living area and equally large dining room each have two sets of French doors opening to the gardens in the south lawn. Each guest bedroom has a private bath, except for the center bedroom with the oriel window that has become the Milton Hall logo (addition of a bathroom would require a drastic change in the original floor plan, and no one advocates that). Some features include queen-size beds and fireplaces. The second-floor master bedroom suite has a sitting area. One of the original bedrooms in the servants' quarters has been converted into a bath suite with whirlpool and fireplace. Some rooms have telephones; a central hall phone is available to all guests.

Guests guests have the choice of a full English morning meal or a continental breakfast, which can be served in your room. Complimentary afternoon tea is provided, as well. Picnics or elegant basket lunches are available to sightseers, and dinner may be served by special arrangement. Plenty of attrac-

tions are nearby: Lake Moomaw, national forests and state wildlife management areas are just a few. There is also the famous Humpback Bridge, Virginia's oldest standing covered bridge, within walking distance. The bridge is the nation's only surviving curved-span covered bridge.

Children are welcome, with proper supervision. Pets accustomed to an environment such as Milton Hall are also welcome. Smoking is not regulated but left up to the guests to give their opinion.

Hot Springs

CARRIAGE COURT

U.S. 220   (540) 839-2345
$-$$$$

Jim and Patricia Poling are hosts at this lovely getaway on Maple Ridge Farm. The inn is surrounded by pastures and wooded mountainsides, and the area is well-known for its natural warm and hot springs. Carriage Court is a group of five old farm buildings that have been remodeled and converted into a country inn and restaurant. The restaurant is in a converted two-story cow barn; lunch and dinner are served in the downstairs dining rooms or at umbrella tables on the outside deck. On the second floor, the Coach Room & Pub provides a pleasant spot to enjoy a cocktail or a candlelight dinner.

The inn has four spacious guest rooms, each with a distinct decor. Number One, which has a king-size bed and a queen-size convertible sofa, a large bathroom, tiny refrigerator, ceiling fan and a French door that opens to a deck with table and chairs. Number Two has two full-size beds, a sitting area, full bath, ceiling fan, tiny refrigerator and a

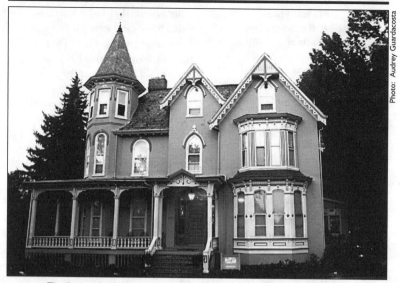

Photo: Audrey Guardacosta

The Joshua Wilton House is a beautifully restored Victorian home.

French door leading to a deck. Number Three has a private stairway leading to the multilevel suite on the second floor, with a separate dressing room, queen-size brass beds, sleeper loveseat and an Old World-style restored bathroom. Number Four is actually a two-room apartment accessible by an outside stairway; a living room, dining area, kitchenette, bedroom with a queen-size bed, two large closets and a bathroom make up this area. The latter two can be joined together as a large apartment to accommodate up to six people.

The world-famous Homestead Resort is a mile away, and the inn is near golf, skiing, skating, riding and hiking trails and hunting and fishing areas. Many fine businesses and restaurants are also nearby. Jim and Patricia will add special touches for important occasions, such as delivering champagne, flowers and breakfast or dinner for two or more.

Millboro and Warm Springs

FORT LEWIS LODGE
Va. 625, Millboro   (540) 925-2314
$$$-$$$$

In 1754 Col. Charles Lewis built a stockade to protect the southern pass of Shenandoah Mountain from Indian raids. This frontier outpost became a vast 3,200-acre farm, situated deep within the Allegheny Mountains. For more than 200 years, this area has remained virtually unchanged. The spectacular scenery and rushing mountain streams are enough to take your breath away. About 15 years ago, John and Caryl Cowden moved from Ohio to manage and operate the farm. Today, they are your hosts at this mountain retreat. They have restored the old red-brick manor house and the Lewis grist mill, dating back to 1850, adding guest lodge.

The large gathering room is framed with massive beams of oak and walnut. The observation tower, which is actually an enclosed stairway leading to the top of an adjoining silo, provides 360-degree views of the grounds; the silo also has three bedrooms. The lodge's 12 bedrooms are decorated with wildlife art and handcrafted walnut, cherry, red oak and butternut furniture, much of it made by local craftsmen from wood cut right on the property. Each guest room has a private or semiprivate bath.

Meals are served in the 19th-century grist mill. Three meals are included in the room rate, and all dishes are homemade and scrumptious. A full country breakfast includes freshly baked breads, eggs, sausage, bacon, fruits and French toast with locally made maple syrup poured over top. Lunch is served in the lodge, or you may opt to take a box lunch along with you. The buffet dinners include fresh vegetables from the farm's garden.

The outdoor activities are abundant here, with more than 2 miles of the meandering Cowpasture River flowing through the valley for swimming, tubing and sport fishing (catch and release) for smallmouth bass and trout. Several state-stocked trout streams are nearby. Miles of marked trails and old logging roads allow you to stroll along or explore. With advance notice, the lodge will outfit overnight campouts anywhere along the property.

MEADOW LANE LODGE

Va. 39, Warm Springs   *(540) 839-5959*
$$-$$$$

Meadow Lane Lodge is the keystone jewel in the crown of heritage tourism country inns. The estate cannot be seen from the road. You must wind your way up a narrow lane, between meadows and woods, finally emerging at a large clearing — and there it is: a white frame house with green and yellow trim. The stone dairy house and the old ice house are right out of the days before refrigeration. The deck behind the 1920s barn is an overlook where guests can see a nature preserve home to almost any plant or animal native to Virginia. Two miles of the Jackson River flow through the property; 1½ miles up the river is a limestone spring, the origin of Meadow Lane's water supply. Peacocks, a pet duck and Japanese Silkies (a type of chicken with black skin and white feathers) roam the grounds.

The history of Meadow Lane goes back to the Colonial days, when the land was part of the original grant given to Charles Lewis, an early Virginia settler, by King George III. An old log cabin, built in 1750, is visible from the west side of the Jackson River, and a stockade built around the cabin during the French and Indian War eventually became known as Fort Dinwiddie. Today, Philip and Catherine Hirsh are the third generation of Hirshes to own Meadow Lane. This year the inn was featured in a nationally-broadcast Tide detergent commercial.

The guest rooms are designed to combine modern comfort and antique grandeur. Choices include double rooms, suites with fireplaces and private cottages. Some rooms have surprising little extras, such as a 19th-century walnut dropleaf table, engravings or a private porch. The Common Room has a fireplace at each end. The Breakfast Room's 1710 oak sideboard is set with a full Southern breakfast each morning.

The Bacova Guild showroom is nearby, as are the Garth Newel Music Center, The Homestead and Lake Moomaw. But many guests just like to stay put and play croquet on the lawn — it's the house specialty! The 1,600-acre expanse allows for hiking, fishing, canoeing and creative loafing. Children older than 6 are welcome. No pets are allowed without prior approval.

Monterey

HIGHLAND INN

Main St., Monterey   (540) 468-2143
$$

Michael Strand and Cynthia Peel are innkeepers of this cozy spot, found in what is fondly called "Virginia's Switzerland." This Victorian home was built in 1904 to serve the lodging needs of tourists escaping from the summer heat of nearby cities. Eastlake porches with gingerbread trim and rocking chairs are so inviting you will want to stay indefinitely.

All 17 guest rooms have their own private baths and are decorated with antiques and collectibles. Choose a standard room (double bed), deluxe room (king-size bed or two beds) or a suite (two rooms). A complimentary continental breakfast is provided each morning, with dinner served in the Monterey Room. The Black Sheep Tavern offers beer and wine every day but Sunday.

Inside
Other Accommodations

After a great day you deserve a great place to stay. The Blue Ridge has a wide selection of comfortable accommodations to fit any budget. In this chapter, we provide a cross-section of motels and hotels. Remember, this is a guide, not a directory. The region is so big that we can't include every option available to travelers. But we can point you toward some of our favorites (see the Resorts, The Blue Ridge Parkway and Skyline Drive, and Bed and Breakfast and Country Inns chapters for additional lodging choices).

Room rates vary widely according to location and degree of luxury, so we've categorized each property by using dollar signs based on the rate for two people per room per night. Unless otherwise specified, major credit cards are accepted.

$30 to $40	$
$41 to $60	$$
$61 to $85	$$$
$86 and up	$$$$

Shenandoah Valley Region

Winchester

HOLIDAY INN
Intersection of I-81, U.S. 50, U.S. 17, U.S. 522
$$ (540) 667-3300

This 174-room motel is a convenient base of operations for exploring historic

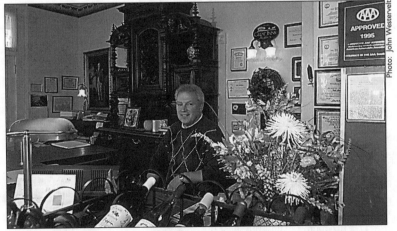

The Hotel Strasburg, a restored and converted 1895 hotel in Strasburg.

Winchester and is close to shopping malls and movie theaters. Amenities include non-smoking rooms, free and pay movies, convenient parking, a swimming pool, tennis courts, a fitness center, restaurant and lounge.

Middletown

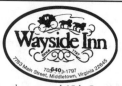

An elegantly restored 18th Century Inn. A place where fine food and lodging is a time-honored tradition. An antique lover's paradise and a historian's delight, offering an atmosphere of casual elegance and romantic charm.

540-869-1797

At the crossroads of Route 11 and I-81 (Exit 302)
7783 Main Street, Middletown, Virginia 22645

WAYSIDE INN
7783 Main St., I-81 Exit 302
$$$-$$$$ (540) 869-1797

Since 1797 this old coach stop has been coddling travelers along U.S. 11, once a major north-south thoroughfare. The restored 29-room stone inn is furnished in period antiques. Allow yourself a couple of hours for examining the artwork and curios in the pub and dining rooms. The Inn serves excellent Southern-style meals in various rooms, including the old stone slave kitchen downstairs. The Wayside Theater is just down the street, and many historical attractions are nearby.

Front Royal

QUALITY INN SKYLINE DRIVE
10 Commerce Ave.   (540) 635-3161
$$$ (800) 228-5151

The 107-room Quality Inn, near the northern entrance to Skyline Drive, is a good overnight stop before going on the scenic highway. It's also convenient for exploring Front Royal or taking part in one of the town's excellent festivals. The motel rooms are comfortable, with cable television and HBO. You can dine in the motel restaurant or at several others nearby. The lounge often has live entertainment. Ask about discounts.

Strasburg

Hotel Strasburg

A charming Victorian restoration, the Hotel Strasburg offers the finest in Southern Hospitalities. Enjoy gracious dining in a casual atmosphere, a drink in our quaint pub, and then relax in one of our finely appointed rooms or Jacuzzi suites, each furnished with period antiques.

1-800-348-8327
Historic Strasburg, Antique
Capital of the World.

HOTEL STRASBURG
201 Holliday St.   (540) 465-9191
$$$-$$$$

This white clapboard structure was built as a hospital after the Civil War. Decorated in antique furniture and folk and fine art, the Victorian hotel is decidedly charming, from the comfortable public rooms to the second-story balcony porch.

The 21 cozy guest rooms have private baths, many with Jacuzzis, and are decorated with period furniture, Victorian wall and floor coverings and classic window treatments. Other special touches are toiletries, fresh flowers, baskets of greenery, telephones and big, fluffy towels. Suites and staterooms also include a sitting area. Three dining rooms and a lounge serve excellent continental meals with a country touch.

This grand old hotel is near the Strasburg Emporium (see Shopping), Hupp's Hill Battlefield Park, Wayside Theatre and Half Moon Beach. Golf packages with nearby courses are available.

Woodstock

RAMADA INN
1130 Motel Dr.   *(540) 459-5000*
$$

Rooms in this 126-unit motel have all the creature comforts, including free satellite television. The Shenandoah Restaurant serves three meals a day. Woodstock is a historic town, containing the oldest county courthouse (1792) in use west of the Blue Ridge Mountains. The town's lookout tower provides a spectacular view of the Seven Bends of the Shenandoah River.

Luray

THE CABINS AT BROOKSIDE
U.S. 211 E.   *(504) 743-5698*
$$$-$$$$ *(800) 299-2655*

Your hosts, Bob and CeCe Castle, oversee a rare sort of accommodation: luxury cabins, with resident peacocks adding a royal touch. These charming cabins have modern baths, queen-size beds, elegant country decor, air-conditioning and heat year round and front porches and private decks overlooking a brook. Some cabins have fireplaces.

The cabins are adjacent to The Brookside Restaurant, where home-style cooking is served in a family-style setting (see our Restaurants chapter). An art gallery and gift shop feature limited edition prints, unique items from local artists and artisans and other mementoes of the Valley.

The Cabins are minutes from the Luray Caverns, Shenandoah National Park, Skyline Drive and New Market Battlefield.

DEERLANE COTTAGES AND CABINS
Off Va. 684, Luray   *(301) 567-3036*
$$$$ *(800) 696-DEER*

The views are outstanding from these quaint, private accommodations minutes from the Shenandoah River and nestled in the Massanutten Mountains. Choose one, two or three bedrooms with fireplaces, decks, kitchens, TVs and VCRs and other amenities. They're close to Skyline Drive and Luray Caverns. Horseback riding, hiking, fishing, golf and canoeing are nearby recreational possibilities. Pets are permitted.

RAMADA INN LURAY
3 mi. east of Luray Caverns
on U.S. 211   *(800) 272-6232*
$$-$$$ *(800) 268-8998*

Of the 100 guest rooms, 15 are furnished with antiques, and many rooms have Jacuzzis. Other amenities include cable television, miniature golf, an outdoor pool, a full-service restaurant, the Presidents' Gallery Tavern and the Presidents' Museum. Luray Caverns and Skyline Drive are minutes away.

New Market

NEW MARKET BATTLEFIELD DAYS INN
9360 George Collins Pkwy.   *(540) 740-4100*
$$ *(800) 325-2525*

On May 15, 1864, Union troops occupied Manor's Hill while the Confederates grouped to the south on Shirley's Ridge. The Confederate troops enlisted the help of young cadets from Virginia Military Institute and pushed the Yankees north. Ninety percent of the battle and casualties occurred on Manor's Hill, where the New Market Battlefield Days Inn now stands. The New Market Battlefield Park Hall of Valor and Military Museum, dedicated to the cadets of VMI, is adjacent to the hotel.

Other attractions in the area include Shenandoah and Endless Caverns and the New Market historic district. A short drive away are Shenandoah National Park, Skyline Drive, Luray Caverns and Bryce and Massanutten ski resorts.

The 92 guest rooms feature king-size or double beds and cable television. Complimentary coffee and pastries are served each morning. The motel has an outdoor pool.

QUALITY INN SHENANDOAH VALLEY
I-81 Exit 264   (540) 740-3141
$$ (800) 228-5151

The Johnny Appleseed Restaurant and Apple Core Village Gift Shop are special attractions at this motel. Extra touches include complimentary sunrise coffee and sunset cider. The 100 spacious rooms have free in-room movies, and the outdoor pool and sauna are good spots for relaxing afternoons. The Inn also has a game room and miniature golf course and is near historic New Market, Luray Caverns and the New Market Battlefield. Discounts are offered.

THE SHENVALEE GOLF RESORT
9660 Fairway Dr.   (540) 740-3181
$$

This 42-room lodge has rooms overlooking the fairway or at poolside. The 18-hole PGA golf course has a practice driving range and a fully equipped pro shop. The resort also has regulation tennis courts, a large swimming pool, a fishing pond and a hair salon. You can take your meals in the dining room or visit the Sand Trap Tavern for a casual evening. To find the resort, take Exit 264 off I-81 and go 1 mile on U.S. 11 S.

Harrisonburg

COMFORT INN
I-81, Exit 247A   (540) 433-6066
$$-$$$

This chain motel has won awards for hospitality. Nonsmoking and handicapped-accessible rooms are available, and the motel serves a complimentary continental breakfast every morning.

There's an outdoor pool on site. Harrisonburg is in the heart of the valley, bordered by Shenandoah National Park on the east and George Washington National Forest on the west. Do as the locals do — head for the woods for fishing, hiking, biking and horseback riding.

SHERATON INN
I-81, Exit 247A   (540)433-2521
$$$-$$$$

The Sheraton's a bit pricier than other area motels, but amenities include nonsmoking rooms, handicapped-accessible rooms, indoor and outdoor pools, a Jacuzzi, sauna, two restaurants and a lounge with live entertainment four nights a week.

Staunton and Waynesboro

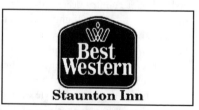

BEST WESTERN STAUNTON INN
U.S. 250   (540) 885-1112
$$-$$$

The newest place for business and vacation travelers in Staunton, Best Western Staunton Inn has the advantage of being beside one of the best restaurants in Staunton, Rowe's Family Restaurant, at Exit 57 off I-81. It's a few minutes driving time to downtown Staunton, Western State Hospital, Mary Baldwin College and the Museum of Frontier Culture. The Inn has 80 guest rooms in a four-story building. An indoor heated swimming pool and protected corridors keep the weather from being a problem. Two double or king-size beds are available, along with nonsmoking rooms on request.

HOLIDAY INN STAUNTON
Va. 275 and I-81, Exit 225
Staunton   (540) 248-6020
$$-$$$$ (800) 932-9061

Historic downtown Staunton is less than five minutes away from this well-endowed 112-room hotel. Also nearby are the Woodrow Wilson Birthplace and the Museum of American Frontier Culture. Nonsmoking and handicapped-accessible rooms are available. Other amenities include tennis courts and an indoor/outdoor heated pool. Guests have golf and tennis privileges at the adjacent Country Club of Staunton, and golf/lodging packages are available. A full-service restaurant in the hotel serves international cuisine, and the lounge features weekend entertainment.

Lexington

BEST WESTERN KEYDET-GENERAL MOTEL
U.S. 60 W.   (540) 464-1500
$$

Best Western is 1½ miles from the Lexington Visitor's Center and is close to Virginia Military Institute, home of the Keydets. This hotel offers a few conveniences not always found at other hotels. For example, they will accept pets, and many rooms have refrigerators and wet bars. Each room is air-conditioned and has a television. You can dine at a restaurant on the property. Senior citizen discounts are available.

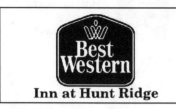

BEST WESTERN INN AT HUNT RIDGE

I-81 and Va. 39	(540) 464-1500
$$-$$$$	(800) 464-1501

To match the beautiful Lexington countryside, this country-themed inn offers 100 guest rooms with a view of the Blue Ridge like no other in the area. You can relax in Hobbies lounge or take a dip in the indoor/outdoor pool. You'll be close to the Virginia Horse Center and historic downtown Lexington, and you can take advantage of G. Willaker's restaurant, which serves all three meals and provides room service. Other extras include in-room coffee makers, electronic door locks, interior corridors and a guest laundry room.

COMFORT INN

Off I-81, Exit 191	
and I-64, Exit 55	(540) 463-7311
$$	(800) 628-1958

Near the Virginia Horse Center and historic downtown Lexington, Comfort Inn offers a complimentary continental breakfast, in-room coffee makers, an indoor pool and free local calls. Children younger than 18 stay free. Several restaurants are next to the hotel. Pets are welcome.

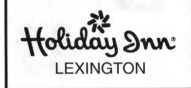

HOLIDAY INN LEXINGTON

I-64 and U.S. 11 N.	(540) 463-7351
$$	(800) 465-4329

Each of the 72 rooms at this Holiday Day, 1½ miles from the Lexington Visitor's Center, has air conditioning and a television. Nonsmoking and handicapped-accessible rooms are available, and the hotel has a full restaurant and pool. Pets are allowed. Ask about the senior citizen's discount.

HOWARD JOHNSON LODGE AND RESTAURANT

I-64 and I-81, Exit 53	(540) 463-9181
$$	(800) 654-2000

This mountain-top hotel is near Washington and Lee University, Virginia Mili-

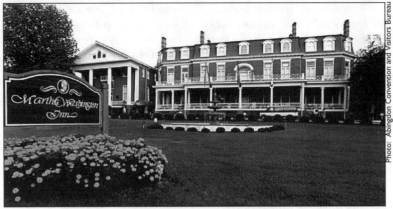

For lodging in Abingdon, the Martha Washington Inn offers top-rated accommodations.

tary Institute and Natural Bridge. A good place for smaller business and social functions, its meeting room can hold up to 135 people. The hotel has 88 regular rooms, 10 nonsmoking and two handicapped-accessible. All have complimentary HBO.

The facility has an on-site restaurant and guest laundry. The gift shop features local hand-crafted items. AARP discounts and group rates are available.

RAMADA® INN
Lexington

RAMADA INN

I-81 at U.S. 11   (540) 463-6666
$$ (800) 228-2828

The business traveler, families and tour groups will appreciate this hotel near Washington and Lee University, Virginia Military Institute and historical sites. The Inn has 80 guest rooms and three suites. The suites or double bedrooms are ideal for families with children. Two of the guest rooms are handicapped-accessible and 12 are nonsmoking.

The Inn's Rockbridge Restaurant (see Restaurants) has a full-service dining room and lounge. Other amenities include an indoor swimming pool and cable TV. The banquet facilities can accommodate up to 200. AARP discounts are available.

Natural Bridge

NATURAL BRIDGE OF VIRGINIA

U.S. 11   (540) 291-2121
$$

Natural Bridge of Virginia, consisting of the Natural Bridge Inn and Conference Center and Stonewall Inn, offers complete accommodations. See the Resorts chapter for more information.

Fancy Hill
Motel

FANCY HILL MOTEL

I-81, Exit 180   (540) 291-2143
$-$$

In the heart of the Shenandoah Valley and near Natural Bridge, one of the seven natural wonders of the world, and the Blue Ridge Parkway and historic Lexington, this motel offers amenities for the traveler in a country setting. Travelers return time and again for its excellent rates, friendly staff and adjacent restaurant with wholesome home cooking. The rooms are extra clean, and smoking and nonsmoking rooms are available. TVs have HBO. It's the best of the small, charming places the Blue Ridge has become noted for.

Roanoke, Troutville and Salem

BEST WESTERN COACHMAN
I-81, Exit 503, Troutville   *(540) 992-1234*
$-$$

Just off I-81, a beautiful hilltop location with panoramic mountain views beckons travelers to this 98-room facility. Seven miles from Roanoke, Best Western also has the advantage of being in beautiful Botetourt County, known for its flowering orchards with bountiful fruit and country scenery. In addition to being clean and offering a variety of accommodation options, the inn has one of the areas' largest outdoor pools. Senior discounts are available.

BEST WESTERN INN AT VALLEY VIEW
5050 Valley View Blvd., Exit 3E
Hershberger Rd., Roanoke   *(540) 362-2400*
$$-$$$$ *(800) 362-2410*

One mile from Roanoke Regional Airport, this new, three-story inn at Roanoke's largest shopping mall, Valley View, has 85 rooms with indoor corridors. The decor follows a country theme with Shaker-style furniture. Nonsmoking rooms and rooms with king-size beds are available. Amenities include cable with HBO, an indoor pool, in-room coffee-makers and a complimentary continental breakfast. Numerous nationally known restaurants are nearby.

COLONY HOUSE MOTOR LODGE
3560 Franklin Rd., Roanoke   *(540) 345-0411*
$$ *(800) 552-7026*

Colony House is 2 miles north of the Roanoke entrance to the spectacular Blue Ridge Parkway. This small, quiet inn specializes in personal service. The 67 rooms are air-conditioned and carpeted and have direct-dial phones, cable TV (with HBO and ESPN) and king-, queen- or double-size beds. A few suites are available, and the Lodge has an outdoor pool. You're close to great restaurants, terrific shopping, the interstate highway and downtown. Colony House is an ideal base for business travelers and tourists. Special discounts and rates also apply.

COMFORT INN — ROANOKE/TROUTVILLE
Off I-81, Exit 150A   *(540) 992-5600*
$$ *(800) 628-1957*

Seventy-two guest rooms are available, each equipped with cable television. Other amenities include nonsmoking rooms, an outdoor pool, enclosed corridors and in-room coffee makers. Senior citizens and other discounts are honored.

COMFORT INN AIRPORT
3695 Thirlane Rd., Exit Hershberger E
off I-581, Roanoke   *(540) 563-0229*
$$

Close to the airport, Valleyview Mall and many major restaurants, Comfort Inn is a good choice for travelers who want cleanliness and ample amenities. Attractive rooms feature king-size beds or doubles, and nonsmoking rooms are available. Cable TV offers HBO, CNN and ESPN. Free local calls and a fax are available for business travelers. Everyone can enjoy an indoor Jacuzzi and outdoor

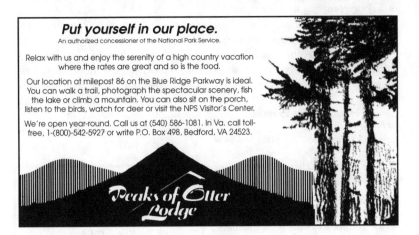

pool in summer, and the Inn offers a fitness center membership and complimentary continental breakfast.

FRIENDSHIP INN

526 Orange Ave., Roanoke   *(540) 981-9341*
$ *(800) 327-5887*

Access to the Roanoke Civic Center is about as simple as it gets from this hotel, since it's just across the street. The Friendship Inn is also less than a mile away from Center in the Square, the historic Farmers Market and the Virginia Transportation Museum. Free coffee is offered each morning. The guest rooms have cable television with HBO. Fax service and shuttle pick up are available. Ask about group, discount and seasonal rates.

HAMPTON INN

6621 Thirlane Rd., I-581 at
Peters Creek Rd., Exit 2-S   *(540) 265-2600*
3816 Franklin Rd. S.W, at U.S. 220
and Va. 419   *(540) 989-4000*
$-$$ *(800) 426-7866 (both facilities)*

Just 3 miles from downtown, close to Roanoke Memorial Hospital and across from Tanglewood Mall, the 59-room Hampton Inn on Franklin Road offers an expanded continental breakfast, HBO

and ESPN, VCRs, direct-dial phones, copier and fax service, king executive rooms, continental breakfast, hair dryers, refrigerator/freezer and microwave and nonsmoking rooms. Hospital and commercial rates are offered. The new Hampton Inn at Thirlane Road is close to the airport and offers the same amenities you would expect with Hampton Inn.

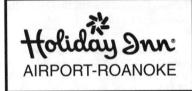

HOLIDAY INN AIRPORT

6626 Thirlane Rd., N.W.
Roanoke   *(540) 366-8861*
$$$

Only minutes from Roanoke Regional Airport, the Holiday Inn Airport offers complimentary transportation for busy travelers and executives. Close to Valley View Mall, the inn offers amenities to help you relax, including Foxes Den Lodge with wide-screen TV, music and dancing. Fox Hunt Restaurant serves traditional favorites. Sunday noon buffet is one of the longest-running in Roanoke, and this also is a popular place for business lunches. King leisure rooms, double rooms, parlor suites and executive suites are available. This inn's longevity says a lot about the service and comfort you can expect.

HOLIDAY INN EXPRESS
2174 Lee Hwy., I-81 S.
 Exit 150-A, Troutville   (540) 966-4444
$$-$$$

The Roanoke Valley's newest accommodation sports all the amenities guests have been asking for at Holiday Inns. All 60 rooms have microwaves, refrigerators, remote control TVs with VCRs and movie rental and complimentary continental breakfast. Local calls are free, and valet service is available. Kids stay free. Pets, however, are not welcome.

Guests can use the outdoor pool and exercise room with sauna. Options are nonsmoking rooms, handicapped rooms and Jacuzzi suites. Business guests can use the fax and copy service and meeting rooms. Golf and tennis are nearby, as are Hollins College, Natural Bridge and the Blue Ridge Parkway.

HOLIDAY INN HOTEL TANGLEWOOD
4468 Starkey Rd., off I-81 Franklin Rd./
Salem Exit, Roanoke   (540) 774-4400
$$-$$$

Close to Tanglewood Mall and just minutes from downtown Roanoke, this hotel's 196 guest rooms are traditionally furnished. Each comes with climate control, color TV (with Showtime, CNN and ESPN), AM/FM radio and two vanity dressing areas. Starkey's Bistro, in the hotel, serves continental breakfast or regional cuisine and also serves up a breathtaking view of the Blue Ridge Mountains. For some excitement, try the Elephant Walk lounge (see Nightlife), which takes its atmosphere from a safari decor.

The hotel offers outdoor swimming and tennis. Complimentary limousine service to the airport is available, as well as rental cars, private limos and taxi service. A concierge level makes this an especially popular place with business travelers whole like personal touches such as a complimentary newspaper and breakfast, hors d'oeuvres and nightly turndown service. AARP rates are available.

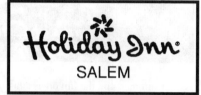

HOLIDAY INN SALEM
1671 Skyview Rd., Exit 137 off I-81
Salem   (540) 389-7061
$$-$$$

Just off I-81 and sitting high on a hill overlooking the Blue Ridge, the Holiday Inn Salem is convenient to the city of Salem and the entire Roanoke Valley. The guest rooms are spacious and comfortable. Executive king beds are available with large double bed for families on vacation. Guests can cool off at the outdoor pool during summer months. The spectacular view is part of the decor in The Knob Restaurant and Lounge, featuring favorite Southern dishes. Expect the same good service, amenities and comfortable accommodations the Holiday Inns have become known for.

HOTEL ROANOKE
& CONFERENCE CENTER
110 Shenandoah Ave.
Roanoke   (540) 985-5900
$$$-$$$$

The landmark Hotel Roanoke & Conference Center lives again after being closed for five years. Built in 1882, this sleeping Tudor-style giant has been revitalized as a Doubletree hotel in partnership with Virginia Tech, an arrangement brought about when the hotel's previous owner, Norfolk Southern Railway, gave the grand dame of luxury hotels to the university in 1989. The re-opening of the hotel, cherished by generations for its service, style and sophistication, is making some of the biggest headlines of 1995 in western Virginia.

Visitors to any of the 332 rooms will be pleased to see that the best was saved and the rest was modernized. The 103-year-old hotel has been completely restored, from its Florentine marble floors to frescos and vaulted ceilings. Visitors can stay in the same rooms where John D. Rockefeller, Amelia Earhart, Gen. Dwight Eisenhower and Elvis Presley looked out upon Mill Mountain. However, both the hotel and conference center have been equipped with 21st-century technology including dual line telephones, voice mail and computer hook-ups in every room.

The conference center can accommodate more than 4,500 people with 20 meeting rooms. A fitness facility and guest services are available. Visitors can have a drink in the Pine Room or dine in style in the Regency Room, famous for its peanut soup.

INNKEEPER MOTEL

815 Gainesboro Rd., Roanoke   (540) 982-0100
$$ (800) 822-9899

The Innkeeper Motel knows that it's the little touches that make a stay more pleasant. Guests at this hotel are treated to a complimentary continental breakfast, coffee, newspaper and ice. The 98 rooms feature firm, extra-length beds, and each room has a sofa, desk, AM/FM clock radio, electronic fire alarm and a remote-controlled color television with cable. Nonsmoking rooms and handicap facilities are available. Some rooms come with Jacuzzis, and guests may use the outdoor pool.

THE JEFFERSON LODGE

616 S. Jefferson St.
Roanoke   (540) 342-2951
$$ (800) 950-2580

The Jefferson Lodge is in the heart of downtown Roanoke, just a few blocks from the main public library, city and federal government buildings, hospitals and shopping. It is only three blocks to the City Market and Center in the Square.

One hundred newly decorated rooms await guests. Free parking, coin-operated laundry and color TV are all provided for your comfort. An outdoor swimming pool and family dining room are on the property. Special group rates are available.

KNIGHT'S INN

301 Wildwood Rd., Salem   (540) 389-0280
$$

Knight's Inn, 3.5 miles west of downtown Salem off I-81, is close to shopping, dining, attractions and major corporations. This clean, efficient accommodation has all ground-floor rooms, TV with HBO, kitchenettes, nonsmoking rooms, complimentary coffee service and free local calls. Senior discounts are available.

QUALITY INN — ROANOKE/SALEM

I-81, Exit 41 and Va. 419
Salem   (540) 562-1912
$$ (800) 228-5151

Quality Inn is great for families with children. At the Quality Park here, kids can swing, play games and enjoy other activities or swim in the children's pool. The 120 rooms have cable TV with HBO, and pets are allowed to stay with you. The dining room, Back to Berkeleys, serves tempting meals from breakfast through dinner. BTB's lounge features live entertainment.

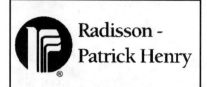

Radisson - Patrick Henry

THE RADISSON PATRICK HENRY HOTEL

617 S. Jefferson St., Roanoke   (540) 345-8811
$$-$$$$ (800) 833-4567

If you're staying in downtown Roanoke, this historic property is a fine choice. It's within walking distance to all the downtown attractions. When the Patrick Henry Hotel opened its doors for the first time in 1925, its 11-story exterior was already a wonder, but visitors and guests were astounded by the beauty of the interior. Today, the hotel, with its ornate decor, has been restored to its previous splendor, and it is one of two operating Virginia Historic Landmark hotels in Roanoke.

To say that the guest rooms are spacious is an understatement. Each has been modernized, but in a way that reflects the hotel's historic heritage. Rooms have kitchenettes. Airport transportation, free parking, complimentary health club facilities nearby, smoking and nonsmoking floors and a first-rate restaurant, Hunter's Grille, are all a part of this hotel's list of amenities. A bonus for woman travelers are special rooms outfitted with amenities such as hair dryers, irons and special bath toiletries.

ROANOKE AIRPORT MARRIOTT

2801 Hershberger Rd. N.W.
Roanoke   (540) 563-9300
$$$

The Roanoke Marriott completed a total renovation in 1994, the year it celebrated its 10th anniversary. It has been ranked by its guests in the top 10 percent of all Marriott Hotels. Situated on 12 landscaped acres, the hotel welcomes its guests in an elegant lobby. The bar, Whispers, is just off the entrance. Nearby are the two hotel restaurants, Lily's and Remington's (see Restaurants). The hotel has 320 guest rooms and suites with numerous amenities, such as individual climate control, AM/FM radio, remote-controlled color cable TV, two direct-dial telephones with message lights, video messages and complimentary personal care products. Twenty-four hour room service, valet service, airport transportation and free parking are other services here.

The Marriott has indoor and outdoor pools, a fitness center, sauna, whirlpool and two lighted tennis courts. For evening entertainment, guests can go to the hotel's lounge, Charades (see the Nightlife chapter).

The grand ballroom, Shenandoah Ballroom and six meeting rooms can accommodate groups of from 20 to 900. Seventeen conference rooms are available, with more than 12,800 square feet of flexible space. Special rates include Two For Breakfast Weekends, Honeymoon Packages, Super Saver and longterm rates.

SHERATON INN ROANOKE AIRPORT

2727 Ferndale Dr. N.W., Hershberger
Rd. Exit off I-581, Roanoke   (540) 362-4500
$$$-$$$$ (800) 325-3535

Indoor/outdoor pools, tennis courts, volleyball and golf are available at this outstanding hotel, which also has a piano bar and a club, Miami's. Oscar's Restaurant offers fine dining in the heart of this elegant hotel. Each of the 150 guest rooms and four suites is equipped with satellite TV, two phones, individual climate control, radio and two double beds or a king-size bed. Pets are allowed in the room with a $25 deposit.

Sheraton has more than 7,200 square feet in meeting and conference facilities. The main ballroom can accommodate events from a small dinner of 20 to a banquet of 350 people. A conference center and luxurious hospitality suites are ideal for business, meeting and social functions. AARP discounts are available.

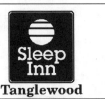

SLEEP INN TANGLEWOOD
4045 Electric Rd., Roanoke (540) 772-1500
$$-$$$ *(800) 628-1929*
The Sleep Inn, in the Tanglewood Mall area off I-581 at the Va. 419 Exit, is the area's new high-tech lodging for business and vacation travelers. The inn has 103 nicely decorated rooms with state-of-the-art security systems. Extras include a large desk in each room, fax service and a fitness program. The oversized showers feature massage shower heads. A complimentary *USA Today* newspaper and in-room coffee service are other amenities. Nonsmoking rooms are available. Each room has a satellite TV with VCR. Associates may charge meals to nearby restaurants including Charley's, Ground Round and Mac & Maggies.

TRAVELODGE — ROANOKE NORTH
2444 Lee Hwy. S., Roanoke   (540) 992-6700
$$ *(800) 255-3050*
Travelodge wants you to feel at home, so they provide a free continental breakfast, free coffee, tea and popcorn and free

You can often book a unique local accommodation for less than the price of a room at a hotel chain. Be prepared for surprises — mostly pleasant ones.

Insiders' Tips

local calls. Rooms offer attractive furniture, cable TV with CNN and Showtime, executive work areas and direct-dial telephones. Children younger than 18 stay free when sharing a room with their parents. Efficiency rooms are available for relocating personnel or longer-term visitors. Pets are welcome, and rooms for the physically impaired and nonsmokers are available.

East of the Blue Ridge Region

Leesburg

CARRADOC HALL/RAMADA INN
1500 E. Market St.   (540) 771-9200
$$$ (800) 552-6702

Carradoc was grand as a historic mansion and is even grander as a full-service hotel. The 122 guest rooms and four mansion suites are elegantly decorated, as is the Black Orchid II Restaurant. The hotel has an outdoor pool and is near sporting and historic attractions. Room rates include an extraordinary continental breakfast.

Warrenton

COMFORT INN
6633 Lee Hwy.   (540) 349-8900
$$-$$$$

Of the 97 rooms in this upscale motel, 59 are king suites. Four suites have whirlpool baths, and four have a kitchen, living area, bedroom and Jacuzzi. All rooms have a refrigerator and coffee maker, with microwaves available on request. Nonsmoking rooms are available. A continental breakfast, newspaper and local calls are complimentary. Other amenities include a laundry, fitness room, basketball court, picnic tables, barbecue grill and an outdoor heated pool.

Charlottesville

BEST WESTERN CAVALIER INN
105 Emmet St.   (804) 296-8111
$$

The 118-room Cavalier is next to the University of Virginia in the center of Charlottesville. Suites, handicapped-accessible rooms and nonsmoking rooms are available. The Inn has an outdoor swimming pool and serves a free continental breakfast to guests. Nearby attractions include Monticello, Ash Lawn and Michie Tavern, and several wineries are open for touring as well.

Special packages are available for families, senior citizens, sporting events and business meetings.

COURTYARD BY MARRIOTT
638 Hillside Dr.   (804) 973-7100
$$$ (800) 321-2211

Shopping, historical sites and the University of Virginia are all close to Courtyard by Marriott. Of the 150 rooms, 120 are nonsmoking. All have color televisions with HBO and ESPN and free in-room coffee. Two handicapped-accessible rooms and 12 suites are available. Guests may use the indoor pool, whirlpool and exercise room. The inn has a restaurant and lounge also. Evening room services is available.

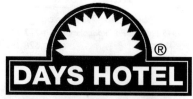

DAYS INN CHARLOTTESVILLE
1901 Emmet St.   (804) 977-7700
$$$ (800) 242-5973

This pleasant hotel is on U.S. 29 just north of Charlottesville, with easy access to the University of Virginia,

Michie Tavern, Ash Lawn and Monticello. The 174 rooms and two suites are modern and comfortably decorated, each with cable television, including HBO. The indoor heated pool has a patio area for relaxing or sunning outdoors in season. Gatwick's Lounge is lively, and Gatwicks's Restaurant features a daily buffet, as well as specialty dishes.

The Inn has 21 king suites, designed with a Queen Anne flair with a sitting room and wet bar. The other 67 rooms are contemporary in style and have two double beds. All rooms have cable TV, AM/FM clock radio, shower massage and automatic wake-up service.

Banquet and meeting facilities are available. A courtesy limousine serves airport travelers.

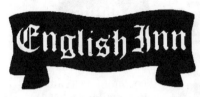

THE ENGLISH INN

2000 Morton Dr.   (804) 971-9900
$$$ (800) 338-9900

Following the centuries-old British tradition, your breakfast is complimentary at this well-appointed chain hotel. Guests are served a continental morning meal in the Conservatory, amid comfortable furnishings, a fireplace and fine art. Other amenities include an indoor pool, a sauna and an exercise room with a Universal weight system, exercycle and treadmill.

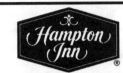

HAMPTON INN

2035 India Rd.   (804) 978-7888
$$$ (800) HAMPTON

Guests in the Hampton's 123 rooms enjoy free airport shuttles, free local calls

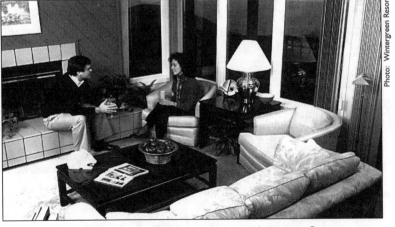

Luxurious mountain condos are available at Wintergreen Resort.

and a complimentary continental breakfast. The rooms are spacious and comfortable, with cable television and air conditioning.

Nonsmoking rooms are available. The Inn has an outdoor pool, and numerous restaurants are nearby. Charlottesville's major attractions — UVA, Monticello, Ash Lawn and Michie Tavern — are within easy reach of the Inn, which is on U.S. 29 north of the city at the Seminole Square Shopping Center.

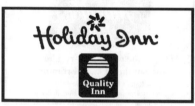

HOLIDAY INN/QUALITY INN

1600 Emmet St.	*(804) 293-9111*
$$$	*(800) HOLIDAY*

This convenient hotel has 201 rooms and three suites, all handsomely decorated and equipped with cable television. The exercise room has a treadmill, universal gym and sauna; outside is a large pool and a landscaped courtyard. The hotel has its own restaurant. Ask about discounted rates.

HOLIDAY INN
CHARLOTTESVILLE/MONTICELLO

I-64 and Fifth St.	*(804) 977-5100*
$$	*(800) HOLIDAY*

This 130-room high-rise is 2 miles from downtown Charlottesville and 4 miles from historical attractions. Meeting and banquet facilities are available for up to 150 people.

HOWARD JOHNSON

1309 W. Main St.	*(800) 654-2000*
$$$	

This hotel, next to the University of Virginia and University Hospital, is favored by football fans because it is handy to the sports complex and stadium. The

Charlottesville historic district, shopping and restaurants are within walking distance. Each studio room has a large living area tastefully decorated for private parties and an adjacent work area with a conference table.

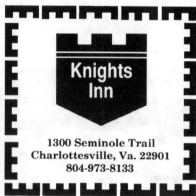

1300 Seminole Trail
Charlottesville, Va. 22901
804-973-8133

KNIGHTS INN

1300 Seminole Tr.	*(804) 973-8133*
$$$	

This member of the clean and comfortable national motel chain is just off U.S. 29 near shopping malls, restaurants and shops and within a five-minute drive of the University of Virginia. Knights Inn's 116 rooms (all on one floor) cater to a largely tourist crowd, along with UVA alums who flock to Charlottesville in the fall for football games and special events at the university. It's an affordable option, but book early for weekends any time of the year.

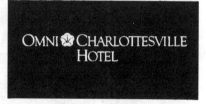

OMNI CHARLOTTESVILLE HOTEL

235 W. Main St.	*(804) 971-5500*
$$$$	*(800) THE-OMNI*

This spectacular hotel is AAA four-dia-

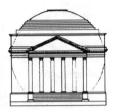
mond rated. The hotel's facilities can accommodate all sorts of events, from a cocktail party for 30 to a conference for 600. Indoor/outdoor pools, a whirlpool, sauna, health club and restaurant are on site. The 208 rooms and six suites are elegantly decorated; three are handicapped-accessible and 36 are designated nonsmoking.

RAMADA INN - MONTICELLO
U.S. 250 E. and I-64   (804) 977-3300
$$

This inn has 101 comfortable rooms with nice features, such as whirlpools, waterbed, king and queen amenitie, nonsmoking options, free HBO and ESPN and free local calling. A restaurant is on the premises, and the meeting and banquet space can accommodate 150. An exercise room, sauna and outdoor pool are available to guests. Senior citizens can get discounts.

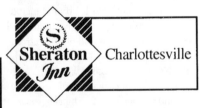

SHERATON INN CHARLOTTESVILLE
2350 Seminole Tr.   (804) 973-2121
$$$-$$$$

This 234-room accommodation on 20 acres offers all the creature comforts — in a palatial setting — after a hard day of sightseeing in Charlottesville. That includes a casual restaurant, Treetop; a formal restaurant, Randolph's; and a fun nightclub, Dooley's. Other amenities include two heated indoor and outdoor pools, whirlpools, an exercise room, tennis courts and jogging trails. This newly renovated property is Charlottesville's largest conference facility.

Lynchburg

COMFORT INN

US. 29 Expressway
at Odd Fellows Rd.   (804) 847-9041
$$ (800) 228-5150

A comfortable and clean room or suite awaits Comfort Inn guests. A free shuttle brings guests from the airport, just a few miles down the road. Other amenities for guests include a free full breakfast, a VIP floor, meeting rooms and fax machines. The Inn is within 5 miles of Liberty University, Lynchburg College and Randolph Macon Woman's College.

DAYS INN

3320 Candler's
Mountain Rd., Exit 8B   (804) 847-8655,
$$ (800) 787-DAYS

Topping the 1,500 Days Inn hotels, Days Inn Lynchburg was awarded the Days Inn chain's top award, Hotel of the Year, in 1994. This hotel has 131 rooms, including queen and king executive rooms and deluxe double rooms, all with electronic card locks. More than 75 percent of the guest rooms are nonsmoking and more than 50 have coffee makers, microwave ovens and refrigerators. The hotel has a large pool and play area. Business travelers will appreciate the hotel's two shuttle vans serving the airport, as well as a guest business center in the hotel lobby with computers, printers, a copier and office supplies.

The hotel's DayBreak Restaurant provides one free hot breakfast per room daily. Dinner discounts to guests are also available in the DayBreak.

HILTON — LYNCHBURG

2900 Candler's Mountain Rd.   (804) 237-6333
$$$$ (800) HILTONS

Families with children should consider the Lynchburg Hilton. In addition to adequate amenities and prompt service, children of any age stay for free when they occupy the same room as their parents. The 168 attractive guest rooms and suites are furnished with large, comfortable beds, color satellite TV and direct-dial telephones. Suites also feature wet bars, refrigerators and double, full-length, mirrored closets. Wake-up service, a gift shop, a newsstand and a courtesy van are other conveniences. The Hilton has an exercise room, a heated indoor pool, spa and sauna.

Johnny Bull's Restaurant serves some of the finest cuisine in Lynchburg, focusing on American, continental and regional dishes. The The Imbibery is the hotel's bar.

HOLIDAY INN

US. 29 and Odd Fellows Rd.   (804) 847-4424
$$ (800) 465-4329

Writing desks, sleep sofas, direct-dial telephones with computer jacks and remote-controlled color television are provided here. If you are enrolled in Holiday Inn's Priority Club, you will also receive a cup of morning coffee and newspaper delivery. The on-site restaurant, The Seasons, offers an interesting menu for breakfast, lunch and dinner, and the luncheon buffet appears to be a hit. Meeting and function space is available. AARP discounts are offered.

Insiders' Tips

If you plan to visit Virginia's mountains during the gorgeous autumn tourist season, book your lodging early — four to six months in advance isn't unrealistic — to be sure you'll have a place to stay during this busy time of year.

HOWARD JOHNSON LODGE

US. 29 N.   (804) 845-8041
$ (800) 654-2000

The 72 rooms here have oversized beds, plush lounge chairs, a writing desk and an extra vanity. Guests get free in-room movies and cable television, and you get great views of the Blue Ridge Mountains from the private patios and balconies. Next door is a Howard Johnson restaurant, which is open 24 hours a day.

INNKEEPER LYNCHBURG

2901 Candler's Mountain Rd.   (804) 237-7771
$$ (800) 822-9899

The Innkeeper offers a free continental breakfast and comfortable, clean accommodations. The guest rooms have extra-length beds, remote-controlled color TV with cable and HBO, desks, sofas and direct-dial touch-tone phones. Nonsmoking rooms and handicapped facilities are available, as are whirlpool baths or shower massages and swimming pools. Children younger than 16 stay free, and roll-away beds are complimentary. Corporate, senior citizen and tour/group rates are available.

Smith Mountain Lake

BERNARD'S LANDING

Moneta   (540) 721-8870
$$$$ (800) 368-3142

Bernard's Landing, a leading resort, is an excellent choice to accommodate travelers (see the Resorts chapter).

Bedford County and Bedford

PEAKS OF OTTER LODGE

MP 86, Blue Ridge Pkwy.
Bedford   (540) 586-1081
$$$

This lodge is like no hotel you've ever seen. Peaks of Otter is surrounded by the beauty of the Blue Ridge Mountains and lush green countryside, with a gorgeous lake nearly at its doorstep. The lodge's interior reflect the natural setting, with wood and subtly blended textures, tones and colors.

The 59 rooms offer double beds and private baths. Three large suites are also available. Each room opens onto a private balcony. The lodge has no telephones, so you can truly unwind and relax away from the rat race. The lodge has a cocktail lounge and dining room. Call ahead for seasonal rates.

Rocky Mount

COMFORT INN

950 N. Main St.   (540) 489-4000
$$

Beautiful Smith Mountain Lake is just 14 miles away from this lovely hotel. The 60 rooms have cable TV with HBO and AM/FM radios. A continental breakfast, sunrise coffee and sunset cider are complimentary to all guests. There is an outdoor pool on the property.

New River Valley Region

Blacksburg

BEST WESTERN RED LION

900 Plantation Rd.   (540) 552-7770
$$ (800) 528-1234

This hotel on 13 wooded acres is an ideal site for a meeting or banquet, since the inn can accommodate up to 400. The 104 guest rooms include two suites and one handicapped-accessible room. Hearty meals are served in the dining room, and the hotel has a lounge with nightly entertainment. The grounds include three tennis courts.

BLACKSBURG MARRIOTT

900 Prices Fork Rd.   *(540) 552-7001*
$$$

The Blacksburg Marriott, in the heart of the city right across from Virginia Tech, has 148 outstanding rooms, including one suite, two handicapped-accessible rooms and 100 nonsmoking rooms. Each room has in-room movies and HBO. Other amenities are an indoor/outdoor pool, tennis courts, a hot tub, children's play area and free access to a nearby health facility. Elegant dining is available in the restaurant downstairs or drinks and conversation in the lounge. Marriott's Sunday brunch served 10 AM to 2 PM is a Blacksburg tradition.

The ballroom and flexible meeting space can comfortably accommodate groups of 10 to 300. It's award-winning landscape creates a gracious setting for all occasions.

HOLIDAY INN OF BLACKSBURG

3503 S. Main St.   *(540) 951-1330*
$$ *(800) HOLIDAY*

Nostalgics will love this hotel for its railroad theme restaurant. The 98 nicely decorated rooms have numerous conveniences. The Inn has one suite, one handicapped-accessible room and 10 nonsmoking rooms. Banquet and meeting rooms can accommodate up to 500. A lounge, coin-operated laundry, game room, pool and satellite cinema are available for guests.

Radford

BEST WESTERN RADFORD INN

1501 Tyler Ave., off I-81
Exit 109   *(540) 639-3000*
$$ *(800) 528-1234*

Classics Restaurant and Lounge makes Best Western *the* place to come in Radford.

The restaurant serves breakfast, lunch and dinner and draws a crowd from all over the New River Valley. The deluxe guest rooms are decorated in Colonial Williamsburg colors. Each room has a color television with cable, a coffee maker, two touch-tone phones, a wall-mounted hair dryer and full bath amenities. King or double and non-smoking rooms are available.

A gazebo-style indoor pool area with whirlpool, sauna and exercise facilities is provided for guests. Free parking, ice and vending machines, babysitters, baby cribs and safety deposit boxes are other amenities. AARP and other discounts are offered.

COMFORT INN RADFORD

1501 Tyler Ave., off I-81
Exit 109   *(540) 639-4800*
$$

Families, business travelers and tourists alike will appreciate the comfort and convenience of Comfort Inn. Thirty-two large rooms with color cable television and tasteful furniture await you. All rooms are nonsmoking and have coffee makers and hair dryers. The hotel is near Radford University, historic Radford Mainstreet, an antiques mall and Virginia's only historic outdoor drama, *The Long Way Home*. AARP and other discounts are available.

EXECUTIVE MOTEL

U.S. 11 W.   *(540) 639-1664*
$

This small motel is clean and comfortable — and very affordable. Its location near St. Alban's Hospital and shopping provides added convenience. Each of the 26 rooms have two double beds, a refrigerator, air conditioning, direct-dial telephones and satellite color televisions.

SUPER 8 MOTEL

1600 Tyler Ave.   (540) 382-5813
$ (800) 848-8888

Super 8 provides a lot of amenities: cable television with the Movie Channel, waterbeds upon request, a 24-hour desk and wake-up call service and free coffee each morning. And the rates are famously affordable. Nonsmoking rooms and business singles are available upon request.

Pulaski County/Dublin

COMFORT INN

Off I-81 at Exit 98
Dublin   (540) 674-1100
$$ (800) 221-2222

A special feature of this hotel is the Emily Virginia's Restaurant. Motor coach groups get a special red carpet greeting, apple cider reception and fresh apple farewell. Each of the 100 rooms has individual temperature control, satellite color TV, AM/FM clock radio and direct-dial touch-tone phones. Some rooms have Jacuzzis. The conference room has a wet bar, and a private banquet room is also available. AARP and other discounts are offered.

Patrick County

DOE RUN LODGE
RESORT AND CONFERENCE CENTER

Mile 189, Blue Ridge Pkwy.
Hillsville   (540) 398-2212
$$$ (800) 325-6189

Just across the border of Floyd County, in Patrick County, Doe Run Lodge Resort and Conference Center and its High Country Restaurant are nestled in the most beautiful part of the Blue Ridge Parkway (see the Resorts chapter).

Alleghany Highlands Region

Alleghany County and Covington

KNIGHTS COURT

I-64, Exit 16, Covington (540) 962-7600
$$ (800) 843-5644

This motel is within a two-block radius of shopping and fine restaurants. The 74 rooms (including nonsmoking) come with amenities such as air conditioning, color TV with HBO and ESPN, direct-dial phones for free local calls and coffeepots. A small conference room is available with advance notice. Truck parking also available.

COMFORT INN

Mallow Rd., Covington   (540) 962-2141
$$ (800) 221-2222

Guests receive a free continental breakfast, and all 99 rooms are equipped with air conditioning, coffeepots, cable TV with HBO and ESPN (VCR available) and direct-dial phones with free local calling. Also available are king-size beds, nonsmoking rooms and two-room suites. Laundry service is available. The hotel has an outdoor pool and indoor whirlpool. A full service restaurant, The Painted Elephant Restaurant & Lounge, is within the hotel, and great shopping is within a two-block radius of the hotel.

HOLIDAY INN COVINGTON

U.S. 220 and 60
Covington   (540) 962-4951
$$ (800) HOLIDAY

The restaurant is especially nice here, and the lounge has nightly entertainment. The rooms are equipped with air conditioning, color TV with HBO and direct-dial phones. Ten nonsmoking rooms are available. The outdoor pool and nearby shopping facilities are other amenities.

Highland County

HIGHLAND INN

Main St., Monterey   (540) 468-2143
$$

Michael Strand and Cynthia Peel are innkeepers of this cozy spot, found in Monterey, fondly referred to as "Virginia's Switzerland." This Victorian home was built in 1904 to serve the lodging needs of tourists escaping from the summer heat of nearby cities. Eastlake porches with

Inside
Restaurants

If you think dining in the Blue Ridge means just country ham, biscuits, fried chicken and apple pie, think again. Sure, there are plenty of old-fashioned restaurants offering hearty, conventional Southern fare. But there are also dining rooms whose chefs have won national and even international reputations for their innovative cuisine.

The latter tend to be concentrated in the Charlottesville area and the northern foothills region east of the Blue Ridge. These highly acclaimed restaurants include the Inn at Little Washington and the Bleu Rock Inn, both just an hour from the "big" Washington beltway; the C and O Restaurant, Clifton Country Inn, and

Memory & Company in Charlottesville; and The Homestead in Hot Springs.

Some of the region's finest restaurants are tucked away inside beautifully renovated country inns — the Joshua Wilton House in Harrisonburg, Prospect Hill in Trevilians and the Valley Pike Inn in Newbern. Others sit smack in the middle of downtown districts and others along the major artery of the Blue Ridge, I-81.

In this vast region, you will find mountaintop restaurants with magnificent views from your table, especially Peaks of Otter Lodge in Bedford, Chateau Morrisette in Floyd County and the historic restaurants inside Shenandoah National Park.

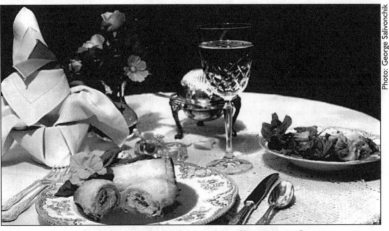

Photo: George Salivonchik

A gourmet dinner in the romantic dining room of The Inn at Union Run in Lexington.

If you have a hankering for exotic ethnic cuisine, try the Maharaja or Saigon Cafe in Charlottesville or one of the fine Brazilian restaurants in Roanoke, such as Carlos' in the downtown market area. Or, if organically grown vegetarian food is your preference, head to the Wildflour at Roanoke's Towers Mall.

The healthy, home-cooked food at Lynchburg's The Farm Basket is wildly popular, with people lining up as early as 11 AM for lunch at one of the few tables. The lunch spot grew out of a fruit stand and vegetable garden; it's famous for its cucumber sandwiches on dill bread and gouda cheese biscuits. Many restaurants throughout the region take pride in relying primarily on local products for their cuisine. The Highland Inn in Monterey specializes in fresh local trout and desserts concocted from Highland County maple syrup.

Many of Charlottesville's restaurants seem to be competing with one another for first place in offering the very finest, freshest and most innovative cuisine. This writer would hate to be the judge of such a contest, because there are so many mouth-watering places to dine in and around town.

We didn't include the franchise and fast-food restaurants in this chapter. However, you'll find just about every kind of national chain represented in every section of the Blue Ridge.

Because of the vastness of the region we have attempted to cover in this guide, we were unable to list every good restaurant in every city, town and village. We hope your favorite is included. But if it is not, drop us a line with your suggestions. We update this book every year and may add your favorite to this list.

Most restaurants accept major credit cards for payment; we indicate those that do not accept credit cards.

Readers may also be able to challenge our pricing guidelines for the restaurants listed below. Personal choices and menu changes will prove us wrong in some cases. Still, we hope to provide you with a basic idea of what you can expect to pay for dinner for two (no fancy desserts, wines or other alcoholic beverages). Price guides also do not include sales tax and gratuities.

Less than $20	$
$21 to $35	$$
$36 to $50	$$$
More than $51	$$$$

Note also that this chapter does not include restaurants in the Shenandoah National Park; those are listed in our chapter on the Blue Ridge Parkway and Skyline Drive.

The restaurants profiled in this guide are listed alphabetically under regional sections, then big cities, such as Charlottesville, Lynchburg and Roanoke. Others are listed by location. As in other chapters of the book, we begin with the northern stretch of the Blue Ridge and work our way south, zigzagging east and west over the mountains and Shenandoah Valley.

Bon appetit!

Shenandoah Valley Region

White Post

L'AUBERGE PROVENÇALE
U.S. 340   (540) 837-1375
$$$

Perhaps Virginia's most celebrated French restaurant, L'Auberge is but an hour's drive west of Washington, D.C., in the gentle hill country of the northern Shenandoah Valley. Expect superb authentic cuisine fashioned from the Provence region of France. An excellent wine selection, including vintages from local vineyards, adds to the upscale experience. The restaurant serves breakfast to inn guests daily and dinner Wednesday through Sunday. Reservations are recommended for weekends.

Winchester

CAFE SOFIA

2900 Valley Ave.   (540) 667-2950
$-$$

This lovely restaurant, open for lunch and dinner, serves the only Bulgarian food in the Shenandoah Valley and some terrific seafood dishes besides. Special decorating touches are handmade tablecloths, eye-catching framed embroidery pieces and an extensive doll collection. It is open for lunch and dinner Monday through Friday and dinner only on Saturday.

EL DORADO

1919 Valley Ave.   (540) 662-6488
$

The Mexican owners aren't shy with their use of hot chili peppers. You can expect generous portions of hearty, spicy food. Four-alarm salsa and tortillas arrive at your table before the meal. The atmosphere is casual: laminated tables and chairs and walls hung with piñatas, Mexican hats and travel posters of the home country. Local Mexicans frequent this place, a sure sign that the food is authentic and good. It's open daily for lunch and dinner.

THE OLD POST OFFICE RESTAURANT & LOUNGE

200 N. Braddock St.   (540) 722-9881
$-$$

This restaurant is inside a Winchester post office building built in 1910. Lunch selections include gourmet sandwiches, salads and pasta, and dinner offerings include fresh veal, pasta and seafood. The restaurant is open for lunch and dinner Monday through Thursday and dinner Friday and Saturday.

Middletown

WAYSIDE INN

7783 Main St.   (540) 869-1797
$$-$$$

This elegantly restored 18th-century inn is the setting for a great dining experience. Regional American cuisine is served in seven antique-filled dining rooms, including the old slave kitchen. Special features on the menu are peanut soup, spoon bread and country ham, a variety of game and seafood dishes and homemade desserts. Wayside Inn is open daily for all meals.

Strasburg

HOTEL STRASBURG

201 S. Holliday St.   (540) 465-9191
$$

Victoriana abounds in this wonderfully restored and converted 1895 hotel. The tables, chairs and paintings are supplied through the nearby Strasburg Emporium, and every item is for sale, so the furnishings are always changing. The restaurant has a strong following in the northern Shenandoah Valley and is known for its generous portions, courteous service and delicious meals. Dinner specialties include Chicken Shenandoah, chicken breast sauteed with country ham, peanuts, apples and an apple brandy cream sauce. The Strasburg salad combines greens and vegetables with pecans, blue cheese, artichoke hearts, eggs and croutons. Reservations are recommended on the weekends. The restaurant is open daily.

Front Royal

THE FEED MILL

500 E. Main St.   (540) 636-3123
$-$$

You can't miss the barn-like building just across from the visitors center, but what's inside will surprise you. Artist Patricia Windrow's trompe l'oeil (literally, "fool the eye") murals of farm animals and Civil War scenes are disturbingly realistic. The simple lunch and dinner meals are well-prepared and presented, from Dixie pork chops to New York strip with a seafood sauce. The Feed Mill is closed Wednesday.

Woodstock

RIVER'D INN

1972 Artz Rd.   (540) 459-5369
$$$$

For fine dining in a classic Victorian country house, River'd Inn is unequalled. Three country-elegant dining rooms, each with its own distinctive fireplace and each with intimate seating for no more than 10 guests, creates a warm ambiance. The refinements of linen, china, silver, soft candlelight and fresh-cut flowers mingle with a varied gourmet cuisine emphasizing fresh ingredients and traditional selections such as filet mignon, lobster tail and chicken Cordon Bleu. Appetizers, soups and salads are equally refined and beautifully presented. The desserts are a delightful mix of traditional favorites with sophisticated twists — sugar cookies with warm caramel sauce, for example, or apple bread pudding with lemon bourbon hard sauce. Fine wines and spirits are served.

The inn itself sits on 25 secluded acres at the base of the Massanutten Mountains, on one of the famous seven bends of the Shendandoah River (see our Bed and Breakfast and Country Inns chapter).

Prix fixe dinner is served Wednesday through Sunday (earlier hours Sunday). There is also a Sunday brunch. Reservations are required.

THE SPRING HOUSE

325 S. Main St.   (540) 459-4755
$$

Word has it there used to be an underground spring on this property, and town folk came to fetch spring water from the lady who lived here. Folks still come here for refreshment, though the spring is now closed. Breakfast, lunch and dinner are served seven days a week. Specialty entrees include Eleanor's Delight (a creamy seafood mixture on an open kaiser roll, with tomato and cheese). Dinners come with a complimentary glass of apple cider, homemade walnut rolls with honey butter and a trip to a huge salad bar.

Luray

THE BROOKSIDE RESTAURANT

U.S. 211 E.   (800) 299-2655
$-$$

The fresh air and natural setting here will give you a hearty appetite, which will serve you well the daily all-you-can-eat home-style lunch and dinner buffets. On the weekend, you can get the breakfast buffet. The salad bar includes goodies you might remember from Grandma's kitchen, and the melt-in-your-mouth breads, pastries and desserts are made fresh daily. Brookside is open daily for breakfast, lunch and dinner from mid-January through mid-December.

PARKHURST RESTAURANT

U.S. 211, 2 miles west
of Luray Caverns   (540) 743-6009
$$$-$$$$

This place is popular with golfers who play Luray's courses in the spring, summer and fall. The atmosphere is casual, although tables are set with cloth napkins, crystal, china and candles. Some of the specialties are escargot, tomato shrimp bisque, fettuccine with shellfish and veal Oscar. Every meal comes with a wonderful relish tray, served with a fresh, light garden dip, homemade breads and more. The Parkhurst is open daily for dinner; reservations are suggested.

New Market

SOUTHERN KITCHEN

U.S. 11   (540) 740-3514
$

If you're hungry for traditional Southern food, nothing fancy, this is the place. There's peanut soup — some say it's the best anywhere — Lloyd's fried chicken, barbecued ribs of beef and the like. It's open daily for breakfast, lunch and dinner.

Lacey Springs

BLUE STONE INN

U.S. 11, Exit 251 off
from I-81   (540) 434-0535
$$ No credit cards

The professors from James Madison University love this place and are willing to stand in long lines for a table, so plan your visit early or late. Specialties are tender steaks and fresh farm-raised fish such as Lacey Spring Trout. The restaurant is open Tuesday through Saturday for dinner.

Harrisonburg

EL CHARRO

1570 E. Market St.   (540) 564-0386
$$

This is a good Mexican restaurant with locations also in Dale City and Fredericksburg. Service is fast and the staff is courteous. El Charro is open every day for lunch and dinner.

HUYARD'S COUNTRY KITCHEN

Va. 42, Dayton   (540) 879-2613
$ No credit cards

Owner David Huyard and his cooks serve up ham, beef, chicken and vegetables buffet-style. The food is homemade and very tasty. The "kitchen" is in the Dayton Farmer's Market, where you can shop for kitchen items, lace, fudge, antiques, fresh cheese, homemade breads and much more. Huyard's opens at 9 AM Thursday, Friday and Saturday and closes in the early evening.

JOSHUA WILTON HOUSE

412 S. Main St.   (540) 434-4464
$$$$

Pricey but worth it, the restaurant inside this beautifully restored Victorian home serves the most exquisite food in town and is easily one of the state's finest dining spots. It's hard to believe the place was once a frat house for James Madison University students. Craig and Roberta Moore gutted the whole building and started over, creating a beautiful, romantic place to have dinner — and spend the night.

The wine list of more than 140 selections includes a variety of American and French wines at very reasonable prices. Appetizer choices include a salmon and scallop mousse and a confit of duck. The smoked-duck salad features carrots, walnuts, raspberries, an artichoke bottom and Boston bib lettuce. Among the entrees are trout with a country ham cream sauce and grilled smoked beef tenderloin with smoked oysters. Also on the menu are creatively prepared lamb, quail, pork, veal, duck, salmon and tuna. Among the many freshly prepared desserts is the creme brûlée — absolutely the best we've tasted anywhere. Dinner is served daily; reservations are suggested. (See our Other Accommodations chapter for information on an overnight stay here.)

L'ITALIA RESTAURANT AND LOUNGE
815 E. Market St.   (540) 433-0961

$$

Owner Emilio Amato's fine restaurants are right off I-81 in Harrisonburg and Staunton. The pasta and sauces are all homemade, and many of the entrees are prepared with a light touch for fat- and cholesterol-watchers. Outstanding offerings are the gnocci (tiny dumplings made with ricotta cheese and topped with a tomato and meat sauce) and the ravioli stuffed with meat. L'Italia has a second restaurant in Staunton, at 23 E. Beverley Street. Lunch and dinner are served Tuesday through Sunday.

PANO'S
Off I-81 at Exit 243   (540) 434-2367
$

Within its French provencial exterior is a cozy, wood-paneled family restaurant offering 65 entrees at lunch, 96 at dinner. All meals are nicely done, and the prices are right too. Pano's is open daily.

THE VILLAGE INN
U.S. 11   (540) 434-7355
$

The dining room at this small, family-owned motel serves simple, delicious meals prepared by Mennonite cooks. The Inn has a gorgeous view of the mountains and is one of the highly rated restaurants in the area (see our Other Accommodations chapter). The Inn serves breakfast and dinner every day except Sunday.

Waynesboro

CAPT'N SAM'S LANDING
U.S. 250 W.   (540) 943-3416
$$ No credit cards

If you love seafood, come dine with the captain. Surrounded by a nautical decor, you can indulge in fish, crab, oysters, lobster, scallops and clams prepared in a variety of ways. The steak and chicken dishes are good too. All entrees are served with a trip to the salad bar (or one hot vegetable) and a choice of french fries, baked potato or rice. Don't miss the week-long Shrimp Feast (held one week every month); all the shrimp you can eat is prepared nine ways, and the meal includes the salad bar, baked bread and fried potatoes.

The adjacent pub serves fresh popcorn and a special menu. Capt'n Sam's is open for dinner every day but Sunday.

THE FOX AND HOUNDS
PUB & RESTAURANT
533 W. Main St.   (540) 946-9200
$$

The Augusta County Court records of March 7, 1798, mention "The First

Main Street in a new town called Waynesborough." In 1837 John and Catherine Long built a house on that street; it would later be used as a hospital for both Confederate and Union troops during the battle of Waynesboro. The building is the second-oldest structure in Waynesboro, and since 1987 has been the elegantly renovated Fox and Hounds, given three stars by Mobil.

The traditional English decor is a spirit-raiser, and the menu includes such favorites as filet mignon, fresh salmon, chuckling oysters and nutty trout. The food is so good that it's hard to save room for delectable desserts such as chocolate mousse, cheesecake and the famous Fox and Hounds Hot Fudge Swan. Only the freshest ingredients are used in the dishes, which are continental and American in style. Lighter dining and imported and domestic beverages (more than 30 beers and five single-malt Scotches) are available in the warm and welcoming Pub. The Fox and Hounds is open Monday through Friday for lunch and Monday through Saturday for dinner. It is closed Sundays.

SCOTTO'S ITALIAN RESTAURANT AND PIZZERIA

1412 W. Broad St.   *(540) 942-8715*
$-$$ *No credit cards*

Join in the casual family atmosphere at Scotto's, where the owners take great pride in their Italian heritage and in the art of true Italian cooking. Their homemade dishes and gourmet pizzas are all reasonably priced and available for takeout or delivery. Lunch and dinner are served every day.

SOUTH RIVER, AN AMERICAN GRILL

2910 W. Main St.   *(540) 942-5567*
$

Open seven days a week for lunch and dinner, South River offers 20 feet of vegetarian salad bar (with homemade salads and fresh fruit) and a varied menu. Favorites include prime rib, St. Louis-style barbecued ribs, hand-patted burgers, homemade soups and an inexpensive children's menu. South River's atmosphere is pure Blue Ridge, with large picture windows, a lot of plants, a fireplace and a full-size hang glider suspended from the ceiling. The restaurant also offers banquet facilities for up to 100 and off-premises catering.

WEASIE'S KITCHEN

130 E. Broad St.   *(540) 943-0500*
$ *No credits cards*

You'll find "nothing fancy" here, according to the owner, but her down-home cooking and laid-back setting draw many regulars and tourists to the kitchen of Mary Eloise Roberts, known as Weasie to her many friends and customers. During the past decade, Weasie has turned the former Dairy Queen at the bottom of Afton Mountain into the major morning hangout in Waynesboro. Breakfast is the big draw, with homemade biscuits and gravy the most requested items. Desserts are also popular, all homemade. Lunch is priced at under $4, including Weasie's freshly made pies, cakes and puddings. On Friday and Saturday the restaurant is open 24 hours a day; it's open daily.

Staunton

THE BEVERLEY

12 E. Beverley   *(540) 886-4317*
$

This restaurant has been around for a long time and is known for its luscious homemade pies and generous afternoon teas. It's a small, family-owned place where you can also get real whipped potatoes and country ham on homemade bread. Traditional English tea is served from 3 to 5 PM on Wednesday and Friday and includes sandwiches, cake, cheese, fruit, scones and other pastries. It's open all day Monday through Friday and Saturday from noon to 5 PM.

THE DEPOT GRILLE

Staunton Train Station   *(540) 885-7332*
$$

This popular dining spot in the old freight depot portion of the restored C & O train station has a 50-foot antique oak bar. On the menu are fresh fish, Black Angus sirloin for two, crab cakes, seafood combination platters, salads and a "lite bites" selection. Daily specials, tasty desserts and a children's menu round out the choices. The Depot Grille has a full bar, including a selection of beers and wines from around the world. The restaurant is open for lunch and dinner seven days a week.

J RUGLES RESTAURANT

18 Byers St.   *(540) 886-4399*
$

Situated in the historic warehouse row, J Rugles is a lively pub with an outdoor patio favored by local businessmen and college students. The upstairs booths offer a more intimate dining area. The menu includes sandwiches, pizzas, pasta, steaks and seafood. Food specials, beverage promotions and special events keep the atmosphere festive. The restaurant is open for dinner seven days a week.

PAMPERED PALATE CAFE

26 to 28 E. Beverley   *(540) 886-9463*
$

This is another great watering hole smack in the middle of the most interesting shopping area in the downtown. Here you'll find gourmet deli sandwiches such

as roast beef and brie on French bread, bagels, stuffed potatoes, iced strawberry tea, and cappuccino served with luscious Italian desserts. You can get a continental breakfast on the second level. The place also sells a lot of wines, including the best Virginia ones, as well as gourmet coffees, gift baskets and imported candies. Wine tastings are offered too. The cafe is open for three meals a day Monday through Saturday and for lunch on Sunday. Hours are extended during the tourist season.

THE PULLMAN RESTAURANT

Staunton Train Station   *(540) 885-6612*
$$$

Step back in time as you enter this authentically restored turn-of-the-century train station that includes a Victorian ice-cream parlor. The building is furnished throughout with antique fixtures and advertising signs. The menu features updated versions of old-time railroad dining car fare, including a variety of steaks, seafood, sandwiches and lighter meals. A lunch soup-and-salad bar is offered six days a week, along with an elegant Sunday brunch buffet. You can sit along the train station concourse and watch the trains pass (Amtrak stops six times a week), and be sure to visit the elegantly appointed bar room. The Pullman is open for lunch and dinner daily.

Greenville

EDELWEISS GERMAN RESTAURANT

U.S. 11 and 340 N. (Exit 213
off I-81)   *(540) 337-1203*
$

Edelweiss offers authentic German cuisine in the rustic setting of a log cabin. Ingrid Moore is hostess at this two-diamond AAA and two-star Mobil-rated restaurant. Dinner menu specialties include German favorites such as sauerbraten (sliced roast beef), knackwurst (German beef frankfurter), rahmschnitzel (thinly sliced pork fillets) and hackbraten (German-style sausage meatloaf). Fresh vegetables are served family style. For dessert the house specialty is schwarzwalder kirschtorte (black forest cake), but the cheesecake, apple cake and tortes are also delicious. If you enjoy beer with your meal, you'll find a nice selection of imported light and dark beers. Attire is casual, and there's a half-price children's menu. The restaurant is open for dinner Tuesday through Saturday and lunch and dinner on Sunday. It's closed on Monday.

Nelson County

LOVINGSTON CAFE

Off Va. 29, Lovingston   *(804) 263-8000*
$

This unpretentious cafe in the heart of Lovingston serves up an array of good, old-fashioned American eats, including great burgers, chicken and soup. It's a nice place to unwind on your way to or from Charlottesville, just a few miles to the north. The restaurant is open daily for lunch and dinner.

RODES FARM INN

Off Va. 151, Nellysford   *(804) 325-2200*
$-$$

The red brick farmhouse run by Marguerite Wade as an inn and restaurant (see our Bed and Breakfast and Country Inns chapter) is legendary in these parts for serving up some of the finest country fare south of the Mason-Dixon Line. The accent is on hearty: roast beef with gravy, fried chicken, pork chops, country ham, fresh garden vegetables, homemade biscuits, pies and cobblers. The down-home

atmosphere attracts some pretty sophisticated palates. Past guests here include such notables as the Earl of Hanover, former President Gerald Ford, Alan Alda, Mick Jagger and John Lennon. Lunch is served daily; dinner, Tuesday through Saturday. Reservations are advised.

WINTERGREEN

Wintergreen   *(800) 325-2200*
$-$$$$

Wintergreen, an 11,000-acre resort, has six restaurants offering varied and delightful dining choices, from sandwiches in the Gristmill lobby of the Mountain Inn to gourmet fare in the elegant Copper Mine. Seasonal restaurants follow the golf and skiing schedules, and three lounges, one with live entertainment, also serve food. See our resort chapter for information on dining at the Trillium House, which lies within the resort.

Lexington and Rockbridge County

HARBS' BISTRO

19 W. Washington St.   *(540) 464-1900*
$

The sophisticated atmosphere, excellent food and fine service at this bistro and gallery make it a popular lunch spot and evening watering hole for students and other locals. Harbs' is the quintessential bistro: an intimate, unpretentious club atmosphere. The cafe's walls are covered with art, and its restroom signs are modeled after a bull and the Statue of Liberty.

During the day, choose from the menu of hearty sandwiches, salads, desserts and other specials. The hero sandwiches are served on freshly baked loaves. The dinner menu changes frequently, but you can count on fresh, delicious bistro fare. Reservations aren't necessary, but you may wish to call ahead for prompt lunch-time service. It is open for breakfast, lunch and dinner Monday through Saturday and breakfast and lunch Sunday.

THE INN AT UNION RUN
Va. 674   *(540) 463-9715*
$$

The Inn at Union Run sits on 12 beautiful acres outside of Lexington, and dining here is a real treat. The romantic dining room seats 22 to 25 guests by candlelight at antique tables. The ambiance is truly memorable, enhanced by gorgeous furniture and such interesting items as Toby mugs dating back to 1755 and 16th-century wine glasses.

The restaurant serves American regional cuisine created with local herbs and vegetables when available. Executive Chef Jim Stewart and his wife, Higgins, are both graduates of Johnston & Wales University in Rhode Island, a top cooking school. The relatively young couple has a great deal of experience in country inn and gourmet cooking. *Gourmet Magazine* is after many of their recipes! The inn is famous for its breakfasts, highlighted by such specialties as gingerbread pancakes and French toast made with English muffins and topped with fresh strawberries. The dinner menu, just as desirable, begins with the Inn's own Union Run country pâté, unique because it's made with pork. Fruits de mer abbink, one of the chef's specialties, consists of scallops, shrimp and salmon with homemade fettuccine and a saffron cream sauce. Grilled quail, braised Greek-style lamb shank and Virginia leg of lamb are given the chef's touch. Desserts include homemade sorbets, French vanilla and cappuccino ice creams and hazelnut torte, and Musician's Pie, loaded with nuts, has

guests calling weeks in advance to make reservations with it in mind. A full wine list is available; in 1993, the inn won the Governor's Wine Award for outstanding sales and promotion of Virginia wines.

The restaurant is open for dinner Tuesday through Saturday and on Sunday and Monday by chance (also see our chapter on Bed and Breakfast and Country Inns).

JASBO'S AT RAMADA INN
I-81 and U.S. 11 N.   *(540) 463-9655*
$$ *(540) 463-6666*

The savory foods served here have been praised as unusually good for a hotel restaurant. The chef presents fresh, contemporary dishes in a comfortable atmosphere where the quality of the food far exceeds the prices. Choose from such dishes as grilled tuna Mediterranean, New Orleans onion bloom, Shrimp Creole and grilled salmon. The pecan-coated chicken with orange sauce is peppery and delightfully rich. Jasbo's has a list of American wines that includes several Virginia varieties. It is open daily for breakfast, lunch and dinner.

SOUTHERN INN
37 S. Main St.   *(540) 463-3612*
$$

This charming historical restaurant has been a tradition in Lexington since the 1940s. The Inn, in the heart of downtown, specializes in Virginia wines. Visit this family restaurant for traditional Southern-style cooking, sandwiches or Greek and Italian dishes. Southern Inn is open seven days a week for breakfast, lunch and dinner.

WILLSON-WALKER HOUSE
30 N. Main St.   *(540) 463-3020*
$$$

The beautiful architecture of this 171-year-old, Greek Revival townhouse sets the scene for an elegant dinner or brunch. But you are welcome, whether you're wearing coat and tie or shorts and loafers. The interior, recently remodeled, has period antique furniture and artwork. Opening off of the foyer are the two main dining rooms, each with a fireplace with a faux-marble mantel and two portraits, c.1840.

The menu of creative American cuisine lists such tempting dishes as Virginia Lacey Springs's trout sauteed, paired with local Rockbridge Chardonnay, veal medallions, poultry, pasta, pork and beef. Desserts are scrumptious and include homemade Bailey's Irish Creme cheesecake and frozen chocolate-and-peanut butter mousse. There's also a children's menu. Second-floor banquet rooms are available for private parties. You can also dine outdoors in the veranda from May to October. The restaurant serves lunch and dinner Tuesday through Saturday. Lunch is not served on Saturday from January to March. Reservations are recommended for lunch and dinner.

LEE HI TRUCK STOP RESTAURANT
U.S. II N.   (540) 463-3478
$

Locals and the trucking crowd appreciate the substantial, hearty fare served at this friendly spot. Order the daily special and go away happy. They're open 24 hours a day every day.

MAPLE HALL
U.S. II N.   (540) 463-4666
$$$$

Fine dining in an elegant atmosphere describes the Maple Hall experience. This antebellum mansion is full of gorgeous antiques and restorations. The seasonal menu allows for the freshest and most delicious cuisine imaginable. It's open

seven days a week for dinner only. Reservations are required.

NATURAL BRIDGE RESTAURANTS
THE COLONIAL DINING ROOM
U.S. II S.   (540) 291-2121
$$

An oasis of good family food, the Natural Bridge Village restaurants are as popular with the locals as they are with visitors at this gigantic tourist attraction. Known for their Friday night seafood buffet and Sunday brunch, The Colonial Dining Room serves quality food daily, including breakfast Monday through Saturday.

Roanoke, Salem and Catawba

ALEXANDER'S
105 S. Jefferson St.   (540) 982-6983
$$$

Excellent food and renowned service make this restaurant well worth the trip into downtown Roanoke. The menu includes such dishes as chicken scampi, grilled breast of duck with raspberry butter and veal Alexander; bread and desserts are freshly made. Lunch is served Wednesday; dinner is served Thursday, Friday and Saturday. The restaurant is also open for private parties seven days a week. Dinner reservations are recommended.

ARTURO'S ITALIAN KITCHEN
5236 Williamson Rd. N.W.   (540) 563-2260
$

Proprietor Paul Dasalva, who gained fame for opening a New York Pizzeria in Ironto, has opened his second restaurant on busy Williamson Road. Its fame is growing just as rapidly. Showcasing real Italian food, daily specials really are special in both quality and price. There aren't many places in town where you can get lunch, including a salad, for less than $5.

Pizza, of course, is the main attraction. Not just any kind, but a choice of nearly 15 types! In addition to the usual pizza delights, there is a gourmet pizza menu featuring bianca pizza (white cheese sauce), stracotto, millenzane and veggie delight. No other place in Roanoke can make such a claim to such a wide variety of pizza. If you're going to have dinner, start with appetizers such as roasted peppers Parmegiana or baked clams. Arturo's has six types of salad, including chef's, pasta and antipasta. For the main course, expect all the mouthwatering standard Italian fare — chicken, veal or shrimp Parmegiana — and the not-so-familiar fare such as broccoli stuffed shells. All food is made to order, so the wait may be longer than at other places, but the results are well worth it.

The chef notes that the only cooking methods used are baking and sauteeing. No microwaves, steam tables or other devices are used to cook food fast. A wine list also is available. Desserts such as cannolli are available, along with surprises including a root beer float.

ASIAN FRENCH CAFE

32 Market Sq.   (540) 345-5593
$$

If you are looking for the best Vietnamese cuisine in the Roanoke Valley, then look no farther. This cafe, in the food court of historic Market Square, has a versatile menu, thanks to the chef's two separate kitchens. You can choose from Asian-, French- or American-style cuisine, such as grilled sesame chicken, quiche Lorraine or fresh fruit plates with honey dip. You may eat in either the elegant dining room or the large, neon star-decorated food court. The dining room is opens for lunch and again for dinner sittings Monday through Saturday; however, if you're just hopping in for a quick bite, the cafe operates two counters in the food court. Dining room reservations are suggested on Friday and Saturday.

AWFUL ARTHUR'S SEAFOOD COMPANY

108 Campbell Ave.   (540) 344-2997
$$-$$$

Seafood lovers, cast your anchor at Awful Arthur's, one of the four seafood restaurants in Virginia using the recipes of the real Arthur who lent his famous Urbanna (home of the Oyster Festival) beach recipes to this successful group. The decor is nautical and basic, just like the food. The main attraction is the large raw bar serving an assortment of items you'd expect on visit to the ocean. Captain's Sampler is the most popular, with oysters, shrimp, clams, crab legs, crawfish and mussels. Fresh is the only language spoken here by the chef, and you can expect everything to taste like it just arrived from the dock.

To ensure quality, all orders are delivered as they are prepared, so all items may not arrive simultaneously. Appetizers include the standard oysters Rockefeller and fried calamari. Also expect surprises such seafood pizza. Seafood pasta salad and tossed Thai salad are out of the ordinary. Pasta dishes complement the array of seafood, such as seafood Alfredo and linguine with clam sauce. If dinner isn't on your agenda, you can get a terrific sandwich of fresh fish of the day; the Awful Burger, which you can build yourself; shrimp Louis; or your basic fried oyster and crab cake sandwiches. A full wine list specializes in Virginia varieties such as Prince Michel Chardonnay, but California and Oregon

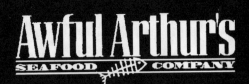
are represented too, and you can get a pricey French vintage.

In addition to quickly becoming one of Roanoke's favorite restaurants, Awful Arthur's is also becoming one of the favorite night hang-outs with popular groups.

BILLY'S RITZ

102 Salem Ave. S.E.   (540) 342-3937
$$

Housed in a century-old hotel building, this traditional American grill is just one block from Roanoke's historic Farmer's Market. You can join the happy-hour crowd at an oak bar and dine in casual elegance in any one of four unique rooms amid a collection of art and antiques — or have your meal in the open-air courtyard.

Although known for its great steaks, grilled fish and teriyaki dishes, Billy's Ritz excels at a variety of other cuisine as well. The Pasta Raphael is sure to please, and don't miss the prime rib on weekends. If you're in town for just the day, lunch with the downtown business crowd on freshly made soups, hearty sandwiches and a wide variety of salads. Wine is available by the

bottle or glass from an extensive list. The star of the dessert list is ice cream cake.

Lunch is served Monday through Friday, dinner Sunday and Saturday. Reservations are recommended for large groups.

CARLOS BRASILIAN INTERNATIONAL CUISINE

312 Market St.   (540) 345-7661
$$

Hundreds of faithful feijao preto (black bean) lovers come from all over the Shenandoah Valley to partake of the magic that is Carlos Amaral's international cuisine. Carlos' time spent working in 28 different restaurants has manifested itself in a menu quite unlike anything even lovers of Brazilian food have seen. What Carlos does with simple fare, such as black beans and angel hair pasta, spiced with international flavor, packs the place for both lunch and dinner on Roanoke's bustling city market. He and his sister, Iima, co-owner of Carlos, have become some of the best-known supporters of the market's continuing renovation.

Carlos is open for lunch Monday

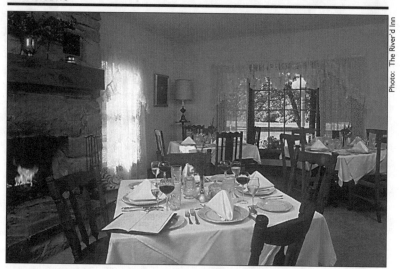

Photo: The River'd Inn

One of the three country-elegant dining rooms at the River'd Inn in Woodstock.

through Saturday, reopening for dinner Monday through Thursday. Dinner only is served on Sunday.

CHARCOAL STEAK HOUSE
5225 Williamson Rd.   (540) 366-3710
$$$-$$$$

Voted "Roanoke's Best Restaurant Overall" and "Best Steak" by *Roanoker Magazine* readers, Charcoal Steak House has been a Roanoke institution for fine dining since 1957. The taste-tempting menu lists more than 50 savory entrees including prime rib, charcoaled choice steaks, poultry, veal, fresh seafood, rock lobster tail and authentic Greek dishes. In addition to individual dining, the restaurant is popular for large family and business gatherings since many families consider the Charcoal Steak House staff family as well. In the evening, live entertainment is offered in the cocktail lounge. Reservations are definitely recommended on weekends.

CORNED BEEF & CO.
107 Jefferson St.   (540) 342-3354
$$

Probably the most successful deli operation in town, Corned Beef & Co.'s hearty fare, served up by three former frat brothers who graduated from Roanoke College, is known both for its great food and downtown atmosphere. The name says it all — don't look for anything pretentious here. What you will find is good, basic deli sandwiches served quickly in a first-class atmosphere. They're open for lunch and dinner Monday through Saturday ('til 2 AM Thursday through Saturday, for the wee-small-hours crowd).

EL RODEO MEXICAN RESTAURANT
4301 Brambleton Ave.
Roanoke   (540) 772-2927
4017 Williamson Rd.
Roanoke   (540) 362-7919
260 Wildwood Rd.
Salem   (540) 387-4045
$

This popular family restaurant will whisk you away to Mexico with its south-of-the-border decor, Mexican food servers learning English who don't always get your order totally correct (but who cares, it's all good!) and ethnic foods. Ingredients are printed on the menu for those unfamiliar with Mexican food. Expect the cuisine — fajitas, taquitos Mexicanos, La Chicana, enchiladas de polo (chicken enchiladas) and more — to be on the mild side. Select from vegetarian, children's and lunch-only menus as well. The chef is always willing to accommodate your substitutions. El Rodeo is open for lunch and dinner Monday through Saturday.

THE HOMEPLACE

Catawba   (540) 384-7252
$$

"Down home cooking that makes you want to eat all your veggies," is the slogan in this grand old farmhouse *cum* family restaurant just outside Roanoke. Thursday is Barbecue Night; you can still order regular fare. The home-style food is served family-style in bowls placed right at your table. Fried chicken, mashed potatoes and gravy, pinto beans, baked apples and hot biscuits are menu staples here. A neighborly and courteous staff will make you feel right at home. Always plan on a wait of at least 20 minutes, since Roanokers pack the place on weekends. But you won't mind it on the big front porch, where you can pet the farm felines while you wait. Dinner is served Thursday through Sunday.

LA MAISON DU GOURMET

5732 Airport Rd.   (540) 366-2444
$$$-$$$$

Here, close to the Roanoke Regional Airport, is fine dining in a gracious 1929 Georgian mansion. Readers of *Roanoker Magazine* voted La Maison the city's Favorite Restaurant for Special Occasions and

Best Restaurant Interior and Exterior. This is a popular spot, where business deals are closed and special events in the Southern tradition are held, including outdoor weddings in the lovely boxwood garden. Proprietor Rance Marianetti oversees the preparation of superbly prepared cuisine, which can be served with private label wines from the Barboursville Vineyard. Homemade Virginia seafood sausage is a house specialty.

Lunches are popular among the business crowd, especially the fresh fruit salads and a flaming spinach salad prepared at your table, as well as sandwiches. Entrees include Maryland crab cakes, beef peppercorn and catch of the day.

Dinner is exquisite. Appetizers might be fettuccine carbonara or escargot à la Bourguingnonne; onion soup grantinee or lobster citrus salad with brandy mayonnaise could be the start of your meal. Specialties du Maison include roast rack of lamb for two, Chateaubriand bouquetiere for two, steak Diane and gourmet seafood. For dessert, the array is tempting: pastries, Baked Alaska, Cherries Jubilee or sorbet with fresh fruit. The service matches the all-around excellence.

La Maison is open for lunch and dinner Monday through Friday; Saturday for dinner only.

THE LIBRARY

3117 Franklin Rd. S.W.   (540) 985-0811
$$$$

The Library, one of the most elegant and exclusive restaurants in the Roanoke Valley, is rated among the top seven restaurants in Virginia and is a memorable dining experience. French cuisine, served by candlelight, includes such classics as veal Princess, beef Admiral and English Dover sole. The decor of the restaurant is that of a well-stocked library. Dinner is served Monday through Saturday. Reservations are recommended.

LILY'S
At the Roanoke Airport Marriott
I-581 at Exit 3-W   *(540) 563-9300*
$$

This casual family restaurant in the Roanoke Airport Marriott serves a full range of moderately priced menu items, as well as popular buffets and children's menus. Prime rib is the feature Friday and Saturday nights, and Lily's has a champagne brunch on Sunday. Reservations are suggested; it's open daily.

LUIGI'S
3301 Brambleton Ave.   *(540) 989-6277*
$$

This Italian gourmet restaurant was established after the tradition of Mama Leone's restaurant in New York City. Naturally, the spaghetti is wonderful; coupled with the other pasta selections, it's an Italian gourmet's delight. Some of their special treats: veal Luigi's, shrimp scampi and the popular Cappuccino L'Amore, a blend of gin, brandy, rum, creme de cacao and Galliano liquor topped with a cinnamon stick, clove and whipped cream.

Homesick Northerners can get real Italian desserts too, such as cannoli and spumoni ice cream. Luigi's is definitely a cut above any other Italian restaurant in town, both for food and service. Each dish is prepared by your special order, so count on a leisurely dinner with a lot of attentive service. Dinner is served daily; they're open until midnight Friday and Saturday.

MAC 'N' BOB'S
316 E. Main St., Salem   *(540) 389-5999*
$-$$

Mac 'N' Bob's is without a doubt *the* place to eat in Salem, whether among the Roanoke College student crowd or the locals. The menu is unpretentious, the service is good and you can get your basic burger and sandwiches fixed the way you want, along with wholesome salads and terrific desserts which appeal to everyone.

MACADO'S
120 Church Ave.   *(540) 342-7231*
$$

The decor is as interesting as the food at Macado's, where both keep the restaurant packed with a younger crowd. A big hot-air balloon drops from the ceiling, and pictures and keepsakes from local or nationally known bands decorate the walls. You'll see the Three Stooges riding in an airplane, a section of a real classic car on the wall, old toys, posters, nostalgic collectibles and antiques. The extensive menu could take your entire lunch hour to read. It specializes in a delicious array of hot and cold deli sandwiches; the salads and chili are exceptional too.

The owner of the Macado's restaurant chain lives in Roanoke and has another downtown restaurant, as well as others in cities throughout the area, including Blacksburg, Charlottesville, Harrisonburg, Salem and Radford. Macado's is open daily for breakfast, lunch and dinner, and stays open until the wee hours.

MEDITERRANEAN ITALIAN & CONTINENTAL CUISINE
127 Campbell Ave. S.E.   *(540) 345-5668*
$

A Turkish touch by owner Ihsan Demirci has turned this out-of-the-way place on the Roanoke City Market into one of the busiest restaurants on the block. Pasta is the main attraction. It is delicious, plentiful and inexpensive. Lovers of fettuccine Alfredo and stuffed shells will be delighted to see their favorite Italian dishes prepared just right. Health food lovers also are treated to a wide array of pasta dishes with fresh vegetables, seafood and chicken. The chicken Saltimboca, a tender breast of chicken with proscuitto and mozzarella cheese smothered in a light sauce of Marsala wine and onions, makes watching your weight bearable in this den of delights. Veal dishes are another attraction, especially the veal Frances, tempting filets of veal dipped in a light egg batter and pan-browned in white wine and lemon sauce. Spaghetti is the side dish, of course. The Mediterranean is open Monday through Thursday for lunch and reopening for dinner; dinner only is served on Saturday and Sunday.

MOUNTAIN COFFEE AND TEA

112 Campbell Ave. S.E.
Roanoke   *(540) 342-9404*
17 E. Main St., Salem   *(540) 389-7549*
$

Success breeds success, and nowhere is this more true than with restaurants. Although Mill Mountain Coffee and Tea really isn't a full-service restaurant, it is one of the most popular hangouts in the Roanoke Valley, with a new Salem location. Both copy the famous Seattle coffeehouse concept — a laid-back atmosphere for mingling — which Roanoke Valley restaurant patrons have enthusiastically embraced. The draw, of course, is the multitude of coffee, tea and Italian soda flavors readily available for refill. The other appealing aspect is having a quiet place to go to talk or conduct business. All you have to do is place your order, sit down and enjoy the company.

REMINGTON'S

At the Roanoke Airport Marriott
I-581 at Exit 3-W   *(540) 563-9300*
$$$$

Remington's has a superb menu of distinctive American cuisine, complemented by superior service and a fine selection of wines. This top-rated restaurant serves dinner Monday through Saturday. Reservations are recommended.

THE ROANOKER RESTAURANT

Colonial Ave. at I-581
and Wonju St.   *(540) 344-7746*
$$

This restaurant has held high standards for more than 50 years, and it shows. It's busy day and night, every day of the week, filled with loyal customers whose parents and grandparents ate here. Run by the Warren family all these years, The Roanoker is frequented by customers who have come to expect quick service and farm-fresh quality food. Owner E.C. Warren received the 1995 Tourism Ambassador award for Roanoke.

The Roanoker was voted Best Place to Eat With Your Mother, and it is! Breakfast is a crowd pleaser; menu favorites include red-eye gravy and ham with biscuits and grits.

The restaurant serves breakfast, lunch and dinner daily.

ROANOKE WEINER STAND

25 Campbell Ave.   *(540) 342-6932*
$ *No credit cards*

In 1916, when prohibition caused the decline of Salem Avenue by forcing its saloons to close their doors, brick-paved Campbell Avenue took over as Roanoke's main thoroughfare. The road was exciting and new, with streetcars and electric street lights. The Municipal Building on Commerce Street and Campbell Avenue opened to the public. And, the Roanoke Hot Weiner Stand opened for business at the location where it would remain for more than 75 years. Harry Chacknes opened the stand with a six-burner stove, a kitchen that measured 13 feet by seven feet (including counter space) and six stools. And, right in the heart of the Magic City, you could get a steaming, plump hot dog for just a nickel.

Almost eight decades later, times have changed. What once cost you five pennies now runs you $1.05. The original six stools increased to 19 in 1988 when the Weiner Stand became a part of Center in the Square. The place even traded up for a more modern stove after using the old one for 72 years. But some things haven't changed a bit. The stand is still in the Chacknes family. Harry's wife, Elsie, ran it in the 1960s. Now his nephew, Gus Pappas, is the owner. Elsie's nephew, Mike Brookman, works in the kitchen. And, while John Liakos is not actually a blood relative, he is certainly a part of the family after working here for more than 30 years. You can still get that delicious, plump hot dog. And we don't think the friendly conversation and warm, honest smiles will ever leave the kitchen of the Roanoke Weiner Stand. It's open for breakfast, lunch and dinner Monday through Saturday.

SUNNYBROOK INN RESTAURANT
7342 Plantation Rd.   (540) 366-4555
$-$$

In 1983 Howard and Janet Schlosser found the perfect place that would create the right atmosphere for their home-style cooking. Sunnybrook Inn, a large farmhouse built in 1912, was the homestead of a 150-acre dairy farm. Each day, the Schlossers bake homemade pies, cakes and rolls in their kitchen. Their menu is a compilation of recipes — some 100 years

old — from all over western Virginia. The peanut butter pie here is legendary. Diners also love their oysters, fresh from the Chesapeake Bay and served year round.

Every Friday and Saturday Sunnybrook Inn serves a spectacular seafood buffet, with crab legs and fried oysters. There are separate children's prices. The restaurant is open for breakfast, lunch and dinner daily. Reservations are required for large groups.

TEXAS TAVERN
114 W. Church Ave.   (540) 342-4825
$ No credit cards

As soon as you open the door to this 64-year-old white brick Roanoke landmark, you can smell the hamburgers and hot dogs sizzling on grill. You will notice that the countertop is dented and dull, and some of the stools are long overdue for attention. Men in industrial-white T-shirts, work pants and aprons shout "hello" to newcomers over the bubbling chili and chattering customers. The staff is neighborly and will shoot the breeze with you — that is, if they have the time. A sign reads, "We serve 1,000 people 10 at a time." Nevermind. You didn't come here for pamperin' — you came for some of the best chili this side of Texas!

The Tavern is a great place for a quick, hot lunch or a midnight snack. It serves all the standards: hot dogs, hamburgers and, of course, chili. And if you order a nice cool drink, you won't get a Styrofoam cup or even an aluminum can. Only glass soda bottles and straws found here. Texas Tavern is near three (pay) parking lots, which is a bonus, since they have little parking space of their own. It is also just a few blocks away from the Farmer's Market and Center in the Square. The restaurant is open 24 hours a day, seven days a week.

309 FIRST STREET

309 Market St.   (540) 343-7017
$$

Dining at 309 First Street is like having your favorite meal with an old friend. If there's one thing that stands out about this place, it's the repeat business it enjoys as a downtown Roanoke favorite on the historic City Market. It's especially popular as a lunch spot for urban professionals.

309 serves lunch and dinner in a sunny, contemporary-style dining room under a skylight filled with green plants. Menu specials include seafood salad and chicken fingers. A popular choice is one of the gourmet hamburgers, such as the Burgundy Burger, a daily special with a hint of fine wine; the Tex-Mex Burger, well-seasoned with jalapeños, hot sauce and cheese; or the First Street Favorite, a top-of-the-line gourmet burger with bacon and Swiss.

Dinner selections include traditional favorites, such as filet mignon, as well as chicken teriyaki and sauteed seafood supreme (a combination of fish, crab, scallops and shrimp sauteed in herbs and butter). Also available to please the vegetarian taste is a popular ratatouille and vegetable and rice medley. All dinner selections include hot bread and butter, fresh steamed vegetables or seasoned rice, and baked potato, onion rings or fries.

They're open for lunch Monday through Saturday. Dinner is served until 2 AM Tuesday through Saturday.

WARD'S ROCK CAFE

109 S. Jefferson St.   (540) 343-CAFE
$

Shake it up, baby! Ward's Rock Cafe features such groups as Cravin Melon, Sick Bugs and Tomorrow's Party. Ward's has helped make a Jefferson Street section of restaurants become *the* hangout for young Roanokers. It features a rooftop section where the latest hot groups are featured. Ward's serves appetizing food made from the freshest ingredients available, with an entertaining atmosphere and service with a smile. Rock 'n' roll's greatest stars provide the menu theme: Costello's Chicken Salad (a tangy concoction of all white chicken breast with walnuts, red onions and tarragon) or The Orbison (roast turkey with Swiss cheese, Thousand Island dressing, coleslaw and spicy mustard on whole wheat). Dessert might be homemade brownies or buttermilk spice cake. Beverages include juices, hot chocolate and domestic and imported beer.

It's open for lunch Monday and Tuesday and lunch through dinner and late-night munching Wednesday through Saturday.

WILDFLOUR CAFE AND CATERING

Towers Mall   (540) 344-1514
$$

If you're going to eat at Wildflour, which everyone in Southwest Roanoke off I-581 at the Colonial Avenue Exit appears to do, be sure and get there before 11:30 AM. This small operation with limited seating makes what many say is the best healthy and homemade-style food in Roanoke. The folks here cook from scratch early, so the smell of fresh baking bread lures people who've been thinking about eating there since morning. The breads du jour are arranged in a flower pot at the cash register for all to smell and admire. The best red beans and rice we've ever eaten comes out of this place — we could eat it every day and not tire of it. As a nice touch, the young owners take the time to chat and get to know everybody, yet run an extremely efficient operation. Wildflour is open Monday through Saturday.

East of the Blue Ridge Region

Loudoun County

ASHBY INN & RESTAURANT
U.S. 50, Paris   (540) 592-3900
$$$-$$$$

Paris, Virginia, (population 47) was not as exotic as it sounds until Roma and John Sherman abandoned the metropolitan fast lane (though John still writes speeches for special clients in Washington and New York) in 1984 and bought a c. 1829 Paris house across the street from the original Ashby Tavern. They turned the place into one of the finest restaurants in Virginia and, with the acquisition of several other buildings, created a bed and breakfast inn that has finicky Washingtonians swooning in luxury and comfort (see our Bed and Breakfast and Country Inns chapter).

More than 100 diners turn out for the Shermans' delightful Sunday brunches, which are held hunt breakfast-style on the back patio overlooking the foothills of the Blue Ridge. The cozy taproom occupies what was once a country kitchen and is a particular favorite of local foxhunters (and followers of the hunt) after a day riding to the hounds.

The menu undergoes a complete change every day to make room for the Shermans' ingenuity, and the specialties of the house are legion. Ashby Inn crab cakes are world-famous but barely outshine a plethora of winter game dishes, gravlaks of Atlantic salmon, gumbo with duck and oysters, seared Virginia bluefish, mushroom tart, corn chowder with backfin crab and so on. You can count on the eggs

and vegetables being local, and the tomatoes being fresh from John's garden, which is also the source of herbs and exotic peppers used in the inn's dishes. The rustic restaurant serves sumptuous breakfasts to its guests and is open for dinner Wednesday through Saturday. Reservations are necessary.

BACK STREET CAFE
Federal St., Middleburg   (540) 687-3122
$-$$

Tutti Perricone reigns over this tiny eatery a block off Main Street and makes sure that her patrons are well-fed and undisturbed, no matter how famous they are. Actor Robert Duvall frequents the place, as do many political notables from Washington. The mostly Italian menu contains some wonderful fish and pasta dishes, and the daily specials are innovative and tasty. The outside deck is great for people-watching in good weather. On Friday and Saturday nights, Tutti engages one or two jazz musicians and can sometimes be persuaded to sing with them. Back Street Cafe serves lunch and then opens again for dinner Monday through Saturday; lunch only is served Sunday.

THE GREEN TREE
15 S. King St., Leesburg   (540) 777-7246
$$$

This famous watering hole, surrounded by the enchanting homes, historic buildings, shops and museums of Leesburg, specializes in authentic 18th-century recipes and does its own baking. Try a house specialty such as Robert's Delight (choice beef rolled in sweet herbs and spices) or Jefferson's Delight (liver presoaked in milk, sauteed with onions on top) while listening to 18th-century music.

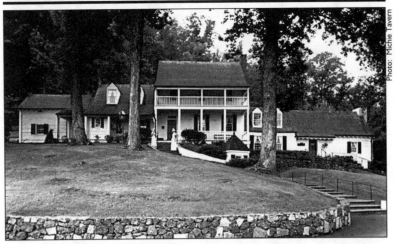

Photo: Michie Tavern

Michie Tavern's The Ordinary, a 200-year-old converted log house, is a restaurant specializing in Southern cuisine.

THE RED FOX TAVERN

2 E. Washington St.
Middleburg   (540) 687-6301
$$$

The Red Fox serves delicious traditional Virginia fare such as peanut soup, pheasant and crab, along with continental seafood and beef dishes. The tavern, believed to be the oldest continuously operating dining establishment in the Old Dominion, sits in a lovely 18th-century stone building in the middle of Middleburg, Hunt Country's premier antiquing and equine center. The restaurant serves lunch daily.

1763 INN

U.S. 50, Upperville   (540) 592-3848
$$-$$$ (800) 669-1763

Uta and Don Kirchner have decorated their historic inn (which is as old as the name implies) with treasures found in their travels, including a Czechoslovakian chandelier and Meissen china from Uta's native Germany. The restaurant is divided into small, intimate dining rooms, one over-looking a lake where swans reside. The cuisine, naturally, is German-American and nicely done, right down to the freshly made desserts. It's a delightful place to stay as well as dine (see our Bed and Breakfast and Country Inns chapter), and history buffs can browse through the Civil War memorabilia in the sitting room next to the bar. The dining room serves breakfast to inn guests every day. It's open daily for dinner and lunch on weekends. Reservations are requested.

Rappahannock County

BLEU ROCK INN

U.S. 211, Washington   (540) 987-3190
$$$$

Owned by brothers Jean and Bernard Campagne, who also operate La Bergerie in Alexandria, the Bleu Rock Inn is situated on 80 acres about an hour from the Washington, D.C., beltway. The Inn's three dining rooms have fireplaces, and in warm weather the terrace is a wonderful place to have dinner, drinks or dessert. From November through April, the chef offers a five-course, fixed-price menu on the weekends and a three-course, less expensive dinner on Wednesday and Thursday. The rest of the year, the restaurant serves dinner à la carte Tuesday through Sunday and is closed on Monday. The duck foie gras on a crisp potato cake receives rave reviews, as do the grilled sea scallops, blackened grouper, loin of lamb with Madeira and rosemary sauce, and desserts. Reservations are suggested. For more information about an overnight stay at the Inn, see our Bed and Breakfast chapter.

FOUR & TWENTY BLACKBIRDS
U.S. 522 and Va. 647
Flint Hill   (540) 675-1111
$$$

This wonderful restaurant is on the border of the Shenandoah Valley region and East of the Blue Ridge, a short drive from Front Royal on U.S. 522 S. Owners Heidi Morf and Vinnie DeLuise prepare creative American cuisine at reasonable prices. The menu changes completely every three weeks so that the cooks can take advantage of the best available seafood and local produce. The first-floor dining room is small but offers privacy for romantics; the tables are in nooks with screens of lace or floral prints.

For dinner, guests can select from four appetizers, seven entrees and three desserts. Appetizers might include corn crepes filled with morels and shiitake mushrooms and served with a smoked red pepper sauce. One acclaimed entree is the beef filet kebabs in a red wine sauce sparked with blue cheese and walnuts and served with lemony sauteed potatoes and snow peas. Morf is the former dessert chef at the highly ac-

claimed Inn at Little Washington, and her work is sensational. Chocolate pecan tart, mango mousse, pecan shortcakes with sauteed apples and maple cider cream are a few of her creations.

The restaurant serves brunch on Sunday and lunch and dinner Wednesday through Saturday. Reservations are suggested for dinner.

THE INN AT LITTLE WASHINGTON
Middle and Main Sts.
Washington   (540) 675-3800
$$$$

This highly acclaimed country inn is a favorite of Washington, D.C., media stars and politicians, being only a little more than an hour's drive from the city. Be prepared to spend big money here for exquisite regional American cuisine. The Mobil Five-Star restaurant has been praised by Craig Claiborne, the dean of food writers and restaurant critics, and in numerous publications, including the *Relais & Chateau*, a sort of Bible for the sophisticated European traveler. The menu changes daily, and guests are served a seven-course meal for a fixed price. Here's what one Richmond food critic rhapsodized over: the "fragrant, plump, explosively juicy little rabbit sausages" and the filet of salmon, wrapped in strudel pastry flavored with mushroom duxelle and accompanied by a delicate watercress butter.

On Saturday, dinner costs $98 per person, not including tax, tip or wine. Sunday through Thursday the price is $78, $88 on Friday. The restaurant is open for dinner every day except Tuesday, but during the busy months of May and October, dinner is served every day. Reservations are required. See our chapter on Other Accommodations for information about the inn.

Madison County

THE BAVARIAN CHEF

Madison   (540) 948-6505
$$-$$$

This restaurant a few miles north of Charlottesville serves huge portions of German cuisine family-style. The food is extraordinary, especially the sauerbraten and homemade desserts, which include a Bavarian nutball and Tiroler apfelstrudel with vanilla sauce. You can also order conventional American seafood dishes. Reservations are suggested. The restaurant serves dinner Wednesday through Saturday, lunch and dinner Sunday.

THE LITTLE CHEF

Va. 29 S., Madison   (540) 948-6908
$$

Regional American cuisine prevails at this popular restaurant, best-known for its family buffets. Ten entrees, numerous sandwiches, pizza and other dishes are complemented by soups and salad. Desserts are freshly made; the Brownie Delight is big enough for two. The Little Chef is closed Monday and Tuesday. Buffets are available for lunch Wednesday through Sunday and for dinner Thursday through Sunday, plus a Sunday brunch buffet.

PRINCE MICHEL RESTAURANT

Va. 29, between Culpeper
and Madison   (540) 547-9720
$$$$ (800) 800-WINE

The owners of Prince Michel de Virginia, the state's leading winery, operate this exquisite French restaurant. Its fixed-price menu emphasizes contemporary versions of traditional French cuisine and includes a choice of several imaginatively presented dishes for each course.

The restaurant offers the extraordinary cuisine of Alain Lecomte, a Frenchman who took first place in the prestigious Concours

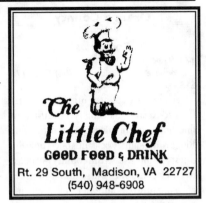

National de France des Chefs de Cuisine in 1990. He re-creates his highly acclaimed French specialities using local products and pairs these dishes with Prince Michel and Rapidan River wines.

Guests enter through Prince Michel's wine shop where they may taste wine at the attractive wine bar and browse the wine museum. The stairway leading to the restaurant sets the stage for a unique experience. Styled by Parisian designer Ariane Pilliard in collaboration with local artist Marie Taylor, the decor focuses on trompe l'oeil effects, including floor-to-ceiling murals that transport guests to the Bordeaux region of France. Opulent table settings with French linen add to the atmosphere of elegance.

The restaurant is open for lunch Thursday through Sunday and dinner Thursday through Saturday. Reservations are required for dinner.

Travelers coming from the north will find the Prince Michel Restaurant ideally situated at the gateway to about half of the state's 40-plus wineries. The smart dinner guest will arrive early to tour the winery (which closes at 5 PM) and enjoy the fascinating displays of its wine museum.

Orange County

ROCKLANDS
17439 Rocklands Dr.
Gordonsville   (703) 832-7176
$$$$

A gracious country inn in a historic Classic-Revival mansion is the setting for fine dining, surrounded by views of the Blue Ridge Mountains. Rocklands offers only the finest cuisine, from a full country breakfast to an elegant four-course dinner. Dishes are a mixture of Southern favorites and international flavors that include selections of seafood, pork tenderloin, beef and poultry. A variety of wines is available from the inn's own cellar. Call for hours and reservations (see our Bed and Breakfast and Country Inns chapter).

WILLOW GROVE INN
14079 Plantation Hwy.
or U.S. 15 N., Orange   (540) 672-5982
$$$-$$$$ (800) 949-1778

Limoges china, crystal chandeliers, Chippendale chairs . . . get the picture? This elegant plantation home, built in 1778, is now a bed and breakfast inn with a sensational restaurant. The regional American cuisine is the most contemporary thing about this magnificent place. The menu changes frequently depending upon the season but includes such items as bourbon molasses-glazed quail with herbed sweet potato cakes or smoked Rag Mountain with horseradish cream. Truly scrumptious desserts include dark chocolate cake with mocha creme and warm chocolate sauce, French lemon tart and white chocolate praline mousse.

The friendly (and handsome) bartender will help guests select an appropriate wine for dinner. The menu also suggests a particular wine for each entree and offers a full range of dessert wines, after-dinner liqueurs and dessert coffees. This is the ideal setting for dinner after a full day of touring Montpelier and other Orange County sites. Reservations are recommended. Dinner is served Tuesday through Sunday, with brunch also offered on Sunday.

Charlottesville

ABERDEEN BARN
2018 Holiday Dr., across from
Holiday Inn North   (804) 296-4630
$$-$$$

This is a well-established restaurant known for its roast prime rib and charcoal-grilled steak. But you can also have Australian lobster tail, crab cakes, shrimp scampi and other seafood delights here. The atmosphere is candlelit and intimate, and the Sportsman's Lounge has live entertainment nightly. Reservations are suggested. Dinner is served Monday through Saturday, lunch and dinner on Sunday.

AWFUL ARTHUR'S SEAFOOD COMPANY
333 W. Main St.   (804) 296-0969
$

This casual seafood restaurant down the street from the UVA campus specializes in fresh seafood and has an awesome raw bar. The menu includes steaks, salads, pasta and sandwiches. The restaurant has an English basement with billiards and darts. Awful Arthur's serves lunch and dinner daily. Reservations are accepted.

BAJA BEAN CO.
1327 W. Main St.   (804) 293-4507
$

In The Corner near the Rotunda, this California-style Mexican restaurant serves up lighter meals than your typical Tex-Mex fare. When owner Ron Morse moved here from San Diego, he brought the healthier California sensibility with him. The vegetarian specialities for lunch and dinner are especially popular. A full bar offers 12 Mexican beers and 15 brands of tequila. All dishes are freshly made, including hot and mild salsas. The festive restaurant is decorated with banners and T-shirts from Puerta Vallarta, Cancun, Cozumel and other Mexican hot spots. Baja Bean Co. is open seven days a week, with live music almost every night.

BILTMORE GRILL
Elliewood Ave.   *(804) 293-6700*
$-$$

One of the most attractive things about this restaurant is the wisteria-covered arbor that shades an outdoor dining area during the warmer seasons. A popular restaurant for UVA students, the place serves creative pasta dishes and other entrees, white gourmet pizza, unusual and hearty salads and much more. You'll find a wide selection of imported and domestic beer and an outdoor bar. The dessert menu includes such yummy items as apple maple pecan tart and the great American chocolate brownie. The Biltmore is open daily for lunch and dinner.

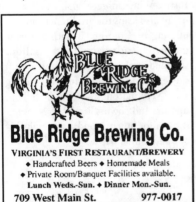

Blue Ridge Brewing Co.
VIRGINIA'S FIRST RESTAURANT/BREWERY
◆ Handcrafted Beers ◆ Homemade Meals
◆ Private Room/Banquet Facilities available.
Lunch Weds.-Sun. ◆ Dinner Mon.-Sun.
709 West Main St.   **977-0017**

BLUE RIDGE BREWING COMPANY
709 W. Main St.   *(804) 977-0017*
$$

If this friendly, casual place smells like a brewery, that's because it is one. In fact, it's Virginia's first brewery restaurant, having opened in 1988. The home brews are named for Blue Ridge mountain peaks, such as Humpback stout, Hawksbill golden lager and Afton red ale. The eclectic menu includes such dishes as bourbon steak, smoked trout wontons, pesto lasagna, Thai pork chops and blackberry cobbler. The bar's open every night until 2 AM, and reservations are suggested.

BLUE BIRD CAFE
625 W. Main St.   *(804) 295-1166*
$-$$

Enjoy the "Best Food in C'ville" in a casual atmosphere at this charming cafe near the historic downtown area. Whether you choose to dine outdoors on the patio or inside, you'll find the experience enjoyable. A diverse menu includes fresh seafood, hand-cut prime beef, veal, poultry and pasta dishes. This is the home of what the menu touts as "World Famous Blue Bird Crabcakes." Fine French, American and Virginia wines are served, as are domestic, imported and microbrewery beers. Full bar service and cappuccino and espresso complement your meal, which simply must include one of the delicious desserts, baked on the premises. The Blue Bird is open for lunch and dinner daily. Dinner reservations are accepted. Ample parking is available on the premises.

THE BOAR'S HEAD
INN AND SPORTS CLUB
U.S. 250 W.   *(804) 296-2181*
$$$$ (Old Mill Room)
$$ (Racquets)

The Boar's Head Inn's Old Mill Room is a restored 1834 grist mill serving regional fare; it has a nationally recognized wine list. Some of the chef's specialties are cider-marinated pork loin, seared Outer Banks tuna steak and local leg of lamb with quinoa, roasted fennel and sauce Provençale. A popular dessert is the chocolate pecan tart with bourbon ice cream.

The less formal Racquets restaurant and lounge offers inn guests a healthy, all-American menu for lunch and weekend dinners, plus a weekday evening light-fare lounge menu.

Sunday brunches here are impressive: omelets and Belgian waffles made to order, pastries, breads, cheeses, smoked fish, breakfast meats and egg dishes, among other dishes.

Reservations are required in the Old Mill Room for dinner and are suggested for lunch.

BRASA RESTAURANT AND TAPAS BAR
215 W. Water St.
next to Omni Hotel   (804) 296-4343
$$-$$$

Mediterranean cuisine is the specialty here, an amalgamation of Spanish, French and Italian influences with an emphasis on wood-cooked seafood and beef dishes. You haven't lived until you've tried wood-fired grilled shrimp! Although intended to be appetizers, the delicious beef, chicken and seafood tapas also make for a meal on their own. Brasa, named for the embers of its wood-fired brick oven, is owned by the same folks who run Boston's L'Espalier Restaurant, so they obviously know a thing or two about fresh seafood. The restaurant is open for lunch and dinner daily. On weekends, the tapas bar stays open until midnight, if there is enough demand.

C AND O RESTAURANT
515 E. Water St.   (804) 971-7044
$$$$ (upstairs dining room)
$$ (Bistro)

"I can confidently assure you that not since Jefferson was serving imported vegetables and the first ice cream at Monticello has there been more innovative cooking in these parts than at the C and O Restaurant," said William Rice, editor-in-chief of *Food and Wine Magazine*.

This celebrated restaurant is proudest of its upstairs dining room, with a menu that features such French cuisine as Coquilles St. Jacques au mangue and smoked duck breast with apricots. Desserts on a typical Saturday night include mint chocolate cheesecake and lemon strawberry torte. Reservations are required upstairs but not in the downstairs Bistro. While more casual, the Bistro's menu also leans toward French cuisine, offering beef tournedos with red wine mushroom glaze and sea scallops steamed with grapefruit dijon cream sauce. Hundreds of wines, including some very old ones, are available both upstairs and downstairs. The restaurant is open for lunch Monday through Friday and dinner daily.

Insiders' Tips

If atmosphere is as important as cuisine to you, the Blue Ridge has many historic inns that serve meals.

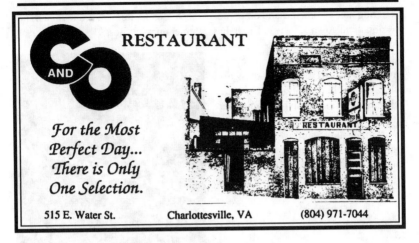

THE CLIFTON COUNTRY INN

Va. 729, off U.S. 250 E.   (804) 971-1800
$$$$

This elegant, historic inn also has a restaurant that serves a prix fixe dinner daily and luncheon by private arrangement. Craig Hartman and Jennifer Wilson-Devaney, award-winning chefs and graduates of the Culinary Institute of America, are considered masters in the kitchen. Craig's reputation, in fact, has earned him two invitations to prepare dinner as guest chef at the famous James Beard House in New York City.

A typical winter dinner might start with smoked duck, move on to a soup of pureed winter vegetables and salad of organic greens, continue with a passionfruit ice and choice of either rack of veal with wild mushrooms or grilled swordfish and end with a chocolate terrine.

Reservations are required.

THE COFFEE EXCHANGE

120 E. Main   (804) 295-0975
$

This bakery/cafe on the downtown mall is a classy place to hang out, sip coffee and read the paper or spy on attractive grad students. Coffees from around the world are served all kinds of ways, from cappuccino to frozen mochaccino. This is also a popular lunch spot, serving what some say is the best potato soup money can buy. The cafe also has salads, sandwiches, light meals, beer, wine and desserts. Be forewarned: The cookies and pastries often sell out by early afternoon (the demand is clearly as high as this establishment's reputation). The cafe is open until 5 PM daily.

COLLEGE INN

1511 University Dr.   (804) 977-2710
$$

This University Corner landmark serves up a wide assortment of continental, Greek, Italian and American dishes. As the name suggests, it's a popular dining spot and watering hole among the university set but also caters to a loyal following of Charlottesville natives and savvy tourists. The restaurant is open daily.

COURT SQUARE TAVERN

Fifth and Jefferson Sts.   (804) 296-6111
$ *No credit cards*

This bar on historic Court Square is a

watering hole for lawyers and other professionals in town. No wonder. It has more than 130 imported bottled beers and Bass, Guiness, Sam Adams and Spaten on tap. You can also order roast beef chili, grilled bratwurst and homemade cheesecake. The British pub atmosphere features antique mirrors and engravings, a stained-glass window and copper-topped bar. The tavern is open from lunchtime until midnight Monday through Saturday.

COUPE DE VILLE'S

9 Elliewood Ave.   (804) 977-3966
$

This is a hip place that attracts scores of UVA students. The food is inexpensive but sophisticated. You can get fresh pasta that's made locally, along with sandwiches, seafood and homemade soups. An acoustic rock band pumps up the volume at 10 PM, except on Wednesday nights, when a country music singer performs; there's never a cover charge. You can dine indoors or outdoors on the garden terrace (even in the rain, since there's an awning). Coupe de Ville's is every day but Sunday.

DURTY NELLY'S PUB

2200 Jefferson Park Ave.   (804) 295-1278
$ No credit cards

Sandwiches are the attraction here. One of the tastiest is the Lady Godiva, a pita stuffed with turkey, bacon, Muenster, lettuce, tomato, onion and pepper-Parmesan dressing. The pub also serves beer, wine and champagne. It's open for lunch Monday through Friday, lunch and dinner on weekends.

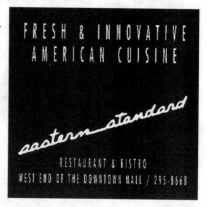

FRESH & INNOVATIVE AMERICAN CUISINE

eastern standard

RESTAURANT & BISTRO
WEST END OF THE DOWNTOWN MALL / 295-8668

EASTERN STANDARD RESTAURANT

Downtown Mall   (804) 295-8668
$-$$

This popular restaurant, next to the Omni Hotel, serves American cuisine with Asian and Mediterranean accents and includes vegetarian dishes and fine aged meats complemented by an extensive wine list. Upstairs is a warm, comfortable dining area overlooking the mall, while the downstairs is devoted to a lively bistro, ES Café.

The Eastern Standard reopened in the fall of 1994 under new management. Co-owner Sean Concannon is a graduate of the Johnson and Wales Culinary Arts School; chef Jannequin Bennett honed her culinary skills while working in New York and Virginia and on travels in South America and Europe.

The restaurant serves dinner Tuesday through Sunday.

GREENSKEEPER RESTAURANT
1517 University Ave.   (804) 984-4653
$-$$

A popular college and "townie" hang-out (it's open until 2 AM every night), the Greenskeeper defies categorization. The menu is all over the map, from pita-pocket sandwiches and grilled eggplant to pastas and burgers on whole-grain buns. Live musical entertainment keeps the place buzzing on the weekends. The restaurant opens at 11 AM.

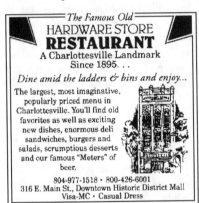

THE HARDWARE STORE RESTAURANT
316 E. Main St.   (804) 977-1518
$-$$

The Grand Old Hardware Store Building, a city landmark since 1895, houses this restaurant that offers an astounding variety of foods. You enter the restaurant from either the downtown mall or Water Street. Inside the central dining area, you'll see the same ladders and shelves that belonged to the old hardware store, which operated continuously from 1895 to 1976. This was the original sales area. On the Water Street end of the restaurant, the hardware store's offices have been transformed into dining rooms, and you can see the original typewriters and adding machines used by the store's clerical workers decades ago.

The restaurant, open for lunch and dinner daily, is known for its generous portions in beverages, sandwiches and salads. The menu's backbone is its array of marvelously concocted sandwiches, such as the Pavarotti, a robust hoagie stuffed with several types of ham, Genoa salami, provolone, onions and peppers. The restaurant also serves barbecued ribs, pasta, mesquite-grilled meats and a variety of crepes. If you simply want to satisfy your sweet tooth, there is a vast selection of pastries to choose from, or you can order a malt from the old-fashioned soda fountain.

You'll find plenty of free parking at the Water Street door. For more information about the shops in the Hardware Store building, see our Shopping chapter.

HOT CAKES
37-A Emmit St.   (804) 295-6037
$-$$

No, it's not a pancake house. Hot Cakes, in the Barracks Road shopping center, serves up an array of homemade breads, pastries, pies and cakes. The bakery also has gourmet lunch and dinner items, including tasty pasta dishes, and a full catering service. Hot Cakes is open daily.

KAFKAFE
20 Elliewood Ave.   (804) 296-1175
$-$$

This airy place is a sophisticated restaurant-cafe-bookstore in one. And a gallery too, considering its changing exhibits of works by local artists. You can dine indoors or on the patio and order as little as a cappuccino or an appetizer. For the latter, we highly recommend the rich, creamy pâté served with olives, capers, cornichons, red onions and French bread.

Salads are both creative — combining meats and diverse vegetables, nuts, cheeses or fruits — and generous, a rare combination. One of the most popular entrees is the chicken satay and Szechuan shrimp served with a hot peanut sauce. Desserts are made daily and include English trifle, Kahlua cheesecake, carrot cake and a lot of wicked treats made with Callebaut chocolate from Belgium. The Chocolate Regal, a rich, dense cake served on a pool of raspberry puree, will make your toes curl, it's so devilish.

Daily newspapers from Madrid, London, Hamburg, Frankfurt and other great cities of the world are also available here. Kafkafe holds fiction and poetry readings at night on a regular basis.

LITTLE JOHN'S
1427 University Ave.　　(804) 977-0588
$

Be it lunchtime or the middle of night, Little John's is the place to go if you've got a hankering for a New York-style deli sandwich. Open 24 hours a day, Little John's is on The Corner, a short walk from the Rotunda at UVA. Specialties are the Nuclear Sub (a combo of coleslaw, turkey, barbecue and mozzarella) and the Baby Zonker (a bagel with cream cheese, bacon, tomatoes and onions).

MAHARAJA
Seminole Square　　(804) 973-1110
$$

If spicy, rich Indian cuisine is your desire, this is the place to dine. The restaurant has a cozy but Spartan atmosphere. You'll find a variety of curries and chicken, shrimp and fish tandoori (which means it's marinated in herbs and spices and grilled in a clay oven) and more. Ginger, tamarind, cashews, almonds and yogurt are some of the ingredients blended

together and served with meats, fish or vegetables, making this cuisine exciting to the palate. You can ask for your food to be chili hot, medium or mild. Maharaja is open daily for dinner and serves lunch every day but Monday. Reservations are suggested for dinner.

MACADO'S
1505 University Ave.　　(804) 971-3558
$

Like its sister restaurants in Roanoke, Farmville, Radford and elsewhere, this is a casual place to have a sandwich and beer or sundae made with Haagen-Dazs ice cream in the candy shop. It's on The Corner, close to the campus and UVA Hospital. It's open until the wee hours daily.

MARTHA'S CAFE
11 Elliewood Ave.　　(804) 971-7530
$

This is a popular place on The Corner, and it's no wonder. The food is freshly made, interesting and reasonably priced, and the atmosphere is casual but never boring. Martha's has been around since 1976 and served cappuccino long before it was in vogue in this city. The menu emphasizes chicken and fish, and nothing is deep fried. It's known for its crab cakes, but other popular items are barbecued shrimp, jambalaya and spinach lasagna. All desserts are made at the restaurant, and they include white chocolate mousse with Frangelica and chocolate decadence cake. Children's portions are available. The cafe is situated in an old house with an enormous elm tree out front. You can dine indoors or, in spring or summer, outside on a cobblestone patio under the elm tree.

Inside, weavings from around the world and musical instruments hang from the walls. A fireplace and bathtub full of goldfish add to the decor in the front room. Owner Ken Waxman loves to play old jazz on the stereo system. Though the cafe is within walking distance of the UVA campus, it does not necessarily cater to students. The clientele is older — a lot of grad students, doctors and professors. As with most of the restaurants on crowded Elliewood Avenue, you need to park in the centrally located parking garage. Martha's is open daily for lunch and dinner.

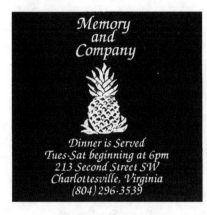

Memory
and
Company

Dinner is Served
Tues-Sat beginning at 6pm
213 Second Street SW
Charlottesville, Virginia
(804) 296-3539

MEMORY AND COMPANY

213 Second St. S.W.   (804) 296-3539
$$$

Founded as a cooking school in the early 1980s, Memory and Company continues as one of the finest restaurant traditions in the city. The restaurant is situated in a historical landmark, c. 1840, ad-

jacent to 200 Second St. and within walking distance of downtown Charlottesville. Executive chef and owner John Paul Corbett trained at the California Culinary Academy in San Francisco and has extensive wine, food service and culinary experience. He has catered to the likes of Robert Mondavi, Silver Oak Cellars and Iron Horse Vineyards in California wine country.

A choice of dining rooms is available, including an exhibition cooking/dining area, a quaint and quiet dining room with wine racks and art displayed by local artists and, when weather permits, outside seating in the herb garden or patio area.

The menu, which changes seasonally, features country French and classical Italian, with accents of Southwestern and California cuisines. The four-course prix fixe meal includes a selection of appetizers, entrees and desserts, all created daily from fresh ingredients. Dinner is served Wednesday through Saturday. An à la carte brunch is served Sunday. The restaurant is nonsmoking; reservations are suggested.

MICHIE TAVERN

Thomas Jefferson Pkwy.   (804) 977-1234
$

At Michie Tavern, a 200-year-old converted log house called The Ordinary serves a sumptuous lunch buffet of fried chicken, black-eyed peas, stewed toma-

So what exactly is Blue Ridge cuisine? Insiders claim it's everything made in, intended for and consumed by Virginians. Virginia country ham is a good place to start, but you can also get Virginia peanut soup, Virginia applewood smoked turkey, chicken, pheasant and trout and, of course, succulent pork barbecue.

Insiders' Tips

toes, coleslaw, potato salad, green bean salad, beets, homemade biscuits, cornbread and apple cobbler every day of the year. Lunch costs $9.50, not including beverage, dessert or tax.

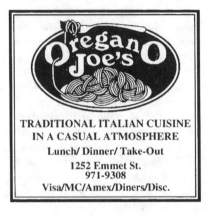

TRADITIONAL ITALIAN CUISINE IN A CASUAL ATMOSPHERE

Lunch/ Dinner/ Take-Out

1252 Emmet St.
971-9308
Visa/MC/Amex/Diners/Disc.

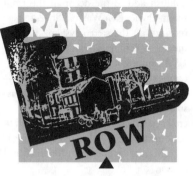

OREGANO JOE'S

1252 Emmet St.   *(804) 971-9308*
$-$$

This is a popular, informal Italian restaurant one block north of Barracks Road shopping center. Owners Carl and Victoria Tremaglio and Roberta Corcoran use fresh local ingredients and imported Italian products, making all sauces, soups and dressings from scratch. Daily specials often include such seafood as salmon, swordfish, tuna and red snapper. You can have cappuccino, espresso and international coffees and Virginia and Italian wines from the full bar. Children are welcome and so are take-out orders.

Oregano Joe's serves lunch on weekdays and dinner seven days a week. Reservations are advised for groups of eight or more for lunch or dinner. Tremaglio's catering business, Festive Fare, handles everything from formal wedding receptions to picnics and business meetings.

RANDOM ROW

247 Ridge McIntire   *(804) 296-8758*
$$

This eclectic restaurant has been a hometown gathering spot for three decades. The menu is loaded with classic and down-home favorities served in generous portions and followed by heavenly desserts. Specialties include Albuquerque nachos, the black bean tortilla stack and lime chicken salad. The restaurant is open daily for lunch and dinner.

RISING SUN BAKERY

109 14th St. N.W.   *(804) 296-2233*
$ *No credit cards*

This family-owned full-service bakery with deli has been serving freshly made goodies to a faithful clientele since 1977. Everything is freshly made from natural ingredients, which makes for delightful lunches and dinners in this relaxed, family-oriented atmosphere. Coffee and pastries are popular in the morning hours, and the espresso bar draws coffee devotees. The bakery's fantastic cakes — seven kinds! — have several times been voted Best in Charlottesville. The bakery is open daily.

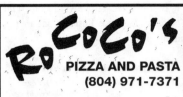

PIZZA AND PASTA
(804) 971-7371

Mesquite Grilled Seafood
Cappucino
Extensive Wine List

Corner of Hydraulic Rd. & Commonwealth
Drive in the Village Green

Brunch, Lunch, Dinner • Serving All Day

ROCOCO'S

Hydraulic and Commonwealth Rds.
in the Village Green (804) 971-7371
$$

The quest to find the restaurant favored by locals would bring many a visitor to Rococo's, an elegant but casual Italian restaurant featuring homemade ravioli, fettuccine, stromboli, calzone, gourmet pizza and more. Since 1988 Rococo's has emphasized the freshest ingredients and creative interpretations of traditional Italian dishes. Some of its specialties are white cheese and pesto pizza and mesquite-grilled half chicken marinated in balsamic vinegar and rosemary. Another favorite is chocolate toffee ice-cream pie. The restaurant has an extensive wine list and a full-service bar. It's open for lunch Monday through Friday, brunch on weekends and dinner every night. The restaurant accepts reservations for parties of five or more and welcomes families.

SAIGON CAFE

1703 Allied Ln. (804) 296-8661
$

The atmosphere is relaxed and comfortable at Charlottesville's first Vietnamese restaurant. Some of the specialties of the house are the Vietnam egg rolls, grilled lemon chicken and shrimp Saigon-style. The soups

are especially noteworthy. Saigon Cafe is open daily for lunch and dinner.

SILVER THATCH INN

3001 Hollymead Dr.
at U.S. 29 N. (804) 978-4686
$$$$

The menu changes every six weeks or so at this exquisite, candlelit restaurant in a beautiful old inn, c. 1780. The Silver Thatch serves regional American cuisine, with an emphasis on fresh produce. Two typical entrees are the peppered and charred veal carpaccio with asparagus and mushroom compote and grilled lamb chops with minted apple and roasted corn relish. The wine list is all-American, with an emphasis on California and Virginia. Desserts are homemade, beautifully presented and mouth-watering. Reservations are recommended. Dinner is served Tuesday through Saturday.

SOUTHERN CULTURE

633 W. Main St. (804) 979-1990
$$

This is a hip cafe and restaurant serving delicious Gulf Coast cuisine. Fettuccine Claire, with artichoke hearts, green chilies, red peppers, ricotta and roasted pecans, is a real hit here, along with crab and corn chowder and sweet potato fries. The atmosphere is dark and artsy, an exciting place for dining and chatting with good friends or a loved one. The bar is a lively gathering place for intellectuals and artists of all sorts. The restaurant and bar are open daily for dinner and drinks, and Sunday for brunch.

ST. MAARTEN CAFE

1400 Wertland Ave. (804) 293-2233
$$

This is a favorite of UVA students, a place to forget your troubles and imagine you're far away on a tropical island. It has a late-night menu until 1 AM. The cafe serves a lot of fresh seafood and burgers. All the soups are made from scratch, and cheese-cakes are also made on the premises. St. Maarten Cafe, on The Corner near the college campus and hospital, is open every day until the wee hours.

STARR HILL CAFÉ

320 W. Main St. (804) 295-4456
$$$

This is an intimate, casual restaurant with a country French atmosphere. The cuisine is mainly classic French, with specialties that include escargot, Caesar salad, salmon with pistachio butter, roast duck with damson plum glaze, and homemade ice cream and sorbet. The wine list is extensive. Reservations are recommended, and jackets are required. The restaurant serves dinner Monday through Saturday.

TASTINGS

502 E. Market St., next to downtown parking deck (804) 293-3663
$$-$$$

This restaurant, wine bar and wine shop combo is run by William Curtis, who also owns the popular Court Square Tavern nearby. You can stop first at the bar and sample a wine to order with your dinner or simply drink and munch on a few crackers.

The wood grill adds a delicate flavor to meats and fish. Foods are straightforward, fresh and deeply satisfying. All year-round entrees include crabmeat casserole, grilled salmon with Béarnaise sauce and herb-crusted rack of lamb, and in the summertime, strawberry rhubarb pie is the seasonal favorite. You can select your dinner wine from more than 1,000 in the shop or order a half or full glass from a list of about 125 wines. Better yet, Curtis will prepare a flight of three wines to sample

during dinner. The wine list has received the Best of Excellence award from *Wine Spectator* magazine. Reservations are recommended.

THE TEA ROOM CAFE AT THE 1817

1211 W. Main St. (804) 979-7353
$ *No credit cards*

For a sunny setting, try lunch at the Tea Room Cafe, which is open only on weekends. It's in the solarium, overflowing onto the gallery-style back porch, of the beautifully appointed 1817 Antique Inn. You'll choose from gourmet dishes at reasonable prices.

Other Restaurants near Charlottesville

PROSPECT HILL

Trevilians (800) 277-0844
$$$$

This historic plantation inn, 15 miles east of Charlottesville, houses a beautifully decorated, candlelit restaurant that serves classic French cuisine with Provençale and American accents. The spring dinner menu lists, among its many entrees, tenderloin of beef tournedos served with a port wine, sun-dried tomato and morel sauce. Or, for lighter fare, there is Volaille Farcie au Provence, a chicken breast stuffed with spinach and boursin cheese and served with Provençale sauce. Desserts are also French and include a chocolate cappuccino mousse and classic mille feuille, which means "a thousand layers."

The fixed-price, five-course dinners cost $40 a person, not including wine, taxes or gratuities. With advance notice, the chef will cater to people whose diets are restricted. Innkeepers Michael and Laura Sheehan invite dinner guests to arrive at 6:30 PM for a half-hour wine tasting and to stroll the grounds or sit by the crackling fire. Dinner is served daily; reservations are required.

Lynchburg

BATEAU LANDING

Main at 12th St.   (804) 847-1499
$ No credit cards

Lynchburg's historic community market, Bateau Landing, offers an array of country fare — fresh eggs, country ham and homemade jams and jellies — with breakfast and lunch. Produce changes seasonally. After having a piece of homemade cake, pie or a cookie, you can browse the market and whet your appetite for shopping. This is a fun place for the whole family, with ever-changing vendors and seasonal goods. The market is open 7:30 AM to 2 PM Monday through Saturday.

CAFE FRANCE

3225 Old Forest Rd.   (804) 385-8989
$$$

Jazz helps create an upbeat atmosphere in the fresh and original setting marked by an art deco decor and a wine bar. Lunch and dinner menus are extensive. Lunch calls for sandwiches, soups and burgers. An additional menu is available with the day's specials, which could include a French dip, soft-shell crab sandwich or seafood au gratin. There is also a soup, dessert and coffee du jour. The dinner menu is even more varied: Jamaican prime rib and Cornish game hen are standards, and other favorites include rack of lamb with Pommery mustard and seasoned bread crumbs and Virginia jumbo lump and backfin crabmeat served with buerre blanc sauce. A menu of dinner specials offers alternatives. A deli take-out menu is available, as well. Lunch is served

Monday through Friday, dinner Tuesday through Saturday. Deli take-out is available Monday through Saturday. Reservations are suggested for dinner.

CHARLEYS

3405 Candler's
Mountain Rd.   (804) 237-5988
$

There is always something special going on at Charleys. A new calendar comes out each month listing special happenings, including karoake on Saturday night. Tuesday is seniors day, when anyone 55 or older receives 15 percent off of an entree. The menu is as varied as the entertainment and includes fajitas, seafood fettuccine, chicken cordon bleu and beef stroganoff, all freshly made. You can dine in the greenhouse dining room or in the more elegant back room. The restaurant is open for lunch, dinner and late-night dining daily. Reservations are suggested for parties of six or more.

CLAYTON'S

3311 Old Forest Rd.   (804) 385-7900
$

Clayton's is a casual restaurant with table service by a friendly staff. You can have breakfast and lunch daily and dinner twice a week. Choose from chicken Tina, grilled marinated shrimp, grilled vegetable sandwich or one of their other tasty sandwiches, plus two hot specials daily. The restaurant is open for breakfast and lunch daily. Dinner is served on Wednesday and Friday.

EMIL'S

Boonsboro Shopping Ctr.   (804) 384-3311
$$ (cafe), $$$ (rotisserie)

Whether you dine in the informal surroundings of the cafe or in the more elegant rotisserie, Emil's is an excellent choice for fine dining. Each area has its own special menu and atmosphere. The cafe is casual and bright with plenty of green plants. Its menu is full of dishes such as G'Schnatzlets, roestis, seafood au gratin and crabmeat imperial. The rotisserie is elegant, with candlelight and a white-table-cloth setting. Here you can enjoy Veal Zurich, roast rack of lamb, Chateaubriand maison, Norwegian salmon and entrees flambéed tableside. Emil's also has a special lunchtime menu. Indulge yourself and try one of the many delicious desserts made in the in-house bakery. Emil's is open Monday through Saturday for lunch and dinner.

THE FARM BASKET
2008 Langhorne Rd.   (804) 528-1107
$ No credit cards

Don't miss The Farm Basket while you're in Lynchburg! Regardless of your age or nature, it's the kind of place that will fascinate you for hours with its shopping opportunities. Then it will amaze you once again with its tiny restaurant that's always packed with locals and others who keep coming back for the homemade food prepared by cooks who look like your Grandma. The cucumber sandwich on dill bread melts in your mouth; Gouda cheese biscuits and Brunswick stew are other famous items. Have a dessert of lemon bread with cream cheese and then go shopping! A lot of Lynchburg matrons stop by this beautiful neighborhood to get box lunches. It's open daily except Sunday.

THE LANDMARK
STEAKHOUSE AND LOUNGE
6113 Fort Ave.   (804) 237-1884
$$

The Landmark allows you to have an elegant dinner in a casual atmosphere. The rustic decor will make you feel at home, while special touches such as linen table-cloths make dining here an occasion. The steak and ribs have a hickory charcoal flavor. You can also choose from chicken and seafood dishes. The restaurant has a full bar and an extensive wine list. A nonsmoking section is also available.

The Landmark is open for lunch Monday through Friday. Dinner is served nightly. Reservations are suggested on weekends and during busy seasons, such as Christmas and prom time.

RED LOBSTER RESTAURANT
3425 Candler's
Mountain Rd.   (804) 847-0178
$$

A nautical American theme perfectly matches the name of this seafood restaurant, which also has a Roanoke Valley location. Although the restaurant is casual, it is still well-suited for business, banquets or special occasions. You can select from a traditional array of fine seafood, including 18 dinner entrees at less than $10. Fragrant, freshly baked garlic cheese bread is include with all meals. Desserts are creative, including Sensational 7 Cake, made with seven different chocolates; the Fudge Overboard, a brownie pie topped with French vanilla ice cream, whipped cream and Hershey's chocolate syrup; and Key lime pie. Red Lobster is open daily for lunch and dinner. Reservations are not accepted, but call-ahead seating is available.

TEXAS STEAK HOUSE
4001 Murray Pl.   (804) 528-1134
$

A real Texas dinner awaits you at this steakhouse, where a casual setting and a Lone Star State theme set the stage. There choices are vast, but steaks dominate the menu with seven- and nine-ounce filets. Try a Yellow Rose of Texas or a Hershey

Brownie for dessert. It's open for lunch and dinner Monday through Friday and dinner only Saturday and Sunday. Reservations are not accepted, but call-ahead seating is offered.

Smith Mountain Lake Area

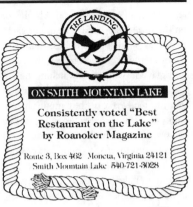

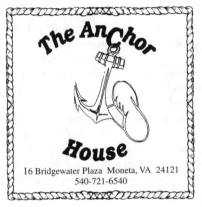

THE ANCHOR HOUSE
Va. 122, Bridgewater Plaza   (540) 721-6540
$$

When you hear the music, you'll know you're near The Anchor House. You'll be in the middle of all the action, day and night, at this lively place on the lower level of Bridgewater Plaza, the hub of activity at Smith Mountain Lake. This is a great place to dine, relax and meet people. It has an outdoor cafe, weekend entertainment and buffet and salad bar, and cocktails in the evening. The food is good, too: your basic tacos, burgers, salads and snacks, plus an extensive list of spirits.

THE LANDING RESTAURANT, CHEF'S INC. AT BERNARD'S LANDING
Va. 940, Moneta   (540) 721-3028
$$

If you want the finest dining and best view on the lake, Bernard's Landing Restaurant has it all! It's truly a special place, well worth the 45-minute drive from Roanoke or Lynchburg. Everything on the menu is a delight, cooked to perfection by Chef Howard Wilcox. Whether you want a sandwich (try the chicken salad) or a seafood platter of shrimp, scallops, flounder and deviled crab, you can expect a gourmet twist to your order. The Friday night seafood buffet is special, and there probably isn't a soul on the lake who hasn't been to Sunday brunch, with waffles and fluffy omelets served to your precise instructions.

If you're going to the lake to experience it the way lake fanatics do each weekend, don't miss this dining opportunity. Nothing can match the gentle lake breezes and nautical decor as a pleasant distraction from the everyday world. Bernard's Landing is open for lunch and dinner Tuesday through Saturday; lunch only is served Sunday.

PADDLE WHEEL CRUISES
Va. 853, Moneta   (800) 721-3273
$$$

Glide across gorgeous Smith Mountain Lake while enjoying some of the best food around. You can ride on the luxurious *Vir-*

ginia Dare, a 19th-century sidewheeler, or on the *Blue Moon*, a 51-foot motor yacht perfect for smaller groups. Bask in the sun on an afternoon cruise or relax with a cocktail or favorite wine while watching the sun set across the lake. Seafood buffets and gourmet food make up the tempting menu. Many trips feature live entertainment. The cruises run year round, but times vary. Call the company for specific information, since they're at a new location close to Smith Mountain Lake State Park. This is a wonderful experience for lake lovers. Reservations are required.

COOPERS CORNER
Va. 608 and 626
Huddleston   (540) 297-7104
$$

A pleasant restaurant specializing in family fare, Coopers Corner has a complete salad bar, special seafood and country and breakfast buffets. Lunch features deli sandwiches, including German hot dogs. For dinner, try the great charbroiled steaks, pasta dishes and fresh seafood such as grilled tuna steaks, rainbow trout almondine and shrimp scampi. Desserts are freshly made and includes such temptations as rice pudding, cheesecake and coconut pies. Coopers Corner is open daily for breakfast, lunch and dinner.

DUDLEY MART & RESTAURANT
Va. 670 and 668
Wirtz   (540) 721-1635
$ No credit cards

Frequented by locals and close to the Smith Mountain 4-H Center, this revamped country school built in 1931 is now home to one of Smith Mountain Lake's most delightful dining surprises. The homemade barbecue and roasted chicken are worth the trip here, and it's a great place for a quick meal while you're touring the lake. You'll find all kinds of odds and ends and groceries as well. Stop by daily for breakfast, lunch and dinner.

SAL'S PIZZA RESTAURANTS
Fairway Village Shopping
Center   (540) 721-8904
South Lake Plaza
Union Hall   (540) 576-2263
$

Homesick Northerners will feel right at home at one of the best restaurants on the lake. Sal's is a family place that folks seem to keep coming back to for the spaghetti and pasta specialities and fantastic salad bar. The pizza is everything you'd hope for in authentic Italian cuisine, and an adequate wine list complements your meal. Kids have a separate menu and can choose their favorite pasta dishes at a reduced price. When you visit on weekends, don't miss the $5 breakfast buffet for a tasty value. Sal's is open seven days a week, breakfast through dinner.

Franklin County

OLDE VIRGINIA BARBECUE
108 Meadowview St.
Rocky Mount   (540) 489-1788
$

Come discover the most succulent pork, beef ribs and chicken barbecue in the county. This restaurant, a local landmark, has created its own Olde Virginia Barbecue Sauce and is a favorite hangout for the Franklin County crowd. You've just never tasted better barbecued chicken and ribs anywhere else, and people who don't even like coleslaw can't believe how Olde Virginia's real Southern variety tastes. Children have their own menu as well, with $3.95 specials. It's open seven days a week for lunch and dinner.

New River Valley Region

Blacksburg

ANCHY'S
1600 N. Main St.   (540) 951-2828
$

A relaxing family atmosphere surrounds you as you dine in this college-town favorite. The menu consists of Euro-Asian favorites and treats such as fresh seafood and steaks. Anchy's is open for lunch and dinner Tuesday through Friday and Sunday; dinner only is served on Saturday. Reservations are suggested.

BOGEN'S
622 N. Main St.   (540) 953-2233
$

Probably the most popular local restaurant with the college crowd and business people, Bogen's slogan is "Casual with Class." The food is inexpensive and the atmosphere, great. The menu features gourmet sandwiches, charbroiled steaks, spicy barbecued ribs and chicken and tempting seafood. To top it off, get cappuccino and one of their outrageous ice-cream desserts — sky high and wonderful! Bogen's opens for lunch and serves until late night daily.

JACOB'S LANTERN
At the Marriott
900 Price Fork Rd.   (540) 552-7001
$$

Whether you are having a light meal or a complete dinner, you'll find both the food and service consistently good at this restaurant, which is open for breakfast, lunch and dinner seven days a week.

PEKING PALACE RESTAURANT
235 N. Main St.   (540) 552-4400
$

For authentic Chinese cuisine in an elegant setting, you can't beat this restaurant in the heart of Blacksburg. Sample some of their delicious dinners, such as Hunan Double Delight, Dragon & Phoenix, General Tso's Chicken and Orange Beef. Also on the menu are special selections for health-minded diners, prepared from guidelines of the American Heart Association. These designated dishes, which are lower in fat, cholesterol and calories and contain no MSG, include Hawaii Chicken, Sizzling Triple Delight and Honolulu Scallops. Peking Palace is open for lunch and dinner weekdays and dinner only on weekends. Reservations are necessary for large groups.

SUNRISE HOUSE CHINESE RESTAURANT
1602 S. Main St.   (540) 552-1191
$

Another top-notch Chinese restaurant in Blacksburg, the Sunrise has a relaxing atmosphere and a varied menu. You can feast on Crabmeat Lagoon, General Tso's Chicken, Triple Delight and Hawaii Five "O." Prices are very reasonable. Sunrise House is open seven days a week for dinner. Reservations are accepted but not necessary.

Check the Annual Events and Festivals chapter for fairs and festivals honoring foods such as apples, beef, cantaloupe, chicken, garlic, mushrooms, strawberries or wine. You're likely to find dishes you've never tasted before.

Insiders' Tips

VICKER'S SWITCH

At the Holiday Inn Blacksburg
3503 S. Main St.   *(540) 951-1330*
$

Vicker's Switch, the hotel's comfortable restaurant with a friendly staff, has a varied menu that includes St. Louis barbecued pork, prime rib and bacon-wrapped scallops. It opens for lunch and again for dinner Monday through Saturday. On Sunday, breakfast is served in addition to lunch and dinner. Reservations are suggested on special dates.

Christiansburg

THE FARMHOUSE

Cambria St.   *(540) 382-4253*
$$$ *(540) 382-3965*

Exceptional service is a trademark of this authentic farmhouse-turned-restaurant that seems to continually expand. The farmhouse was part of an estate built in the 1800s and opened as a restaurant in 1963; and an old train caboose was added in the early 1970s. The staff extends Southern hospitality to its diners, who include families, corporate executives and college students. The rustic setting, decorated with both antiques and country furnishings, adds to the ambiance. The menu is full of such favorites as prime rib, jumbo ocean shrimp cocktail, steak and the famous Farmhouse onion rings. A separate children's menu is available. The Farmhouse is open seven days a week for lunch and dinner.

THE HUCKLEBERRY

2790 Roanoke St.   *(540) 381-2382*
$$$

Convenient and luxurious, this restaurant is near I-81 and several hotels in the Christiansburg area. Two lounges, Whispers and Sundance, offer top-40 and country and western entertainment. The succu-

lent barbecued items are slow-cooked in "the finest hickory-smoking oven money can buy." The restaurant also guarantees the high quality and freshness of its beef. You can choose from baby back ribs, dijon chicken, filet mignon and broiled lobster tail. There is also a special children's menu. Senior citizens receive a 15 percent discount on all entrees. It's open daily for breakfast, lunch and dinner.

STONE'S CAFETERIA

1290 Roanoke St.   *(540) 382-8970*
$ *No credit cards*

A longtime favorite with locals and tourists alike, Stone's gives you real country food as fast as you can go through the cafeteria line to get it. Lovers of dishes such as fried chicken, greens, mashed potatoes and pinto beans will be in their glory, both when they taste and when they pay. Stone's is open for breakfast, lunch and dinner Monday through Saturday.

THE OUTPOST

U.S. 460 and Va. 11
off I-81   *(540) 382-9830*
$$$

Since 1960, lovers of Lebanese food have been flocking to The Outpost every Wednesday for Lebanese Night. Other nights, The Outpost is full of people ordering their chicken, seafood, spaghetti and real Italian pizza. Imported beer, wines and cocktails top off a fine meal. Service is excellent. The Outpost is open for dinner Tuesday through Saturday.

Radford

GALLERY CAFE, BOOKS AND MORE AND HOT CHILIES RESTAURANT AND BAR

1115 Norwood St.   *(540) 731-1555*
$$

Radford's trendiest restaurant, Gal-

lery Cafe attracts crowds of professionals and students who enjoy artfully prepared international cuisine in a casual
and memorable gallery setting. The
Gallery Cafe, Books and More offers
fresh ground and brewed gourmet
coffees, as well as pastries, fancy foods
and a great selection of magazines and
books. Downstairs, Hot Chilies has a
southwest accent with an eclectic flair.
The menu features selections by a vegetarian chef and owner Charlie
Whitescarver, a three-time winner of
the Virginia State Championship Chili
Cookoff contest. Diners get three types
of hot sauces to challenge the meek or
satisfy the bold.

The Norwood Room is elegantly appointed, and the Garden Room is a
charming open area where diners can
get a buffet lunch Monday through
Friday. The restaurant is open for
lunch Monday through Saturday,
opening again for dinner Wednesday
through Saturday. Brunch is served on
Sunday.

MACADO'S RESTAURANT
AND DELICATESSEN

510 Norwood St.   (540) 731-4879
$$

One of a chain of family-owned res-
taurants throughout the Blue Ridge, in-
cluding Roanoke and Blacksburg,
Radford's restaurant offers a fun dining
alternative in the New River Valley.
Macado's is popular both with students
and professionals for its overstuffed sand-
wiches and unique, antique- and col-
lectibles-filled decor. The deli is full of
international gourmet items, including
cheeses, wine and fine candies. Macado's
is open from midmorning to the wee
hours daily.

Giles County

MOUNTAIN LAKE RESORT RESTAURANT

Va. 700, Mountain Lake   (540) 626-7121
$$$ (800) 346-3334

If dining in absolutely gorgeous surroundings is your idea of a great evening,
as it is for many from nearby Virginia
Tech, then you should drive the 7 winding miles up the mountain — the second-highest in Virginia — to Mountain
Lake. This 2,600-acre paradise was the
setting for the movie *Dirty Dancing*, and
that glorious scenery wasn't designed in
the prop room. For miles all you see are
tall trees, rolling hills, beautiful wildflowers and a clear mountain lake. And as if
that weren't enough, the dining is out of
this world.

The elegant atmosphere matches the
outstanding cuisine, which changes daily
and may include chilled blackberry soup,
sauteed shiitake mushrooms, London
broil Madeira or red snapper with pecan
butter. Breakfast could be a Giles County
Platter of country favorites or Appalachian
buttermilk pancakes. Sunday brunch is
popular for special events from May to
October, when Mountain Lake is open.
The prices are low for the high quality of
the food you receive. Reservations are important, since guests dine there too as part
of resort stay.

Floyd County

BLUE RIDGE RESTAURANT INC.

113 E. Main St.
Floyd   (540) 745-2147
$ No credit cards

Lunchtime regulars and those just passing through will find plenty of friendly faces
here. The generous servings and honest-
to-goodness *real* food — real mashed po-

tatoes, not instant, and pinto beans that are always soaked, dried beans, not canned — are well-known in the area. Choose from such delicious country-style favorites as hotcakes, country ham, grilled tenderloin and fried squash. Children have their own dinner menu at a reduced price. The restaurant is open daily for breakfast, lunch and dinner May to November and shorter hours through the winter.

LE CHIEN NOIR

At Chateau Morrisette
Meadows of Dan   *(540) 593-2865*
$$

Chateau Morrisette, a family-owned winery in the Rocky Knob growing district, produces world-class Virginia wines. Founded in 1978, the winery is small enough to remain in the family and yet large enough to produce several varieties of award winning wines. The winery's restaurant serves both American and international cuisine in an elegant Old World atmosphere. Their Jazz on the Lawn events are reminiscent of a Monet painting of a French picnic, and the price is right at $5 a plate. Visitors are welcome to tour the facilities, sample the wines and enjoy a light meal surrounded by the magnificent Blue Ridge Mountains.

Le Chien Noir is open for lunch Wednesday through Sunday. Dinner is served on Friday and Saturday evenings. Reservations are requested.

PINE TAVERN

Floyd   *(540) 745-4482*
$$ *No credit cards*

Live music and theater are reasons enough to lure you to Pine Tavern, where dinner theater is performed on Tuesday evenings for an additional $4 on the price of your meal. Dinner is served before the show, and dessert and coffee are available during intermission or after the show. Special nonsmoking evenings are set aside for those who would not be able to attend otherwise. Area bands play in the dining room on Saturday evenings and the Dave Figg Quartet plays jazz here several times a month.

The menu sparkles with delectable dishes such as lasagna, eggplant parmigiana, Szechuan tofu and baby ganouj. The chef uses organic and locally grown vegetables in season. Vegetarians may select from a special meatless menu that includes vegetable stir-fry, black bean chili and French onion soup. The chef even uses separate cutting boards for vegetables and a separate deep fryer with vegetable oil for veggies only. Pine Tavern is open Wednesday through Friday for dinner, Saturday for lunch and dinner and Sunday from 2 to 9 PM. Reservations are suggested on Friday, Saturday and holidays.

THREE LEGGED COW CAFE

110 N. Locust St.   *(540) 745-2201*
$

The name might be a little odd, but there's nothing strange about the rave reviews for this Floyd restaurant. As the proprietors say, "We're Udderly Delicious!" Surrounded by Floyd's nostalgic downtown, Three Legged Cow Cafe serves seafood, steaks, burgers, pizza, vegetarian choices and even escargot. They also have Cajun and Mediterranean foods. The Buffalo Room upstairs is done in art deco reminiscent of an old ice-cream parlor starring an original soda fountain amidst the bright colors. Stop in for live music from 5 PM to midnight Thursday through Saturday. Every second Saturday the cafe hosts a coffeehouse in the main restaurant.

The Three Legged Cow Cafe is open

for lunch and dinner every day except Wednesday and Sunday.

Pulaski County

NEW RIVER CRUISE COMPANY
Howe House Visitors Center Dock
Claytor Lake   (540) 674-9344
$$$

Take a ride on the *Pioneer Maid* across stunning Claytor Lake and enjoy authentic foods made with recipes from our Colonial past. Due to its size — 60 feet long by 18 feet wide — this vessel can provide a fully enclosed deck and an open starlit one. Each day, the boat departs from the visitors center dock and cruises down the New River at approximately 5 miles per hour. A narrative of historical points along the world's second-oldest river enhances your trip. Lunch cruises feature deli sandwiches and fresh salads. The moonlight dinner/dance cruise is called Virginia is for Lovers, with local talent providing the music for dancing under the stars. On the dinner menu are George Washington Ham, Thomas Jefferson Fried Chicken, cooked greens with garlic and tomato and Virginia spoon bread.

The cruises are two hours of drifting through the fantastic Blue Ridge Mountains. Office hours are 9 AM to 5:30 PM Tuesday through Sunday. Reservations are required.

THE RENAISSANCE
55 W. Main St.   (540) 980-0287
$

Part of historic downtown Pulaski and its beautifully revitalized Main Street, The Renaissance offers fine dining and a full-service bar in a casual atmosphere. Specialties include prime rib, seafood, chicken, pasta and steak. The Renaissance is across from the old courthouse — a convenient spot

for sightseers — and is famous for its terrific atmosphere and service. Lunch and dinner are served Monday through Saturday; Sunday hours are 11 AM to 3 PM.

VALLEY PIKE INN
Old Wilderness Tr.
Newbern   (540) 674-1810
$

The charm and history of this beautiful old inn is reason enough to come visit. Built before 1839, this stagecoach inn and tavern was a welcome stop for weary travelers on the Old Wilderness Trail. This center of hospitality was once known as the Famous Haney Inn, named after its owners, John "The Jolly Irishman" Haney and his wife, Cornelius. It changed hands several times before Marilyn Rutland, a prominent Louisiana belle, fell in love with the area and bought the structure in 1989. She decorated with sconce lights, a chandelier and dried Virginia wildflowers. Church pews were used to make the tables, and all the doors and windows are from a structure built in 1834.

All meals are prepared and cooked from scratch, and the menu includes fried chicken, roast beef, country ham, spiced apples and homemade biscuits. You can also sample Virginia wines with your meal. Dinner is served Thursday through Saturday; Sunday hours are 11:30 AM to 6 PM. Hours vary slightly by the season.

Alleghany Highlands Region

Alleghany County

THE CAT & OWL
STEAK AND SEAFOOD HOUSE
Low Moor Exit off I-64   (540) 862-5808
$$

Antiques create the scene as you dine in this beautifully remodeled home. This steak and seafood restaurant has a Victorian atmosphere that will please the eye and a wide selection of tasty dishes that will delight the palate. Popular selections are charbroiled shrimp, filet mignon and fresh tuna steak. Finish off your meal with delicious banana fritters. The restaurant is open Monday through Saturday for dinner. Reservations are suggested.

LAKEVIEW RESTAURANT
AT DOUTHAT STATE PARK
Va. 629, Clifton Forge   *(540) 862-8111*
$ *No credit cards*

This historic landmark is a vision of rustic beauty. The casual dining area has high beamed ceilings and a large gorgeous fireplace. The porch overlooks a 50-acre lake stocked weekly with trout. Try their sandwich menu for lunch; buffet on Friday, Saturday and Sunday evenings; and the pleasing à la carte Monday through Thursday. Lakeview Restaurant is open daily for lunch and dinner.

EAGLE'S NEST RESTAURANT
4100 Kanawha Tr.
Covington   *(540) 559-9738*
$$$

At Eagle's Nest, established in 1930, you can have a gourmet meal on a deck overlooking a waterfall, somewhat like dining in Frank Lloyd Wright's private home! The nature lover and adventurous tourist will love this place in the middle of practically nowhere (about 1½ hours from Roanoke west, 20 minutes from White Sulphur Springs, West Virginia, east) and one of the most intriguing in the entire Blue Ridge. In an ancient log cabin decorated with antiques, beside that breathtaking waterfall outlined in purple irises and a pool filled with trout and ducks, you'll see chubby felines (the restaurant's charity cases) roaming the mountain crags 70 feet

straight up. The scenery alone makes this place one you won't forget. But nothing about the food is forgettable either!

Served on country-blue speckled metal plates, dinners may be international in flavor one day, with a cucumber and mint salad, or fresh brook trout the next. Salads may be mandarin orange with pecan and the soup may be cream of leek. Select from a full complement of house wines, including their own Virginia table wine under the Eagle Nest Label with Horton Wineries. They have also won the Virginia State and Wine Marketing Program for a Three Cluster top award for the last three years. The service by fresh-faced waitresses is impeccable.

This is an experience anyone in love with the Blue Ridge shouldn't miss. Fidgety children might not do well here, since the pace is leisurely. The restaurant is open for dinner seven days a week. Reservations are requested.

HOLIDAY INN
Va. 60 and 220, Covington   *(540) 962-4951*
$$

A relaxing atmosphere and top-notch service accompany a meal at this restaurant. Choose from steak, seafood and other American favorites. It's open seven days a week, breakfast through dinner.

IMPERIAL WOK
348 W. Main St., Covington   *(540) 962-3330*
$

A Chinese restaurant of high caliber, Imperial Wok is a favorite of Covington residents and is known miles around for its quality. The more popular dishes include the Seafood Delight, chicken and shrimp combo and mixed vegetables with shrimp. Another favorite is the Happy Family meal, which is made with chicken, beef, pork, shrimp and fresh vegetables. It's open daily for dinner.

JAMES BURKE HOUSE EATERY
232 Riverside St.
Covington   (540) 965-0040
$

Stop in here for breakfast or lunch. They serve soups, sandwiches, salads and desserts and are closed Sunday.

MARION'S CAFE
804 S. Highland Ave.
Covington   (540) 962-5022
$ No credit cards

Marion's serves terrific home-cooked meals in a comfortable atmosphere. Their specialties are homemade pies and German dishes. The cafe opens very early every day and serves through dinner.

Bath County

CAFE ALBERT
Cottage Row, Hot Springs   (540) 839-5500
$$

Come discover this small, intimate cafe in Hot Springs. Continental breakfasts and light lunches are on the menu, as are a wide assortment of freshly baked breads, pastries and cookies from The Homestead kitchens. You can start off your day with fresh berries, sliced banana with cream or melon. Then try the scrambled eggs Western style with cheddar cheese and fresh fruit, served with toast. Or sample the Cafe's Crepe Albert, paper-thin crepes with fluffy scrambled eggs and tomato butter sauce served with smoked, sugar-cured ham.

Cafe Albert's lunch menu is just as tasty. While waiting for your lunch, the cafe offers you its own strawberry spritzer or Virginia apple cider cooler. You have a choice of sandwiches, such as hot corned beef or chicken salad, all served on rye, white, whole wheat, brioche or croissant, according to your preference. You will also receive your choice of macaroni, potato, fruit or tortellini salad, coleslaw or cottage cheese. Lunch entrees include Spinach Salad Supreme; Virginia's Highland County smoked beef frank with chili, sauerkraut and relish; and the Cafe's Shenandoah Croissant, a thinly sliced breast of turkey with spinach leaves on a Homestead croissant, with watercress spread, pepper jelly and potato salad. Desserts include a soda float and banana split. The cafe is open year round for lunch and early dinner; outdoor service is available in warm weather.

THE CASINO
Homestead Grounds
Hot Springs   (540) 839-5500
$$$$

You can dine out on the lawn in view of the beautiful tennis courts or indoors at this elegant restaurant. Treat yourself to the buffet luncheon, sandwich service or a Sunday champagne brunch while relaxing in style. The Casino is open daily April through October.

THE GRILLE
The Homestead
Hot Springs   (540) 839-5500
$$$$

If you want to get all dressed up and go — coat and tie for men are required here — you'll appreciate the fabulous setting and gourmet dining at The Homestead, which serves delightful fare for lunch, dinner or late supper daily from April through October. Reservations are required.

THE HOMESTEAD DINING ROOM

The Homestead
Hot Springs   (540) 839-5500
$$$$

The world-renowned Homestead (see our Resorts chapter) offers exquisite dining and dancing with a decidedly sophisticated ambiance. Ladies and gents are expected to dress for dinner, which is served daily. Reservations are required. You can also have breakfast here.

SAM SNEAD'S TAVERN

Main St., Hot Springs   (540) 839-7666
$$

For a taste of Colonial Virginia, visit this tribute to Hot Springs' living legend and native son. A historic old bank building houses the tavern. Lunch and dinner are served with a golf theme: Chip Shots (appetizers), From the Halfway House (sandwiches, burgers and light offerings), Water Hazards (fish), The Main Course (meat entrees), Handicaps (desserts) and From the 19th Hole (beverages). Appetizers include lump crabmeat cocktail, spinach salad and chili con carne. For light fare, select a seafood taco salad, the "Sam" burger or a golden-fried breast of chicken sandwich. Fresh Virginia Allegheny Mountain rainbow trout from Highland County and fresh swordfish steak are examples of the fish menu. The medallion of veal or the hickory-smoked barbecued spareribs and chicken are other good choices. Desserts include parfait creme de menthe, fudge fantasy and a chocolate nut sundae. Seasonal entertainment is offered. Homemade meals are served daily.

THE WATERWHEEL RESTAURANT

The Inn at Gristmill Square
Warm Springs   (540) 839-2231
$$$

Continental cuisine is served in the setting of an old mill here. This area, composed of restored 19th-century buildings, is full of rustic beauty. The restaurant's fresh trout is a favorite. Dinner is served daily; there's also a Sunday brunch.

Highland County

HIGHLAND INN

Monterey   (540) 468-2143
$$

This historic inn is a memorable setting for dinner. Formerly the Hotel Monterey, this three-story landmark is one of the few mountain resorts of its size still in operation in Virginia. Lace curtains, candlelight and classical music set the mood. Local fresh mountain trout and grilled Brace of Quail are just two of the creative choices. Be sure to leave room for their maple pecan pie, made rich with Highland County maple syrup — simply delicious. The Inn is open for dinner Wednesday through Saturday and for brunch on Sunday.

Inside
Nightlife

People don't come to the Blue Ridge of Virginia for the nightlife. Instead, they come to get away from big crowds, noise and smoke-filled rooms. A survey of community leaders pretty much bears this out. Nobody seems to miss night prowling because there's so much to do and see during the daytime.

However, there are those who would argue with this premise. One chatty, trendy monthly publication, *V Magazine*, covers the nightlife in the middle Blue Ridge area. You'd do well to get a copy by calling (540) 343-5138 before visiting Charlottesville, Lexington, Roanoke,

Richmond, Staunton, Lynchburg or the New River Valley. You'll also find *V* at most of the "in" places.

Exceptions to the in-bed-at-a-reasonable-hour syndrome are clubs in the college towns of Charlottesville and the New River Valley metropolitan areas of Roanoke and big resorts such as The Homestead, The Greenbrier, Wintergreen and the Boar's Head Inn, which offer something for everyone. Another exception is Cockram's General Store in Floyd County, where everybody from miles around comes on Friday nights for a real hoedown.

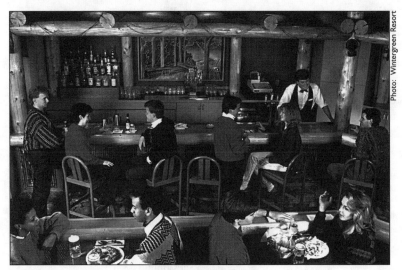

Photo: Wintergreen Resort

Nightlife at Wintergreen Resort.

Shenandoah Valley Region

Harrisonburg

Night owls will find happiness at **Clayborne's**, 221 University Boulevard, where the decor is palm trees and skylights. This restaurant and bar engages a disc jockey on Friday and Saturday nights to keep its dance floor hopping. Occasionally, Clayborne's following among the James Madison University students is treated to a live band. In the Sheraton Hotel on E. Market Street, the action is at **Scruples**, a lounge offering disc jockey-guided music every night except Thursday, when it hosts a popular comedy club, and Sunday, which is karaoke night. If you're not yet familiar with this form of entertainment, it's when common folk like us get to stand on stage and make fools of ourselves singing solo to popular hits.

Staunton

In Staunton evening entertainment takes on a more refined, relaxed tone at the **Belle Grae Inn**, a restored Victorian mansion on Frederick Street which has received the Historic Staunton Preservation Award and a AAA four-star rating. The **Bistro Bar** in this historic downtown inn and restaurant has classical and jazz music on Friday and Saturday nights. The decor is sophisticated and so is the service. We can't say enough about the Belle Grae — you'll want to experience this gem for yourself.

For more action try **McCormick's Pub and Restaurant**, on Augusta and Frederick streets. This restaurant has a small dance floor and occasional live music. **Mulligan's Pub & Eatery** in the Holiday Inn offers live bands every Friday and Saturday night and karaoke night every other Thursday. In the downtown area, try the **Mill Street Grill**, a cozy restaurant in an enchanting old converted grist mill, the historic White Star Mill Building.

Lexington

In Lexington and Rockbridge County, local night owls like **The Palms**, a rowdy downtown bar and restaurant with a big screen TV and juke box. This is a popular college hangout, but locals also feel at home here.

A quieter, more sophisticated alternative is **Harbs' Bistro**, on W. Washington Street, which serves wine, beer, cappuccino and extraordinary desserts, as well as a full menu. The patio is a perfect place to sip a cool drink on a hot summer night.

These days, a younger crowd flocks to **Sharks**, on E. Nelson, for a night of pool.

Without question the most exciting nightlife in Lexington in the summer happenings at the outdoor **Lime Kiln Theater** (see our Arts and Culture chapter). The Sunday Night Concert Series draws huge crowds to hear reggae, bluegrass or folk music. Most every other night, Lime Kiln Theatre stages a play the theme of which relates in some way to the culture of the Southern mountains. Lime Kiln has great picnic spots for dining before the performances.

Visitors should also check with the Lexington Visitors Bureau to find out about other plays and concerts at Washington & Lee's **Lenfest Center** and other sites around town.

Roanoke Valley Region

Things definitely start getting livelier if you drive an hour south to the Roanoke Valley. Forget the bedroom communities of Botetourt and Craig counties, though. Everybody's home with their families, sleeping or else moved here to get away from noise. However, you can find others with insomnia, rub shoulders with young people on dates or meet the newly single seeking to be double at a variety of nightspots in this area.

A real gem, unique to the Blue Ridge, is **Roanoke Comedy Club**, a comedy club that has hosted some of the biggest names in comedy since it opened a decade ago. In downtown Roanoke on the City Market, it is a fun place where you can get rid of the week's stress. Every Thursday night is ladies' night, and the club has a show for nonsmokers every Friday night.

If you're going bar hopping in Roanoke, you'll find some nicely appointed ones, such as **Charades**, at the Marriott off I-581 on Hershberger Road, an action lounge with dancing, promotions and a hungry-hour buffet. **The Elephant Walk**, at 4368 Starkey Road, close to Tanglewood Mall, is also very popular. **Scooch's**, 5010 Williamson Road, is one of Roanoke's oldest rock 'n' roll bars; it's close to Hollins College. (But, fellas, you can forget about picking up a Hollins girl here because most of them are at private fraternity parties at the all-male enclaves of VMI or Washington & Lee and Hampden Sydney.) Scooch's has a karaoke contest every Thursday. Jazz lovers congregate at **Lowell's Restaurant and Lounge**, 2328 Melrose Avenue N.W. At Lowell's, you'll think you're in New York City when you hear the R&B, soul and jazz, with a DJ to spin out the music on Friday and Saturday. For real atmosphere, don't miss the **Iroquois Club**, 324 Salem Avenue downtown, where the action includes a variety of music and foot stomping or slam dancing. Big counterculture names are frequently booked here. It's considered to be one of the hippest places in town with the younger set.

The latest addition is **Awful Arthur's**, 108 Campbell Avenue, with its Thursday bands and long lines on weekends. Also new is **Star City Diner**, which you can't miss! Its skyline at 118 Jefferson Street is a conglomeration of curiosities such as a lighted sign ticking off the national debt per citizen (your share should be up to about $25,000 by 1995-96) to the old-fashioned Big Boy Restaurant statues so popular in the '50s and '60s. Across the street is **Ward's Rock Cafe**, 109 S. Jefferson Street. College students and other fun seekers have been known to line up around the block just to get in! **Confetti's**, 24 Campbell Avenue S.E., is a popular hang-out in the Roanoke City Market Building. And **309 First Street**, found at 309 Market Street, is popular with the artsy crowd downtown. Here you can catch such local favorites as Anastasia Moon and Cows in Trouble (great names, eh?). Speaking of art, try the Art By Night events, which follow First Fridays the first Friday of every summer month downtown. More young and unattached people show up here than for any other event all year. Scheduled the first Sunday of every month is the Jazz Jam at **Henry Street Music Center**, where Roanoke rocked with jazz and blues in the days before desegregation.

You can enjoy a quiet, inspirational moment (no children allowed) at the **Third Street Coffeehouse**, in Old Southwest at the lower level of Trinity Methodist Church, Third Street and Mountain Avenue. It's a throwback to the coffeehouses of the '60s, and you'll find many people from that era soaking up the good karma amidst guitar plucking and poetry readings. Another quiet place — shades of Seattle — is **Mill Mountain Coffee & Tea**, in the heart of the downtown City Market at 12 Campbell Avenue S.E., as well as Main Street in Salem. They've got the best coffee and tea du jour in the Blue Ridge, along with yummy desserts. Everybody who's anybody meets here for both business meetings and fun. Also try **Full Moon Cafe**, 107 Market Square, for relaxation and good conversation. Bet you can't finish the yard-high beer stein beverage. Few ever make it to bottoms up and when they do, it's a real splash!

For an alternative experience, do **The Park**, 615 Salem Avenue S.W., and mingle with Roanokers both gay and straight. Many consider it the best place in town to dance due to a Saturday 5 AM closing time and spacious dance floor. You'll find people from your office right alongside the drag queens and teen-agers with yellow, red or purple hair and black nailpolish (good luck telling who's who).

In Salem, you can go to **Cheers**, 419 and Braeburn Drive, voted Roanoke's Best Bar. If country and western dancing is your thing, wear your two-step boots to **The Top Rail**, 1106 Kessler Road. You also can go country at **Spurs**, 1502 Williamson Road N.E. Also two-step over to **Valley Country**, 3348 Salem Turnpike, Thursday through Saturday for dancing!

East of the Blue Ridge Region

Charlottesville

Many restaurants in town bring in musicians on weekends and some weekday nights and usually don't charge ad-

mission. The popular **Biltmore Grill**, on Elliewood Avenue, headlines good old-fashioned American food and live music. **The Blue Ridge Brewing Company**, on W. Main, has canned music but wonderful homemade meals and beers. It's Virginia's first restaurant/brewery. **The Terrace Lounge** at the Boar's Head Inn is a piano lounge with live music Monday through Saturday. When the weather's nice, you can sit outside on an open porch overlooking the lake. **Durty Nelly's** is a gritty little joint on Jefferson Park Avenue that serves great sandwiches and has live music Tuesday, Friday and Saturday nights. Schedules often change with the seasons, so call ahead if you're headed their way.

Other places where you'll find action at night in Charlottesville include **Dooley's**, in the Sheraton on Seminole Trail. On Wednesday and Friday nights, Dooley's hosts the only live comedy show in town, bringing in top stand-up comics. After the show, stay for dancing and a buffet. Saturday nights are devoted to top-40 dancing.

Katie's Country Club, on U.S. 29 N. by Office America, is a rocking place with live country music Thursday, Friday and Saturday. A popular place with the Greene County locals and the 29 N. suburban crowd, Katie's has been known to host wrestling matches.

Miller's, in the Downtown Mall, is an excellent jazz club and restaurant with live music Monday through Saturday. You'll also hear blues and country here. There's a big outdoor patio that can be nice in the summer if the heat isn't too withering.

We talked about the **Prism Coffeehouse**, on Gordon Avenue in our Arts and Culture section but mention it again here because it is such a great place to hear live bluegrass, folk and other acoustic music. The coffeehouse sometimes brings in nationally known musicians, but it also provides a forum in which the area's top folk, acoustic and traditional musicians can perform.

Two large nightclubs are back to back in the building at 120 11th Street S.W., close to campus: the country-oriented **Max** and the mostly rock 'n' roll **Concert Music Hall**. Max boasts the largest dance floor in central Virginia. It has DJs on weekday nights and live country music on the weekends. Students pour in Thursday nights for country line dances and Wednesday night for lessons in two step. The Concert Music Hall is the hot spot in town to listen and dance to some nationally known and popular regional artists. A broad mix of acts in 1994 included the reggae sounds of Pato Banton and Yellow Man, plus the popular Soul Hat from Texas and even some hip-hop from Public Enemy. Catch live bands Monday through Saturday and a DJ on Tuesday.

For a calmer, more intellectually stimulating evening, several places around town host poetry and fiction readings from time to time. Contact the **Williams Corner Bookstore**, (804) 977-4858, on the Downtown Mall; **Kafkafe**, (804) 296-1175, a continental/American restaurant/espresso bar/bookstore on Elliewood Avenue; or Lisa Russ Spaar, (804) 924-6675, of the UVA Creative Writing Department to find out about upcoming readings.

Nelson County

Wintergreen Four Seasons Resort, (800) 325-2200, near Nellsyford is a swinging place, particularly during ski season. Its three lounges usually have live entertainment and are often standing room only.

Smith Mountain Lake

When you go to gorgeous Smith Mountain Lake, the action will be at the **Bridge Club**, 133 Long Island Drive. Just look for the Hales Ford Bridge and it will be underneath. A lot of young people and people looking for a good time after boating and getting tan on the lake all day head for the Bridge Club at night. You should too if you want to enjoy beach music and very good fare.

New River Valley Region

One hour south, you'll hit College Town, USA: the New River Valley. If you feel self-conscious around The Young and The Tanned, stay in Roanoke, where the crowd is older. If you don't, head for Blacksburg pronto! There you'll find two major universities, Virginia Tech and Radford, within cruising distance of each other. Where to start? How about Blacksburg, home to 23,000 students, half of whom are likely to be the opposite sex.

Blacksburg

If you want to do something with your hands other than hold a drink, check out the action at a sports bar. **Champions Italian Eatery and Cafe**, 111 N. Main Street, features dart lanes, pool tables, food and drink and some live music. You'll hear such bands as SCUM, Not Shakespeare, Baby Igor, Yams from Outer Space and The Rhinoz. For more sedate music (and band names), try **Jacob's Lounge**, at the Marriott, 900 Prices Fork Road. Or for a quick sandwich, there's **Arnold's**, 220 N. Main Street, where you girls will find the mother lode of guys — a real Fraternity Heaven! Also try the **Cellar Restaurant**, 302 N. Main Street, for good food and mixed company.

If watching a loud, live band isn't your mug of beer, there's always the landmark **Carol Lee Doughnuts**, 133 College Avenue, a nice, quiet place for terrific, albeit fattening, donuts. But who cares? You wouldn't be doing the night life scene in Blacksburg with the college crowd if you were worried about calories, right?

Radford

Actually, there is a place in Radford, a half-hour south of Blacksburg, where you can get nonfattening, super broiled seafood: the **East Coast Raw Bar**, a downtown watering hole for old salts that features everything from stuffed fish to surfers. A wonderful restaurant and gathering place is **Alleghany Cafe**, 1009 Norwood Street, with a long bar, excellent food and terrific music upstairs.

If you just want to sit and chat, and you like espresso and glorious desserts, get to **Radford's Gallery Underground**, a cozy downtown pub under the Gallery Cafe at 1115 Norwood Street. It's a favorite of university professors.

If country music is your thing, you'll fine plenty of it, good and loud, at **The Walton House**, on Va. 663, with first-class country groups who sing with the best of them to leave you crying in your beer.

Floyd County

In Floyd County, you'll do your rollicking and rolling country style at the legendary **Cockram's General Store**'s Friday night hoedowns on Locust Street or at **The Pine Tavern**, where anybody who's anybody hangs out on Saturday night to be entertained. The Pine Tavern, on U.S. 221 N., also has dinner theater Tuesday in June and offers nonsmoking performances part of the time. **Ray's**, also on U.S. 221 N., is another popular hangout for country and western and bluegrass.

Alleghany Highlands Region

The western limits of the Blue Ridge limits its nightlife to the great Homestead and Greenbrier resorts. **The Homestead Club** offers cocktails and entertainment at the prestigious resort. The Tuxedo Junction Orchestra entertains with dance music nightly starting at 9:30. Just as elegant a club life awaits you at The Greenbrier's **Old White Club**, where you can dance under sparkling chandeliers to live bands of the contemporary or Big Band variety. At either resort, it will be a night to remember.

Inside
Real Estate and Retirement

Thinking of buying a house in the Blue Ridge? You've come to the right place for quality of life. On many occasions, visitors passing through the Blue Ridge have spied the home of their dreams and clinched a deal even before finding new jobs.

Homes in the Blue Ridge can be found to fit every taste: modern homes perched atop mountain ridges near resorts such as Bryce, Wintergreen and Massanutten or on the fairway at private communities such as Glenmore and Keswick near Charlottesville. If the classics are more your style, the region is rich in tin-roofed Victorians, such as those in Salem or Edinburg, and New York City-style brownstones in downtown Lexington and Lynchburg. If what you want is a primitive log cabin to fix up yourself, check out Southwest Virginia. And if you're looking for a farm, consider the horse country of Loudoun and Albemarle counties, the wine region of Warren County, gorgeous Catawba Valley near Roanoke or isolated country estates in Loundoun, Fauquier, Allegheny, Highland or Bath counties.

You don't have to go to the ocean to live near the water. A visit to Smith Mountain Lake's Bernard Landing's condominiums or the townhomes at Mallard Point along Claytor Lake's white sand beaches will convince you you're already there.

Virginia, the first, largest and wealthiest of the British colonies in America, has more historic homes than all other states combined. And the Old Dominion zealously guards these treasures, preventing historic structures from giving way to industry and subdivisions. Nearly 100 old homes are open for visitation, and they do change hands. Two real estate companies specializing in historic homes are Mead Associates in Historic Lexington, an affiliate of Sotheby's International, and McLean Falconer in Charlottesville, the chosen city of movie stars and millionaires, who often favor such houses.

Also, *The Charlottesville Area Real Estate Weekly*, issued by the Charlottesville Area Association of Realtors, is a helpful, comprehensive guide to real estate in the seven-county area. Pick one up at any one of more than 400 locations or receive a copy in the mail by calling (800) 845-4114 or (804) 977-8206.

Lucky visitors may stumble upon their dream homes, but your best bet is to let local real estate professionals know that you're looking. Homes in Middleburg, Warrenton, Charlottesville, South Roanoke and Lexington are often sold by word of mouth before they ever see the marketplace. Realtors can also offer guidance on the best schools and shopping areas and the level of satisfaction in the neighborhood you're considering.

Local boards of Realtors can answer questions about major developments and fair market prices. In this chapter, we've included information about these boards for each region, as well as local homebuilder's associations, in case you decide to remodel or build and want reputable contractors. Finally, we offer the average price of a home in each region, as provided by the Multiple Listing Service of the Virginia Association of Realtors. The following organizations can assist you in making regional or state-wide comparisons or answer questions about purchasing or building a home.

• **Home Builders Association of Virginia**, 1108 E. Main Street, Suite 700, Richmond 23219-3534; (804) 643-2797

• **Virginia Association of Realtors**, P.O. Box 15719, Richmond 23227; (804) 264-5033

Shenandoah Valley Region

Winchester

The east end of this northern Shenandoah Valley city and the southern part of Frederick County are growing rapidly. This is in part a result of the westward migration of Washington-based workers, people willing to commute an hour or so to their jobs in order to live in an area that's less crowded and costly. But the Winchester area also has a good number of industries that keep the real estate market healthy.

Much of the historic city's beauty comes from the graceful old homes along tree-lined streets and row houses built before and during the Civil War. Many of these row houses, which are a short walk from the pedestrian-only Downtown Mall, are being restored and remod-

eled. You'll also see a lot of old homes that were built partially of stone.

In Winchester, the average price of a home on the market in June 1995 was $128,700. In Frederick County, which has many developments of modestly priced homes on small lots, the average price of a home was $136,200.

Just to the east, in Clarke County, prices were higher in June 1995. The average asking price of a home in that beautiful, rural county was $197,200. Also in Clarke, an occasional estate in the country was selling for more than $1.1 million. Clarke County boasts quite a few 19th-century manor homes surrounded by rolling pastures, and these have attracted some of the county's wealthiest newcomers, Washingtonians willing to make the long commute to work or wanting a second home for the weekends.

Front Royal and Warren County

Many federal employees and retirees have moved into this area, attracted by the beauty of the land and relaxed pace. The most prized properties here are those with a sense of privacy and clear views of the Shenandoah River or the mountains. While some vacation homes could be bought for as little as $68,900 in the summer of '95, prices ranged as high as $350,000. A historic estate in this county can cost in the millions, but it's rare when one comes on the market. Spacious new homes on the county's two golf courses, Shenandoah Valley Golf Club and Bowling Green, are as high as $400,000, but the average price of a Warren County home in 1995 was $123,600.

For more information on real estate in Winchester, Front Royal and War-

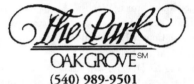
ren, Frederick and Clarke counties, contact:

• **Blue Ridge Board of Realtors**, 181 Garber Lane, Winchester, 22602; (540) 667-2606.

• **Top of Virginia Building Association**, 18 E. Piccadilly Street, Winchester 22601; (540) 665-0365.

Shenandoah and Page Counties

Shenandoah County encompasses several quaint, historic towns, including Woodstock, Edinburg and New Market, along with the Bryce Resort community in Basye. Page County is more rural, with much of its land tucked between Massanutten Mountain and the Blue Ridge range farther east. Retirees and

young couples are always seeking weekend retreats in both counties. The average price of a home is $90,000, but prices are much lower in Page County, where the average cost is closer to $80,000. Riverfront property is usually more expensive and hard to come by (the south fork of the Shenandoah River runs through Page County, and the north fork winds through Shenandoah County).

For the most part, architectural styles are simple — this is a rural, no-frills kind of region. The county has a few interesting old homes, but brick ramblers, Cape Cods and modest, plainly built homes are more the norm.

Bryce Resort in western Shenandoah County is an entirely different real estate market. The year-round resort community has chalets, condominiums and townhouses near the resort's ski slopes, lake and other facilities. Prices range from $30,000 to $300,000, depending upon the size of the property and its proximity to the slopes.

Bryce Resort includes four timeshare developments but only one, Chalet High, is still selling. Managed by Alexander Properties, Chalet High is a development of chalets and townhouses on the northern end of Bryce Resort's golf course.

For more information about real estate in Shenandoah and Page counties, contact:

• **Massanutten Association of Realtors**, 129-C S. Main Street, Woodstock 22664; (540) 459-2937.

• **Shenandoah County Homebuilders Association**, c/o Harris Thompson, Route 1, Box 1, Edinburg 22824; (540) 984-4136.

Harrisonburg

In the heart of the Shenandoah Valley, Harrisonburg is a thriving university city and the seat of Virginia's leading agricultural county, Rockingham. Housing prices in this area accelerated during the 1980s but began leveling off in the '90s. In 1995 the average price of a home was about $110,000. You could buy a starter home for as low as $70,000 or a more luxurious house for up to $400,000.

It's increasingly difficult to find nice, historic properties in many areas of the Blue Ridge but not in Harrisonburg and Rockingham County, where a good number of old homes, some needing renovation and others already restored, are often available. It is also fairly easy to find farm properties; dairy and poultry farming are the leading agricultural industries.

Massanutten Village, a year-round mountain resort community, is a 15-minute drive east of Harrisonburg. You'll find chalets, condominiums and townhouses near the resort's ski slopes, golf course, tennis courts and swimming pools. A property owners' association maintains the roads, runs the police department and manages the entire 600-home development. Lots are still available here.

Three hundred villas and condominiums at Massanutten are timeshares. The units cost from $8,000 to $16,000 for one week per year at the resort. Owners can also swap that week for one at a condominium in Germany, Key West, the Bahamas or any timeshare development that participates in an exchange program of Resort Condominiums International.

For more information, contact:

• **Harrisonburg-Rockingham Association of Realtors**, 633 E. Market Street, Suite B, Harrisonburg 22801; (540) 433-8855.

• **Shenandoah Valley Builders Association**, 245 Newman Avenue, Harrisonburg 22801; (540) 434-8005.

• **Massanutten Homeowners Association**, (540) 289-9466.

Staunton, Waynesboro and Augusta County

Augusta County is growing by leaps and bounds, especially in the Stuarts Draft area close to Waynesboro. A number of industries have built plants there over the past several years, including Hershey and Little Debbie Bakery, and this has led to a boom in housing. Farther west, more and more people from Washington, D.C., New York and other Northern states are retiring in the Staunton area, drawn to its rich history, pastoral beauty and vibrant downtown.

While the average price of a home in Staunton is about $70,000, it is closer to $90,000 in the Stuarts Draft area. In Waynesboro, a city that's home to such industries as Dupont and Genicom, homes average $80,000.

A great demand continues from newcomers to the county for big old homes and farmhouses, but both are in short supply. It isn't that they don't exist. They just rarely come on the market.

Two major residential developments in Staunton are worth mentioning. Ironwood, a private community next to the Staunton Country Club, is characterized by spacious, red cedar homes with private gardens. Baldwin Place is a planned community in Staunton's north end, where the homes, streets and even flora are reminiscent of early American villages. Numerous small, well-maintained developments throughout the county offer five to 20-acre parcels.

Staunton's downtown area is being developed into a major tourist area worthy of many repeat visits. Developers and families have grabbed up many of the charming, architecturally sound commercial buildings and homes, but a few may still be left.

For more information contact:

• **Staunton-Augusta Association of Realtors**, 1023 N. Augusta Street, Staunton 24401; (540) 885-5538.

• **Waynesboro Board of Realtors**, 531 W. Main Street, Suite 15, Waynesboro 22980; (540) 949-4904.

• **Augusta Homebuilders Association**, P.O. Box 36, Waynesboro 22980.

Lexington

In Lexington, known for its historic downtown and rolling pastures, the average price of a home is estimated at $87,000, according to local real estate professionals. Naturally, there are wide disparities in the cost of farmland estates, which can run anywhere from $200,000 to a cool million, to the historical homes downtown that can go for $370,000 on Marshall Street. Forty percent of Rockbridge County is farmland.

Lexington's historic downtown has long been popular for filming period movies. In 1938 Lexington's Virginia Military Institute was the site for scenes in *Brother Rat*, and, in the summer of 1992, dirt was poured on the streets for the Civil War film *Sommersby*. Lexington has numerous buildings and homes that represent most of the architectural styles prevalent in American communities during the 19th century. You will find Victorian cornices and stoops on Main Street, turreted Gothic buildings at VMI, Roman Revival, slender Tuscan columns and bracketed pediments. The town even has an Italianate villa at 101 Tucker Street dating to the late 1850s; a central bell tower surmounts its bracketed overhanging roof. Many of these gems are open for a Christmas holiday tour and again in the spring during Historic Garden Week.

The price of land in the Blue Ridge is considerably lower than in other parts of the country, especially the Northeast and West Coast.

Insiders' Tips

Lexington's proximity to the state's Virginia Horse Center has attracted many would-be gentleman farmers, whose presence has driven up the price of farms. A restorable 1820 brick residence and cottage on 82 acres sold for about a half-million dollars, but small family farms are still available for $100,000 (no house). With a house, you'll probably pay at least $50,000 more. Many such homes are sold by Mead Associates, Realtors, in the historic Jacob Ruff House at 21 N. Main Street.

Lexington has average family developments with above-average prices. Homes in the suburban, family-oriented neighborhoods of Birdfield, Mt. Vista and Country Club Hills start at $100,000, with many $150,000 and up. If you're looking for something in the price range of $80,000 to $100,000, neighboring Buena Vista offers some nice neighborhoods.

For more information, contact:

• **Buena Vista-Rockbridge Board of Realtors**, P.O. Box 311, Buena Vista 24416; (540) 261-2176.

• **Lexington-Buena Vista-Rockbridge Association of Realtors**, P.O. Box 797, Lexington 24450; (540) 464-4700.

Roanoke Valley

The average price of a home in the Roanoke Valley runs $80,000. In the nearby Smith Mountain Lake area, populated by retirees and second-home owners, the average price is determined by whether or not a home is waterfront. Lake homes easily average $250,000. The nearby growing bedroom community of Botetourt County averages $80,500, and finders' fees are often offered for farmland. Others choose to live farther out in rural Craig County and the Catawba Valley, where a wide variety of homes aver-

aging $60,000 and large spreads are easier to find.

Roanoke's neighborhoods are well defined, often bound together by civic leagues and The Neighborhood Partnership, an energetic organization uniting neighborhoods for the past dozen years, encouraging pride and fellowship. Popular areas of town range from pricey Hunting Hills in Southwest Roanoke County, with an average sales price of $270,000, to up and coming Wasena, where an average family home in a nice neighborhood can be purchased for $60,000. South Roanoke remains a favorite, with minuscule turnover in homes ranging from $100,000 to $450,000. More affordable but equally nice are such family favorites as Raleigh Court and Penn Forest, where neighborhood block parties and nightly strolls are the norm. Nearby Salem offers everything from downtown-area, tin-roofed Victorian-style homes with stained glass that can cost as much as the highest bidder offers (and we mean on the high side, not low!) to Beverly Heights, where young families congregate in ranch homes valued from $80,000 to $125,000. The adjoining town of Vinton offers pricey subdivisions such as Falling Creek, with homes costing more than $150,000, and charming downtown wonders you can still buy for less than $60,000.

For more information, contact:

• **Roanoke Valley Association of Realtors**, 4504 Starkey Road S.W., Roanoke 24014, (540) 772-0526.

• **Roanoke Regional Home Builders Association**, 1626 Apperson Drive, Salem 24153; (540) 389-7135.

East of the Blue Ridge Region

On the eastern side of the Blue Ridge Mountains between Front Royal and

Charlottesville lie five counties — Rappahannock, Madison, Greene, Orange and Albemarle (home of Charlottesville) — with some of the prettiest land on the East Coast.

Rappahannock, Madison, Greene and Orange Counties

Generally speaking, prices are higher in Rappahannock County because of the growing number of affluent residents who commute to Northern Virginia to work. Prices drop farther south in Madison County, then rise again in Greene County, which is becoming a bedroom community for fast-growing Charlottesville and Albemarle County. Orange County, just to the east of Greene and north of Albemarle, has some grand old estates and large farms.

In this region, some of the most beautiful historic properties have been transformed into bed and breakfast inns, more than doubling their number in a decade.

In Rappahannock County, the minimum requirement for developing land is 25 acres. Madison County's rules are more relaxed: Three acres is the minimum. The median price of a home in Madison County was $90,000 in 1995; in Rappahannock County, it was closer to $125,000. It is difficult to find historic Victorian or Colonial homes on the market in Madison and Rappahannock counties. Instead, the predominant styles are the brick rambler and simpler homes with vinyl siding.

The real estate market in Orange County, home of James Madison's Montpelier and the Barboursville Winery, is more upscale. You will find a diversity of residential properties and prices that are generally lower than in Albemarle County. But the gap is closing. The median price of a home in Orange County is roughly $100,000. Generally, the homes are scattered across the county, because the local government does not allow the growth of residential neighborhoods.

More than 95 percent of Orange County is zoned agricultural, and land cannot be subdivided into more than four parcels in any five-year period of time. Thus, it is practically impossible to rezone agricultural land to residential. This is precisely what makes it such a desirable place to live for people who can afford the prices of some of the stately old estates.

For more information about real estate in Rappahannock, Madison, Orange and, farther east, Culpeper counties, contact:

• **Greater Piedmont Association of Realtors**, 47 Garrett Street, Warrenton 22186; (540) 347-4866.

Charlottesville

Charlottesville has the dubious distinction of being one of the most expensive areas in Virginia in which to live, second only to Northern Virginia. People of great wealth are drawn to the area, captivated by the beauty of the land, its historic estates and the city's cosmopolitan atmosphere. The many hospitals in the area attract doctors, and jokes abound about the number of lawyers per capita — graduates of UVA who refuse to leave the area. In short, there's a lot of money floating around, and the real estate market has risen to the occasion.

This is especially true in the stretch of land west of the city along Barracks Road, toward Free Union and east of the city at the Keswick development. In the western area near Free Union, new homes on three- to six-acre lots in a subdivision named Rosemont cost $600,000 and up. Near the Farmington Country Club, also west of the city, stately homes run anywhere from $500,000 to more than $1 million. Inglecress is another exclusive development along Barracks and Garth roads, where homes on three to five acres cost anywhere from $750,000 to $1 million.

Architectural styles of most of these new homes are similar — white columns and symmetrical porticos abound. Jefferson's Monticello and University of Virginia are architectural models, at least on the exterior. But inside many new homes you'll find contemporary features such as vaulted ceilings, skylights and open spaces.

The Keswick community gives new meaning to the term "exclusive," even by Charlottesville standards. Sir Bernard Ashley, cofounder of Laura Ashley company and founder of Ashley House Inc., is also owner and developer of the 600-acre Keswick Estate. This is a private, gated community with a maximum allowable density of about 100 homesites in two- to four-acre parcels. Amenities include the Keswick Club, a private-membership golf and leisure club with an 18-hole Arnold Palmer signature golf course and Keswick Hall, a 48-room country house hotel (see our chapter on Resorts).

Community services are the Keswick Estate Homeowners' Association, the Keswick Estate Design Review Board, underground utility services (central water and sewage, electricity, natural gas, telelphone and cable television), fire and police protection and a rescue squad. Architectural controls ensure that all homes will be developed to the same high standards of design and construction. Lots are priced at $185,000 to $295,000.

Also east of Charlottesville is Glenmore, a private, gated community off U.S. 250. The 1,144-acre community is wrapped around a championship golf course, swimming facility, tennis complex and equestrian center with 15 miles of bridle trails. The community will have only 750 homes at build-out, with homesites on the golf course, in deep woods, on grassy knolls, overlooking the 2.5-mile frontage on the Rivanna River or with views of Thomas Jefferson's Monticello. Property owners are presently automatically prequalified for membership in the Glenmore Country Club, a privately owned sports and social club with a new $4 million clubhouse and the best in sporting facilities. Elegance prevails, with plans, landscaping and builders subject to approval by the community's Architectural Review Board. Homesites of one-third to one acre are priced at $85,000 to more than $200,000. Homes range in value from $340,000 to more than $1 million. Golf cottages with maintenance-free groundskeeping start at $225,000.

More than 100 homes in the Charlottesville area were built between the early 1700s and the Civil War era. Wealthy families, often using royal land grants, began migrating west from Richmond in the early 1700s. Such estates as Plain Dealing, Estouteville and Edgemont are registered historic landmarks. Because there are so many historic homes in the area, one or two may be on the market at any given time.

Estates with names posted on signs at the road are not limited to rich historic properties. It's become the fashion to name your abode, no matter how new. This is an English tradition, of course. It started when many early settlers in the area (who were either from England or whose parents were from England) gave their new homes a name that often linked it somehow to their ancestral home in the old country.

The city, which has no more room for development, has some beautiful neighborhoods. Gracious old homes are concentrated in the Rugby Road area, but you'll find more modest, rambler-type homes and Cape Cods close to the university. Within a two-block range of Rugby Road are homes that sell for $300,000 to $1 million.

In the city, the median price of a home in early 1995 was $110,000, including condominiums and townhouses. In the county, median prices ranged from the upper $120,000s to the mid $130,000s, not including farms and estates.

Albemarle County is very restrictive in allowing for growth. The local government has targeted Crozet and the Ivy area, a few miles west of the city, as growth areas and is allowing some higher-density development. But the Free Union area and many other parts of the county are to remain as rural as possible, with minimum requirements of one residence per 20 acres.

Some other important numbers:

• **Charlottesville Area Association of Realtors**, 2321 Commonwealth Drive, Charlottesville 22901; (804) 973-2254.

• **Blue Ridge Homebuilders Association**, 2330 Commonwealth Drive, Charlottesville 22901; (804) 973-8652.

Wintergreen Resort

This four-season resort has luxury condominiums and single family homes on the ridges overlooking the ski area, Devil's Knob Golf Course and the surrounding mountains. In the valley is a growing community which has at its center the award-winning Stoney Creek golf course.

Wintergreen is secluded from encroaching development by the Blue Ridge Parkway and Shenandoah National Park on the north and west and the George Washington National Forest to the south. More than half of Wintergreen's 11,000 acres have been set aside as permanent, undisturbed wilderness.

The community has its own preschool and primary school and private police force. Property owners who are members receive benefits and privileges that include special lift lines at the ski slopes and preferred reservations for golf tee times and tennis courts.

Condominiums cost anywhere from $60,000 to $650,000, homes from $100,000 to more than $1 million and land from $25,000 to $300,000 per lot. The posh resort is about a half-hour's drive from Charlottesville.

For more information, call (800) 325-2200 or (804) 325-2500.

Lynchburg

"In the Blue Ridge Mountains of Virginia" is a well-known ballad in Central Virginia, particularly in the Lynchburg area. Certainly, the mountain view is one reason people choose to live in the City of Seven Hills, where the average price of a home is $82,000.

Lynchburg, along with surrounding Bedford County, is one of the most rapidly growing regions in the state. According to Realtor Alice Smith of Smith & Thurmond Inc., spokesperson for the Lynchburg Realtors, the average selling time for a home is only 115 days.

Among the areas of growth are Ivy Hill, a planned community around Ivy Lake and Ivy Hill Golf Course; Poplar Forest, a neighborhood of fine homes on wooded lots carved out of Jefferson's land surrounding his home; Meadowwood, just outside the city on lots averaging two to three acres; and Meadowridge, homes on two- to three-acre lots close to the mountains. Prices in these areas range from $125,000 to $350,000.

Campbell County, which is west and southwest of Lynchburg, continues to stretch out into previously agricultural areas. The largest and best-known subdivision is Wildwood, with mostly wooded lots ranging from one-half to one acre and prices in the $100,000 to $125,000 range.

In Lynchburg, you'll love the tree-lined streets lined with two-story brick Colonials with manicured lawns. Among the most prestigious and desirable are Peakland Place, Linkhorne Forest, Link Road, Rivermont Avenue and Boonsboro Forest. New growth west of the city is due to developable land there.

Lynchburg is proud of its designated historic areas, where many turn-of-the-century homes are being renovated into glorious showcases. Neglected for years, many are being restored to their original condition: high ceilings, winding staircases and beautiful fireplace mantels, among other original features. The most advanced of these historic districts are Diamond Hill and Garland Hill. Close

behind are Federal Hill, College Hill and Daniels Hill.

Lynchburg homes sell well, according to Smith, because of overall good economic conditions, availability of land for new construction, the variety of neighborhoods and wide price ranges (from $40,000 for a small, two-bedroom home to $1 million dollars for the larger homes). She also emphasizes outstanding scenery, the lowest interest rates in 20 years, available mortgage financing and, of course, a warm and friendly atmosphere.

For more information, contact:

• **Lynchburg Association of Realtors**, 3639 Old Forest Road, Lynchburg 24501; (804) 385-8760.

• **Builders & Associates of Central Virginia**, P.O. Box 216, Forest 24551; (804) 385-6018.

Smith Mountain Lake, Bedford and Franklin Counties

The average price of a home in this area varies greatly as you consider waterfront golf communities, second homes and retiree getaways. Most waterfront homes list for around $200,000. Some of the more popular communities are Chestnut Creek, Waters Edge and the Waterfront and Waverly. Condos prices start in the low $80,000s at Bernard's Landing and the $60,000s at Striper's Landing.

It's worth a boat trip around Smith Mountain's 500 miles of shoreline just to

Insiders' Tips

Do your homework before you buy that Blue Ridge mountain retreat. Land values, building restrictions, soil and water conditions, public services and accessibility vary from region to region.

see the architectural, custom-built splendor of some of the homes. One of the most noted builders of cedar lake homes is Smith Mountain Cedar Homes, perennially a high-volume performer, along with its parent company, Lindal Cedar Homes.

Rural farmsteads and homes in Bedford and Franklin counties are more affordable and available than in any of the other Roanoke bedroom communities. The average price of a home is less than in Roanoke, at around $63,000. Naturally, the cost of lake property brings up the median, but some real rural bargains still can be found.

For more information, contact:
• **Builders & Associates of Central Virginia**, P.O. Box 216, Forest 24551; (804) 385-6018.
• **Roanoke Regional Home Builders Association**, 1626 Apperson Drive, Salem 24153; (540) 389-7135.

New River Valley Region

The average price of a home in the New River Valley runs $90,000. In both Montgomery County, Blacksburg and Radford, well-paid university professionals have driven up the price of homes and land, especially premium farmland in Floyd and Giles counties. The New River area is considered one of the five major growth areas of Virginia, according to noted Realtor E.R. Templeton of Raines Real Estate of Blacksburg. Requests for finders are often found posted on bulletin boards in little towns such as Newport.

Potential homeowners will most likely find Christiansburg and Pulaski the least expensive places to buy a home, according to the local Board of Realtors. The average price of a home was $20,000 higher in nearby Blacksburg.

The downtowns of Blacksburg and Radford offer true small-town atmospheres conducive to leisurely evening strolls, breathtaking parks (especially Radford's Bisset Park along the New River) and the likelihood of meeting others who enjoy an academically stimulating lifestyle. They also are packed with apartment complexes and townhouses for the thousands of students here. The majority of apartments are well-kept, and the students are pleasant and add immensely to the area's quality of life and diverse culture.

Popular family developments near Blacksburg are Foxridge, Heathwood, Toms Creek Estates and Westover Hills, where the average price of a home ranges from $90,000 to $95,000. In Christiansburg, the same type of development home will cost between $70,000 and $85,000. Some of Christiansburg's better known developments are Craig Mountain, Diamond Point, Victory Heights and Windmill Hills. In Radford, a family can buy a home in Sunset Village for a price on the low end ($40,000 to $70,000) and in the newer developments of College Park and High Meadows for $100,000 to $150,000.

Many New River Valley residents opt to live in the environs of Giles, Floyd and Pulaski counties, where rural living is prevalent. Farms still aren't inexpensive, since a lot of professionals also like to live out in the country. The quality of farmland varies in each county and is scarce, due to the area's beauty and proximity to the Blue Ridge Parkway. It probably is least expensive in Pulaski County, where good farmland sells for about $1,000 an acre. Much of the land there is devoted to dairy farms and raising cattle and hogs.

Numerous second homes have been built in Pulaski County's Claytor Lake area. One development, Mallard Point, near Dublin, is a luxurious waterfront community of gracious townhomes unique to the popular water playground. The spacious two- and three-bedroom units offer amenities such as a whirlpool, individual lighted boat slips and a private tennis court.

Downtown Pulaski is definitely on the rise, due to its dynamic Main Street Program. Professionals from Washington, D.C., and other metropolitan areas are renovating some of the Prospect Street mansions, notable for their witches' caps and winding front porches. An area short on bed and breakfast inns, Downtown Pulaski probably has more old mansions that would lend themselves to this cause than any other place in the New River Valley. It's the next hot spot of New River Valley tourism!

If you're looking for a nice family development, consider Mountain View Acres or Newbern Heights, with houses priced from $70,000 to $120,000. Oak View is more expensive at $80,000 to $160,000 but considerably more affordable than a similar development in neighboring Montgomery County.

For more information, contact:
• **New River Valley Association of Realtors**, 811 Triangle Street, Blacksburg 24060; (540) 953-0040.
• **New River Valley Home Builders Association**, P.O. Box 2010, Christiansburg 24068; (540) 381-0180.

Alleghany Highlands Region

This area has no organized real estate board, and no Multiple Listing Service records are kept on the average price of a home, but local real estate agents say most homes typically sell for a fourth less than their urban counterparts. Another rule of thumb, from Highland County's Building Permits Office, is that the cost of building a new home there is $40 per square foot compared to $79 in Northern Virginia.

The area also is unusual in that much of the rural, mountainous property is owned by people who don't live there. For example, half of Highland County, the least-populated county in Virginia, is owned by people who live elsewhere but come to vacation in the highest county east of the Mississippi.

The real estate is prized for its proximity to The Homestead, the Potomac and James rivers and hunting and fishing preserves. Here, one can buy farms with miles of split rail fences on emerald-green pastures, maple sugar orchards, wooded tracts, trout farms and cattle farms. It's obvious to visitors that the sheep outnumber the human population five to one. Many look to this area for retirement.

Retirement

Determining the perfect place to retire takes planning, with careful consideration of individual tastes and personal needs. The Blue Ridge has numerous agencies and contacts to help you determine where you would be happiest. Here is a list by region of helpful agencies or programs. They're full of tips about personal care programs and local perks such as Cox Cable Roanoke's free cable TV installation for seniors, "Enjoy the Prime Time of Your Life." Also check with local hospitals, county health departments and social service departments, since many offer ongoing senior services, programs and seminars.

Shenandoah Valley Region

Agencies

**SHENANDOAH AREA
AGENCY ON AGING**
15 North Royal Ave.
Front Royal   (540) 635-7141

**ROCKINGHAM COUNTY PARKS
AND RECREATION DEPARTMENT**
602 County Office Blg.
Harrisonburg   (540) 564-3160

**AUGUSTA COUNTY PARKS
AND RECREATION DEPARTMENT**
P.O. Box 590
Verona 24482-0590   (540) 942-5113

**WAYNESBORO DEPARTMENT
OF PARKS AND RECREATION**
413 Port Republic Rd.
Waynesboro   (540) 949-6505

**THE VALLEY PROGRAM
FOR AGING SERVICES INC.**
325 Pine Ave.
Waynesboro   (800) 868-VPAS

**SENIOR CORPS OF
RETIRED EXECUTIVES (SCORE)**
(540) 886-2351

HOSPICE OF THE SHENANDOAH INC.
(540) 943-6886

MEALS ON WHEELS — STAUNTON
(540) 886-1219

**AMERICAN ASSOCIATION
OF RETIRED PERSONS**
Glasgow/Rockbridge
Chapter   (540) 463-1661

**FAMILY SERVICE
OF ROANOKE VALLEY**
3208 Hershberger Rd. N.W.
Roanoke   (540) 563-5316

LEAGUE OF OLDER AMERICANS
706 Campbell Ave. S.W.
Roanoke   (540) 345-0451

Retirement Communities

BALDWIN PARK
21 Woodlee Rd.
Staunton   (540) 885-1122
   This retirement community close to downtown Staunton has studio and one- and two-bedroom apartments with window boxes and patios or balconies. All services, including meals, are provided.

BRANDON OAKS
3807 Brandon Ave. S.W.
Roanoke   (540) 989-1201
   Several spacious floor plans are available, plus dining, housekeeping, 24-hour security and on-site professional health care. The community has 172 units offered as one- and two-bedroom apartments and two-bedroom cottages.

ELM PARK ESTATES
4230 Elm View Rd.
Roanoke   (540) 989-2010
   Elm Park Estates is near hospitals, medical facilities and shopping (Tanglewood Mall is across the street).

Amenities include a craft room, library, beauty salon and planned daily activities. Studios and two-bedroom apartments are available, and pets are permitted.

ROANOKE UNITED METHODIST HOME
1009 Old Country Club Rd. N.W.
Roanoke   (540) 344-6248

Several types of living arrangements and levels of care are available to people of all faiths. The facility has social rooms, a chapel and a library. Guest rooms are available.

THE PARK-OAK GROVE
4920 Woodmar Dr. S.W.
Roanoke   (540) 989-9501

Seven spacious designs are available, varying in size from studios to one- and two-bedrooms units. A first floor art gallery has been the scene of numerous exhibits, part of The Park-Oak Grove's ongoing Visual and Performing Arts Series. Inquiries are welcomed. Guided tours and complimentary lunches are easily arranged by calling during regular business hours.

East of the Blue Ridge Region

Agencies

THE JEFFERSON AREA BOARD FOR AGING (JABA)
2300 Commonwealth Dr.
Charlottesville   (804) 978-3644

THE SENIOR CENTER INC.
1180 Pepsi Pl.
Charlottesville   (804) 974-7756

ALZHEIMER'S DISEASE AND RELATED DISORDERS SUPPORT GROUP
                          (804) 973-6122

MEALS ON WHEELS
                          (804) 978-3644

CENTRAL VIRGINIA AREA AGENCY ON AGING (SERVES BEDFORD CO.)
2511 Memorial Ave.
Lynchburg   (804) 528-8500

CITY OF LYNCHBURG DEPARTMENT OF PARKS & RECREATION
301 Grove St.
Lynchburg   (804) 847-1640

SOUTHERN AREA AGENCY ON AGING (SERVES FRANKLIN CO.)
433 Commonwealth Blvd.
Martinsville   (540) 632-6442

Retirement Communities

THE COLONNADES
2600 Barracks Rd.   (804) 971-1892
Charlottesville   (800) 443-8457

The Colonnades is on 59 acres, nearly half of which is a nature preserves with maintained walking trails. The community offers concierge and supplemental personal services, including regularly scheduled private transportation to shopping and dining spots.

VALLEY VIEW
1213 Long Meadows Dr.
Lynchburg   (804) 237-3009

Services include meals, housekeeping, transportation, wellness programs and a community center with hot tub and visiting nurse, which are included in the monthly rental fee. The facility has a country store, barber/beauty shop, a games and crafts area and an exercise room.

WESTMINSTER CANTERBURY
501 VES Rd.
Lynchburg   (804) 386-3500

Residents have a choice of eight apartment styles. Services and amenities include a beauty/barber shop, individual climate control, no-scald water control, housekeeping and your choice of dining arrangements (either in your apartment or in the central area).

New River Valley Region

Agencies

NEW RIVER VALLEY AGENCY ON AGING
143 Third St. N.W.
Pulaski   (540) 980-7720

Retirement Communities

WARM HEARTH
VILLAGE RETIREMENT COMMUNITY
2607 Warm Hearth Dr.
Blacksburg   (540) 961-1712
   On a 220-acre wooded site, Warm Hearth has 46 one-level townhomes,

apartments in three low-rise buildings and apartments for assisted living in a licensed home for adults.

Alleghany Highlands Region

Agencies

LEAGUE OF OLDER AMERICANS
Serves Alleghany   (540) 345-0451

VALLEY PROGRAM
FOR AGING SERVICES INC.
Serves Bath and Highland   (800) 868-VPAS

Inside
Airports and Bus Lines

With its beautiful scenic mountains and interesting historical sites, Virginia is second only to Florida as the most popular tourist destination in the South. Airports are an important means for out-of-state tourists to conveniently visit the area.

More than 300 airports serve travelers in Virginia. These range from grass landing strips to large international facilities. Commercial airports generate 35 percent of the air industry's economic impact in Virginia, while general aviation airports account for only 7 percent. Yet the importance of general aviation in the Blue Ridge is recognized by a constant upgrading of the existing air transportation system.

Of the existing system in the Blue Ridge, three large airports — Charlottesville, Roanoke and Lynchburg — receive varied commercial passenger service. They also provide a wide range of general aviation services for corporate and private aircraft. Others, such as Shenandoah Valley Regional at Weyers Cave and Ingalls Field, next to The Homestead Resort in Bath County, have limited scheduled flights. The majority of Blue Ridge airports are designed to accommodate the single-engine and light twin-engine aircraft that represent more than 90 percent of Virginia's aircraft.

In this chapter, we list the commercial airports, north to south, then the remaining scheduled service and general aviation airports.

Commercial Airports

CHARLOTTESVILLE-ALBEMARLE AIRPORT
201 Bowen Loop   *(804) 973-8341*

The Charlottesville-Albemarle Airport is 8 miles north of Charlottesville in Albemarle County. It is accessible via U.S. 29 and Va. 649 and is served by three major airlines: Comair, The Delta Connection, United Express and USAir Express. These carriers provide 28 departures per day to six major hub airports, including Salisbury, Charlotte, Pittsburgh, Greater Northern Kentucky/Cincinnati, Baltimore/Washington and Washington/Dulles international airports. From these points, connections are available to an additional 175 domestic and international destinations. USAir Express also provides daily nonstop service to and from New York's LaGuardia Airport.

The terminal consists of a 60,000-square-foot building with four airline ticket counters, six airline gate areas, baggage claim space, a 500-space parking area, 61-space hourly parking lot and an on-site travel agency.

Ground transportation is available from Avis, Budget, Hertz or National, and on-call taxi service is also provided.

A number of hotels provide courtesy shuttle van service to and from their establishments.

A food vending court and cafe-deli are also available.

The Charlottesville-Albemarle Airport's market includes the cities of Charlottesville, Staunton, Harrisonburg and Culpeper, as well as the counties of Albemarle, Greene, Madison, Culpeper, Orange, Louisa, Fluvanna, Nelson, Augusta and Rockingham.

General aviation services are provided by Corporate Jets of Pittsburgh, with aircraft fueling, hangaring and maneuvering services available. Flight instruction and aircraft rental is available through Blue Ridge Flight School. Navcom Aviation Inc. provides aircraft repair services. Auto rental service is provided at Corporate Jets through Avis, and courtesy vehicles are also available.

• **Major Airlines:** Comair(800) 354-9822; United Express, (800) 241-6522; and USAir, (800) 428-4322.

• **Car Rentals:** Avis, (804) 973-6000; Budget, (804) 973-5751; Hertz, (804) 973-8349; and National, (804) 973-2948

• **Parking:** (804) 973-5145

LYNCHBURG REGIONAL AIRPORT
4308 Wards Rd.   *(804) 582-1150*

The Lynchburg Regional Airport is 6 miles south of Lynchburg in Campbell County. It is accessible via U.S. 29 and is served by three airlines: ASA/Delta, USAir Express and United Express. These provide 23 departures per day to six major hub airports, including Charlotte, Atlanta, Pittsburgh, Philadelphia, Washington and Washington Dulles international airports. From these points connections are available to more than 200 domestic and international destinations.

The facilities at the airport consist of a 35,000-square-foot terminal building, built in 1992, with one airline ticket counter, six airline gate areas, second-level boarding capabilities, a 400-space daily parking area and an on-site travel agency.

Ground transportation is available from Avis, Budget and Hertz, and on-call taxi service also serves the airport. A number of hotels provide courtesy shuttle van service to and from their properties.

The Lynchburg Airport's west central Virginia market area includes the cities of Bedford and Lynchburg and the counties of Amherst, Appomattox, Bedford and Campbell.

General aviation services are provided by Virginia Aviation, with aircraft fueling, hangaring, maneuvering as well as flight instruction services available. Virginia Aviation also provides aircraft repair services, aircraft rentals and charter services, parking and tie-down.

• **Major Airlines:** United Express, (800) 241-6522; and USAir, (800) 428-4322.

• **General Aviation:** Virginia Aviation, (800) 543-6845.

• **Car Rentals:** Avis, (800) 239-3622; Budget, (800) 527-0700; and Hertz, (800) 654-3131.

• **Parking:** Republic Parking Systems, (804) 239-7574.

• **Taxi/Limousine:** Airport Limo, (804) 239-1777.

ROANOKE REGIONAL AIRPORT
5202 Aviation Dr., N.W   *(540) 362-1999*

Roanoke Regional Airport is 3 miles northwest of Roanoke. It is accessible via I-581 and is served by five major airlines (see below), which make 48 departures per day to 8 major hub airports, with nonstop or direct service to 21 cities. From these points, connections are available to all over the world.

The airport's $25 million terminal opened in 1989. The dramatic glass-fronted, 96,000-square-foot building features four Jetway loading bridges, a modern baggage handling system and a panoramic view of the Blue Ridge Mountains. There are 1,038 daily and 227 hourly parking spaces, an on-site travel agency and a First Union Bank ATM.

Ground transportation is available from Avis, Dollar, Hertz and National and three limousine services are on call. A number of hotels provide courtesy shuttle van service to and from their properties. The facility also has a snack bar, restaurant and gift shop, lounge and conference center, as well as a telephone hotel reservation system.

The Roanoke Regional Airport's market includes the cities of Roanoke and Radford and the counties of Alleghany, Bedford, Botetourt, Craig, Franklin, Floyd, Giles, Montgomery, Roanoke and Pulaski.

General aviation services are provided by Piedmont Aviation, including aircraft fueling, hangaring and maneuvering. Piedmont also offers aircraft maintenances, as does Executive Air Inc. and Roanoke Aero Services. Flight instruction services are offered by Star City Aviation. Air charters are offered by Piedmont, Executive Air, Hillman and Saker flying services.

- **Major Airlines:** Delta Connection (ASA), (800) 354-9822; Delta Connection (Comair), (800) 354-9822; United Express, (800) 241-6522; USAir, (800) 428-4322; USAir-Express, (800) 428-4322; and Northwest Airlink, (800) 225-2525.
- **Car Rentals:** Avis, (540) 366-2436; Dollar, (540) 563-8055; Hertz, (540) 366-3421; and National, (540) 563-5050.

- **Parking:** APCOA, (540) 362-0630.
- **Ground Transportation:** Blacksburg Limousine, (540) 951-3973; Cartier Limousine, (540) 982-5466; Roanoke Airport Limo, (540) 345-7710; and Yellow Cab, (540) 345-7711.

General Aviation and Scheduled Service Airports

WINCHESTER REGIONAL AIRPORT
491 Airport Rd.   *(540) 662-5786*

This airport is 2 miles south of Winchester and 42 miles northwest of Washington-Dulles International. The airport and a U.S. Customs Service are open 24 hours a day. All-weather access (AWOW III, Localizer approach, Pan Am Weathermation) is available to pilots, and there is a lighted runway. Executive fax, secretarial services and conference room with audiovisual equipment make business travel easier. There's on-demand air charter/taxi, overnight hangars, aircraft rentals and flight instruction. Crew car and courtesy vans provide transportation to nearby hotels and golf courses. There's a $5 nightly tie-down fee for single-engine aircraft, $8 for larger aircraft.

FRONT ROYAL-
WARREN COUNTY AIRPORT
Va. 4, Front Royal   *(540) 635-3570*

Four miles west of Front Royal, this facility has a new terminal and hangars. A Duat weather system is available for pilots. Local car rental, cab service and maintenance are available. Parachuting trips are also offered. Tie-down is $3 overnight.

SKY BRYCE AIRPORT
County Rd. 836, off Va. 263
Basye   *(540) 856-2121*

This unmanned airport with a 2,300-foot runway is within walking distance of

Bryce Resort, a large, family recreational spot offering a myriad of activities. There is no fuel. Do-it-yourself, no-fee tie-down is available.

LURAY CAVERNS AIRPORT
County Rd. 652, Luray   *(540) 743-6070*

The 3,300-foot paved, lighted runway at the Luray Caverns Airport sells fuel and charges no fees for incoming craft. Between the world-famous Luray Caverns and the Caverns Country Club Resort, this facility offers free transportation to all Luray Caverns facilities.

NEW MARKET AIRPORT
59 River Rd.   *(540) 740-3949*

This airport 2 miles west of historic New Market and the Shenandoah Valley Travel Association Visitors Center has full-time aircraft maintenance, a flight training school, sightseeing rides, soaring, hot-air ballooning, aircraft rental, radio-operated lights and fuel sales at $1.64 a gallon for 100 LL with an after-hours fueling program. Hours of operation are 8 AM to 5:30 PM daily. Tie-down is $3.50 nightly, and cab service is available.

BRIDGEWATER AIR PARK
Va. 727   *(540) 828-6070*

Operated by K&K Aircraft and close to Bridgewater College, this airport sells fuel and has limited overnight tie-down sites at no fee. Hours of operation are 8 AM to 5 PM weekdays, 9 AM to 4 PM Saturday and Sunday noon to 4 PM. Taxi service is available from Harrisonburg.

SHENANDOAH VALLEY REGIONAL AIRPORT
Va. 771 (Airport Rd.)
Weyers Cave   *(540) 234-8304*

Renovations are underway to expand this 10,000-square-foot terminal building, which offers a restaurant and Hertz and Avis car rental services. A general aviation terminal has fixed-base services, including fuel and maintenance. There are air charter, corporate management services and two flight training schools. Information on hot-air ballooning, sky diving and sail planes is available. Parking is free. There are no pilot fees. Free use of Weathermation, Duat and other flight-planning facilities is offered.

EAGLES NEST
Va. 5, Waynesboro   *(540) 943-3300*

Close to Wintergreen Resort, Eagles Nest offers fuel, car rental and mechanical service, with three mechanics on the field. Tie-down fee is $3 nightly. A flying school, rides and glider plane rental are available.

VIRGINIA TECH AIRPORT
1600 Ramble Rd.
Blacksburg   *(540) 231-4444*

Adjacent to the Virginia Tech Corporate Research Center and a mile from the main 24,000-student campus, this airport is situated on the Eastern Continental Divide at 2,134 feet above sea level. The runway is lighted and complemented by full-instrument approach capabilities. Tech Airport offers a full line of mainte-

The larger airports have excellent ground service to area accommodations, many provided by major hotels. And the major metropolitan bus lines offer fine transportation. Call ahead for ground service information and bus schedules.

Insiders' Tips

nance services and refueling. Flight instruction is offered and Ground School students can earn three academic credits from Tech. Hard-surface tie-downs cost $5. Hangar space has a three-year waiting list. Two rental car services (Holiday Ford and Rent-A-Wreck) are nearby, and taxis are available.

NEW RIVER VALLEY AIRPORT
Va. 100 N., Dublin   *(540) 674-4780*

Two miles north of Dublin, New River offers fuel, maintenance and tie-down at $4 nightly. Hangar space is available. One plane is available for rental. A flight school also operates from here.

FALWELL AVIATION INC.
4332 Richmond Hwy.
Lynchburg   *(804) 845-8769*

Falwell, within the city limits of Lynchburg, offers fuel, maintenance, hangar, flight instruction, aircraft rental and turbojet, turboprop and piston aircraft for charter. No landing or parking fees are charged, but the charge is $2.50 for overnight tie-down.

NEW LONDON AIRPORT
Va. 1, Forest   *(804) 525-2988*

Between Lynchburg and Smith Mountain Lake, this airport offers fuel and minor maintenance. There is no tie-down fee.

BROOKNEAL-CAMPBELL COUNTY AIRPORT AUTHORITY
Brookneal   *(804) 376-2345*

This unattended rural airport has a pay phone on the field. Rental cars are available nearby, and there is no tie-down fee.

SMITH MOUNTAIN LAKE AIRPORT
Va. 1, Moneta   *(540) 297-4500*

Adjacent to Virginia's largest lake, with 500 miles of shoreline, Smith Mountain

offers fuel, sightseeing charters, limousine and car rental. Tie-down is $5 nightly.

INGALLS FIELD
Va. 703, Hot Springs   *(540) 839-5326*

Gateway to the world-famous Homestead Resort, Ingalls Field might have no planes one day and look like O'Hare the next, depending on which conventions are meeting. A commuter offers two round trips daily to Washington/Dulles, and other trips are on demand. Rental cars and limo are available to Hot Springs, Warm Springs and other Bath County points of interest. Overnight tie-down is $3, and there's no landing or parking fee.

Metropolitan Bus Lines

Public transportation plays a vital role for major cities in the Blue Ridge. It provides an alternative to tourists or those with their own transportation and also provides the elderly and disabled with a means of getting around town.

Due to increased concern over energy consumption, ozone pollution and other critical issues facing the world today, public transportation is no longer just an alternative but an environmentally responsible way to travel. Major cities in the Blue Ridge offer bus transportation that is clean, accessible and inexpensive.

For a guide to public transportation in Virginia, call the Virginia Division of Tourism at (804) 786-4484. You'll receive an easy-to-read map prepared by the Virginia Department of Transportation.

Roanoke

VALLEY METRO GREATER ROANOKE TRANSIT COMPANY
12th and Campbell Aves. S.E.   *(540) 982-0305*

Valley Metro is Roanoke's regional

transportation system, which tries hard to accommodate everyone from eager tourists to the disabled, who are given special consideration with STAR service.

Valley Metro serves more than 5,500 passengers daily with its fleet of 46 buses. The modern main terminal, Campbell Court, is in the heart of the shopping district, across from First Union Bank on Campbell Ave.

Riders may send for a bus guide in advance. Exact fare or your ticket should be ready since bus drivers carry no change. No smoking, eating or drinking is permitted. The bus operator should be signaled a block before you want to get off.

Charlottesville

CHARLOTTESVILLE TRANSIT SERVICE
425 4th St. N.W.   *(804) 296-RIDE*
UNIVERSITY TRANSIT SERVICE
1101 Millmont St.   *(804) 924-7711*

The City of Charlottesville's Transit Service and University Transit work together to provide dependable, efficient, convenient and safe transportation.

Riders may send for a bus guide in advance. When they ride, they should have exact fare or a ticket. Designated transfer points and routes are clearly marked on the guide in various colors. Eating, drinking and smoking are not permitted.

Two front seats may be reserved for senior citizens or those with disabilities.

Lynchburg

GREATER LYNCHBURG TRANSIT COMPANY
Kemper St.   *(804) 847-7771*

Greater Lynchburg Transit serves both the City of Lynchburg and parts of Amherst County, carrying 3,500 to 4,000 passengers daily. Its fleet of 26 buses radiates from a main terminal at Plaza Shopping Center, the only transfer point, between Memorial Avenue and Lakeside Drive. New bus guides, marked with colored routes, are available by mail, on any bus or at the office on Kemper Street. Exact fare or a pass is required.

Nestled in the heart of the New River Valley is one of Virginia's outstanding universities. Enjoy a world of educational and entertaining activities ... plays, concerts, lectures, exhibits, athletic events and programs.

RU

RADFORD UNIVERSITY

A World of Difference

- **Top-notch cultural entertainment, including national and international groups:**
  College of Visual and Performing Arts, (540) 831-5141

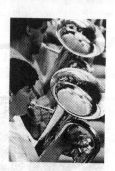

- **Popular entertainment, lectures:**
  Heth Student Center Information, (540) 831-5420

- **Exhibits and outdoor sculpture court:**
  University Art Galleries, (540) 831-5754

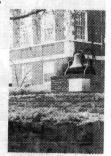

- **Exciting NCAA Division I Highlander sports action:**
  Ticket and sports information office, (540) 831-5211

- **Elderhostels, conferences and adult learning programs:**
  Office of Continuing Education, (540) 831-5845

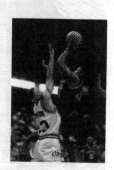

Tours for students and parents:

Office of Admissions, (540) 831-5371

For further information about Radford University, call or write:

Office of Public Information
P.O. Box 6916
Radford, VA 24142
(540) 831-5324 or Admissions, (800) 890-4265

COME VISIT AND ENJOY OUR CAMPUS.

Inside
Education

Some of Virginia's finest colleges and universities can be found in the Blue Ridge region, the foremost being "Mr. Jefferson's University," the University of Virginia in Charlottesville. UVA's School of Law and Colgate Darden Graduate Business School consistently rank in the top 15 nationally, and its undergraduate program is highly regarded nationwide.

Virginia is also known for fine college preparatory schools such as Notre Dame Academy and Foxcroft School in Middleburg. Randolph-Macon Academy in Front Royal has been turning out stellar students since 1892. South of Front Royal is Wakefield Country Day School, where seniors' SAT scores average 1323 points. Charlottesville area prep schools include St. Anne's-Belfield, Woodberry Forest in nearby Orange County and the Miller School of Albemarle, a military boarding school for boys.

Lynchburg has several prep schools, including the Virginia Episcopal School and the Seven Hills School. Lynchburg is also home to five colleges and two business schools drawing more than 15,000 students each year.

Every major city in the Shenandoah Valley has at least one college or university, and the area has several college preparatory, parochial and military boarding schools.

The Roanoke Valley is home to Roanoke College and Hollins. Excellent prep schools include North Cross and Roanoke Catholic.

Harrisonburg, the seat of Virginia's leading agricultural county of Rockingham, bustles with academic activity. James Madison University, Eastern Mennonite College and Seminary, and Bridgewater College are within a few miles of each other.

To the south, in historic Staunton, are Mary Baldwin College, a Presbyterian-affiliated school for women; and Stuart Hall, Virginia's oldest Episcopal preparatory school for girls.

Washington and Lee University and the embattled Virginia Military Institute sit in quaint, historic Lexington. VMI is the only public all-male college in the nation, but an ongoing court challenge could force the cadets to study, drill and sweat side by side with women.

A strict regime is also a way of life at two military boarding schools in the Valley: Fishburne Military School in Waynesboro and Massanutten Military Academy in Woodstock.

In addition to Mary Baldwin College, several esteemed private women's colleges are in the mountains and foothills of the Blue Ridge, including Hollins College in Roanoke, Randolph Macon Women's College in Lynchburg and Sweetbriar College in Amherst. South of Roanoke, the

New River Valley is home to Virginia Tech and Radford University, two of the most popular choices in Virginia higher education.

Listed below in geographic order, north to south and east to west, are four-year colleges and some of the better-known preparatory schools in the Blue Ridge region. Information on two-year community colleges is available from the State Council on Education, (804) 225-2628. Tuition and fees may change slightly; not all schools had released their 1995-96 rates by press time.

Shenandoah Valley Region

SHENANDOAH UNIVERSITY
Winchester   (540) 665-4581

This small university sits on 62 acres on the southeast edge of Winchester. It offers eight undergraduate degrees, the Bachelor of Music being one of the most popular. The school also has a lively music theater program. Graduate degrees are offered in business, music and physical therapy, among others. Tuition at the Methodist Church-affiliated institution is $10,700; room and board is $,264. The school has a satellite campus in Loudoun County.

CHRISTENDOM COLLEGE
Front Royal   (800) 877-5456

This is a tiny college founded in 1977 to inspire and educate Catholic students for church lay leadership. The student body will probably never exceed 450, to retain a close community life. The college is situated on a 150-acre campus of gently rolling land surrounded by the Blue Ridge Mountains. Bachelor of Arts degrees are awarded in English, history, philosophy, political science and theol-

ogy. The college also offers a two-year Associate of Arts degree. Tuition and fees are about $8,880; room and board is $3,600.

EASTERN MENNONITE COLLEGE AND SEMINARY
Harrisonburg   (540) 432-4118

Christian values and global concerns are integrated with the learning process at this private college, which was founded in 1917 to serve the educational needs of the Mennonite Church. The school has about 1,000 undergraduates and 100 seminary students. The most popular majors are business, education, biology, nursing and social work. Tuition is $9,650; room and board is $3,800.

JAMES MADISON UNIVERSITY
Harrisonburg   (540) 568-6147

This is a comprehensive public university offering a wide range of courses on the bachelor's and master's levels. The strongest academic areas include the arts, education, communication and health and human services. The beautiful 472-acre campus is within walking distance of downtown Harrisonburg. Average enrollment is 11,000. In-state tuition is $1,836, fees are about $2,200, and room and board is $4,544.

BRIDGEWATER COLLEGE
Bridgewater   (540) 828-2501

This private, Church of the Brethren-affiliated college is 7 miles south of Harrisonburg. Its average enrollment is 1,000 students, and the most popular majors are business and general sciences for pre-med students. Founded in 1880, Bridgewater was the first coeducational college in Virginia. Tuition and fees is $11,265; room and board is $4,725.

*Come visit the sixth oldest institution
of higher learning in America
characterized as "one of the most dignified and
beautiful college campuses in the nation."*

WASHINGTON AND LEE
UNIVERSITY

Lexington, Virginia

FOR INFORMATION CALL (540) 463-8400

MARY BALDWIN COLLEGE

Staunton   *(540) 468-2262*

This private women's college enrolls about 950 students, more than half Virginians. The students represent 42 states and eight foreign countries. Forty major and minor courses of study are offered, but the top five are art, psychology, sociology, business and education. Also popular is a program of study known as the independent major, a focused, individualized program combining studies from more than one academic discipline. Chemistry and biology majors in pre-med programs at Mary Baldwin maintain a 100 percent acceptance rate at medical schools. The pretty campus is within walking distance of downtown Staunton. Tuition is $11,800.

WASHINGTON AND LEE UNIVERSITY

Lexington   *(540) 463-8400*

Washington and Lee University in historic Lexington was founded in 1749 and enrolls about 1,600 undergraduates and 400 law students. *U.S. News and World Report* has rated W&L one of the top bargains for a quality private school education in America. The university offers both bachelor's and juris doctor (law) degrees.

Its history is rich with historic names. In 1796 George Washington contributed 100 shares of canal stock in the James River Co. to Liberty Hall Academy, a Presbyterian seminary. The grateful trustees changed the school's name to Washington Academy in 1798 and to Washington College in 1813.

Decades later, Gen. Robert E. Lee rode into town on his horse, Traveller, in 1865 and became the college's president until his death in 1870. While there, Lee established the nation's first journalism program and its School of Law. W&L's gracious campus is designated a National Historic Landmark, with neoclassical brick buildings dating back to the generosity of Washington. Lee Chapel, on the tree-line colonnade, is a focal point for students, who gather there for lectures, concerts and special events. Lee designed the beautiful chapel and is buried there.

Although the student body is more diverse than ever, it is largely made up of the sons and daughters of wealthy Southerners and Easterners.

W&L is a charter member of the 14-college Old Dominion Athletic Conference and is a member of NCAA's Division III.

Tuition is $14,500, with a total average cost of $21,500, including expenses.

VIRGINIA MILITARY INSTITUTE

Lexington   (540) 464-7000

Virginia Military Institute joins W&L in Lexington as a national treasure of tradition. Lt. Gen. Thomas J. Jackson, the immortal Stonewall, taught here 10 years before heeding the call of the South in the Civil War. Again this year, VMI leads the nation's publicly supported colleges in endowments per student. VMI has produced some of the most famous military leaders in the world as graduates, including Gen. George C. Marshall, class of 1901, author of the Marshall Plan to reconstruct Europe after World War II. A museum in his honor is next to the 12-acre parade ground. About 40 percent of graduates are commissioned while 18 percent of alumni make the military a career.

This is the school that was portrayed in Ronald Reagan's film, *Brother Rat*, about VMI's infamous Rat Line. However, tradition is being tested in the federal courts, since state-supported VMI doesn't want to admit women but the U.S. Justice Department does. The U.S. Court of Appeals has ruled that VMI may remain all-male as long as nearby Mary Baldwin College offers women a similar leadership program. Nobody's expecting the Justice Department to leave things as they are, so the fight for males-only status undoubtedly will continue.

VMI offers its 1,200 cadets a baccalaureate degree in 13 disciplines and must also take four years of ROTC. They are encouraged to sign a formal contract during their last two years, which normally leads to a commission. Degrees are in biology, chemistry, civil engineering, computer science, economics and business, electrical

engineering, English, history, international studies, mathematics, mechanical engineering, modern languages and physics. Tuition is $2,980 in Virginia, $9,020 out of state. The school has 13 intercollegiate athletic teams in NCAA Division I.

HOLLINS COLLEGE

Roanoke   (540) 362-6451

Founded in 1842, Hollins College was the first chartered women's college in Virginia. Enrollment is 1,070, with 882 undergraduate women and 188 coed graduate students. Hollins awards a bachelor's of arts degree with 26 majors and offers graduate programs in five disciplines: English/creative writing, children's literature, psychology, liberal studies, teaching and a certificate of advanced studies.

Hollins is known internationally for its clinic for stutterers, the Hollins Communications Research Institute; the school also has a clinic for head injury patients, the Hollins College Rehabilitation Research Institute. Hollins emphasizes community outreach through its adult studies, the Women's Center and summer programs for women and rising juniors and seniors in high school.

Hollins enjoys a strong liberal arts focus, with nationally recognized programs in creative writing. Three Pulitzer Prize winners — Annie Dillard, Henry Taylor and Mary Wells Ashworth — graduated from Hollins. Other notable alumna include *Time* publisher Lisa Valk Long, *ABC News* correspondent Ann Compton and Elizabeth Forsythe Hailey, author of the best seller *A Woman of Independent Means*. Hollins has the first graduate program for the writing and study of children's literature and is also noted for its international concentration.

The college hosts more than 200 public events annually.

Lynchburg *is* Lynchburg's College

Offering undergraduate degrees in 51 fields in the liberal arts and professional studies with graduate degrees in business administration, accounting, education, and counseling.

A selective, independent, coeducational, residential college founded in 1903 as one of Virginia's first coeducational institutions.

LYNCHBURG COLLEGE
IN VIRGINIA

Nearly half of its graduates study abroad. One new program is offered through Christie's of London for museum and auction house studies. Hollins' sports programs are also well-known in the NCAA Division III and Old Dominion Athletic Conference. Its Riding Center is popular for women who like to take their horses to college with them. No wonder, since its riding team often wins first place at the Nationals. Tuition is $14,000 for 1995-96.

ROANOKE COLLEGE
Roanoke   *(540) 375-2500*

This Lutheran-affiliated college, the second-oldest American college related to the Lutheran religion, is more than 150 years old. It enrolls 1,700 students and offers bachelor's degrees in 27 majors with a strong commitment to liberal arts and church-related values. After having been named for several consecutive years as the number one Up and Coming Liberal Arts College in the South, Roanoke College was named by *U.S. News & World Report* in 1994 as the number one liberal arts college

in the South. Roanoke has 15 sports in the NCAA Division III. Tuition is $14,100 annually.

East of the Blue Ridge Region

UNIVERSITY OF VIRGINIA
Charlottesville   *(804) 982-3200*

"Mr. Jefferson's University" is the hub of the Charlottesville community. With its neoclassical buildings, white porticos and graceful landscapes, the university's grounds are considered among the most beautiful in America.

A recent survey by *U.S. News and World Report* hailed UVA as the second-best public institution in the nation, next to University of California-Berkeley. In the magazine's "best buys" category, UVA ranked fourth in the nation among both public and private universities.

It should be noted that the university has pretty much succeeded in shaking its reputation of being a party school, notori-

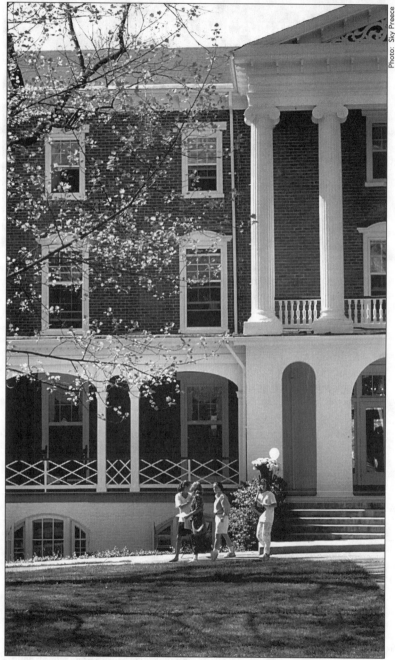

Photo: Sky Preece

Hollins College is an all-women's college in Roanoke.

ous among *Playboy* readers and others for its annual Easter parties and infamous mud slide near Fraternity Row. This is due in part to tougher entrance criteria; the number of applications far exceeds the space available for undergraduates. About half of all in-state applicants get in, and roughly two-thirds of the student body is made up of Virginians. But they are smarter, more studious and harder-working than ever.

The University of Virginia is especially noted for its schools of Law and Medicine and for the Colgate Darden Graduate School of Business Administration.

It's also known across the state for its Center for Public Service, which helps localities by collecting demographic and economic data for use in developing public policy. The University's Center for Liberal Arts provides continuing education for classroom teachers from across the state.

Total enrollment is about 18,000 graduate and undergraduate students. In-state tuition is $3,724, fees are about $800 and room and board is $3,778.

SWEET BRIAR COLLEGE

Sweet Briar   (804) 381-6100

Sweet Briar College is a nationally ranked, highly selective, independent women's college of the liberal arts and sciences, offering the bachelor of arts or the bachelor of science degree. It is 12 miles north of Lynchburg in Amherst County, on 3,300 rolling acres in the foothills of the Virginia Blue Ridge. The college is known for its laboratory-based and equipment-intensive program in the sciences. Its program in international education, which includes study-abroad in France, Spain, Germany, England and Scotland, attracts students from colleges across the country. Poet Mary Oliver, Pulitzer Prize and National Book Award

winner, and celebrated writer John Gregory Brown form the core of the college's distinguished creative writing program.

Sweet Briar's all-level riding program, which regularly snags national championships, boasts one of the best on-campus facilities in the country. About 600 women from more than 40 states and 15 foreign countries choose from Sweet Briar's 39 majors, including interdepartmental and self-designed majors. For women older than 25, the college offers the Turning Point Program. Tuition is $14,990 annually.

LYNCHBURG COLLEGE

Lynchburg   (800) 426-8101

Lynchburg College, an independent, coeducational institution related to the Christian Church (Disciples of Christ), is one of America's top 50 liberal arts schools, according to the *National Review College Guide*. The school serves approximately 1,650 undergraduates and 400 graduate students.

Two teaching innovations at Lynchburg College are the Lynchburg College Symposium Readings course and the Senior Symposium. LCSR incorporates classical reading selections across the curriculum, while in the Senior Symposium, students read selections from the classics and attend weekly lectures to discuss major themes addressed in the readings. The college also offers a leadership development program. Small classes and one-on-one interaction with professors are among the many benefits of an education at Lynchburg College.

Master's degrees are offered in business administration, accountancy, counselor education, curriculum and instruction and educational leadership. The Adult Center for Continuing Education and Special Services (ACCESS) program for adults who want to earn an undergraduate degree is specifically designed to address the special needs of persons age 25 and older. Services include admission, enrollment, advising, transfer arrangements, faculty contacts and program planning. The nursing program offers advanced degrees and specialization.

Tuition is $13,980 annually.

LIBERTY UNIVERSITY

Lynchburg   *(800) 522-6225*

Liberty University is a Christian, comprehensive, coeducational university committed to academic excellence. Liberty serves more than 10,000 students from 50 states and 31 nations at the undergraduate and graduate levels. The school was founded by Dr. Jerry Falwell, the TV evangelist who is also founder of the Moral Majority. Liberty celebrates its 25th anniversary in the autumn of 1995.

The school adheres to strict fundamentalist Christian principles. For example, no modern or classical music is permitted in dormitories, and a demerit system with fines is enforced for students caught listening to anything other than Christian music on campus. Liberty is accredited by the Southern Association of Colleges and Schools and offers 75 areas of study. Liberty Baptist Theological Seminary offers master's degrees in Christian education, divinity, counseling and theology.

Liberty's facilities include a 12,000-seat football stadium and the 9,000-seat Vines Convocation Center, which are used by the Flames athletic teams, who compete on the NCAA Division I level. Prospective students or anyone interested in the school is encouraged to visit. For a free video tape, call the number above. Tuition is $6,000 annually.

RANDOLPH-MACON WOMAN'S COLLEGE

Lynchburg   *(804) 947-8000*

Randolph-Macon Woman's College, a four-year liberal arts college affiliated with the United Methodist Church, serves 725 women from 42 states and 20 countries. It sits on 100 acres near the Blue Ridge, with a 100-acre riding center nearby. For more than a century, women have come to the campus to prepare for a multifaceted life, through rigorous academics, opportunities for cross-cultural experiences and an emphasis on community service and involvement. Individual research and the unique sense of community that draw women to the campus is enhanced further by the student-faculty ratio of 9-to-1.

All classes are taught by professors rather than teaching assistants, and most classes have 18 or fewer students. The college offers approximately 25 majors, as well as many relevant emphases and concentrations. The interdisciplinary First-Year Colloquium emphasizes discussion and debate and frequently draws upon the college's nationally recognized Maier Museum of Art, featuring works by noted American artists including Georgia O'Keeffe, George Bellows and Mary Cassatt, as a resource. The Across-the-Curriculum Writing Program ensures every student has strong writing skills. Also, many students choose to enhance their studies by going abroad. The Prime Time program is offered for women of nontraditional college age.

The value of asking questions and pursuing knowledge clearly is conveyed to Randolph-Macon students, many of whom further their studies. The college ranks in the top 25 percent of private, four-year institutions nationwide in numbers of graduates going on to earn doctorates.

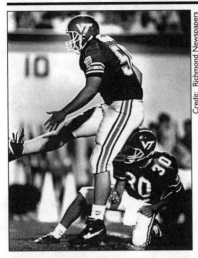

Credit: Richmond Newspapers

The Virginia Tech Hokies compete against the nation's top collegiate powers

The staff of the Career Development Center provides a one-on-one, four-year career preparation program, assisting students with graduate school and career decisions. Tuition is $14,770 annually; the room and board fee is $6,330.

FERRUM COLLEGE

Ferrum   *(540) 365-2121*

More than any college in the Blue Ridge, Ferrum celebrates its ties to local culture and brings national attention to Virginia, Franklin County and a nearly extinct way of life. Situated on 800 acres in Franklin County, near Smith Mountain Lake, Ferrum is a private, coeducational, liberal arts United Methodist Church affiliate founded in 1913. Ferrum offers bachelor's degree in 32 majors, plus a teacher education program, to 1,100 students.

Ferrum is nationally renowned for its Blue Ridge Institute and Blue Ridge Folk Festival each autumn. There, traditional music, crafts, food and recreation are part of the program that brings thousands each year to the college.

While educating students for success in modern society, Ferrum has remained attuned to those cultural traditions which give the region its sense of place and identity. In the early 1970s the Blue Ridge Institute was established to document and interpret that heritage through research, fieldwork and educational outreach. Ferrum even was nominated for a Grammy Award for a recording series exploring Virginia folk music. Concerts have brought together traditional musicians, tale tellers and craftspeople. A Blue Ridge Archive preserves photos, recordings and printed materials important to Virginia folk culture.

Tuition is $14,500 annually. The college is in NCAA Division III; baseball and football are popular sports at Ferrum.

New River Valley Region

VIRGINIA TECH

Blacksburg   *(540) 231-6000*

Virginia's largest and most diverse university, Virginia Tech has a pervasive presence in western Virginia as the largest employer in Southwest Virginia. The school employs 5,800 full-time employees and has an annual payroll of $250 million. Virginia Tech enrolls nearly 24,000 undergraduate and graduate students and has 76 undergraduate and 124 graduate degree programs. Virginia Tech consists of eight colleges: Agriculture and Life Sciences, Architecture and Urban Studies, Arts and Sciences, Business, Education, Engineering, Human Resources, Veterinary Medicine and the College of Forestry. All 50 states and nearly 100 foreign countries are represented in the student body.

Tech's 3,000-acre main campus is in a town of 32,000 residents, in the scenic Blue Ridge Mountains. As you would expect, many students can't bear to leave Blacksburg after graduation, and legions of them stay to make it a top-notch, stimulating university town. Additional facilities include a 120-room conference center, 800-acre research farm, Equine Center, graduate centers in Roanoke, Hampton Roads and the Washington, D.C., metro area and 12 statewide agricultural experiment stations. The newly-reopened Hotel Roanoke Conference Center, 36 miles away, is also partially owned by Virginia Tech.

U.S. News & World Report has ranked Virginia Tech in its top 20 with National Merit Scholars and top 50 nationally in annually sponsored research. Its Corporate Research Center is one of the best-known in the South. As a land-grant university with a statewide mission, Tech is responsible for Virginia's Cooperative Extension, which is carried to 107 Virginia communities. Tech is also a leader among universities in the United States in the use of communications technology. The entire campus is connected with the town of Blacksburg and the world through the unique Blacksburg Electronic Village. The school has gained quite a bit of fame through this bold use of the electronic superhighway. It also is famous for its traditional Cadet Corps.

Tech is a member of the Big East Football Conference and a member of the Atlantic 10 Conference for other sports. It has a 51,000-seat stadium, offering some of the most popular spectator sports in the Blue Ridge. Be prepared for hour-long traffic jams when the Hokies play football at home. Tuition is $4,087 in state and $10,739 out of state annually, fees included.

RADFORD UNIVERSITY
Radford   (540) 831-5371
The New River Valley's other major state-supported educational institution, Radford University, enrolls nearly 9,100 students in this residential community of

14,000. Radford is 45 miles southwest of Roanoke in the Blue Ridge Mountains. In addition to the Graduate College, Radford has five colleges offering bachelor's degrees: Arts and Sciences, Business and Economics, Education and Human Development, Nursing and Health Services, and Visual and Performing Arts. Special pre-professional programs are offered in law, pharmacy, physical therapy, veterinary medicine, sports medicine, medicine and ROTC. A Global Studies program, which internationalizes the university's entire curriculum, begins in 1997.

As with Virginia Tech, many students elect to stay to live and work in this beautiful college town beside the scenic New River. Radford belongs to the Big South Conference and NCAA Division I and offers 17 varsity sports. Annual in-state tuition is $3,114; out-of-state, $7,688.

Southwest Virginia Region

EMORY & HENRY COLLEGE
Emory   (540) 944-4121
This historic (1836), private, liberal arts college enrolling 850 has been cited by *Money Guide* magazine as one of the 100 Best Educational Buys in the United States. *U.S. News & World Report* calls Emory & Henry one of the top 10 regional liberal arts colleges in the South.

Emory & Henry offers 20 majors and special programs, including Appalachian Studies, pre-med and pre-law. It also ranks with the top 1 percent of U.S. colleges and universities in alumnae giving. Faculty-student ratio is 1 to 14. In addition to a small, intensive setting for education, it is ideal if you are interested in spectacular mountain views and easy access to the recreational opportunities they afford, including mountain climbing, hiking and bicycling. The college is close to the historic town of Abingdon. Six varsity sports for men and five for women are in NCAA Division III, with membership in the Old Dominion Athletic Conference.

Tuition is $9,300 annually.

Preparatory Schools

FOXCROFT SCHOOL
Foxcroft Rd., Middleburg   (540) 687-5555

This prestigious boarding and day school for girls in grades 9 through 12 was founded in 1914 by Charlotte Noland, who served as the school's headmistress until she retired in 1955. Miss Charlotte valued such old-fashioned virtues as determination, courage and character, but she wasn't above having a bit of fun. She said she wanted to establish a school that girls "would hate to leave because they loved it." Alumni will attest to her success.

The school is set in 500 idyllic acres of orchards, fields and streams near Middleburg. Local foxhunts meet frequently at the school, and many of the students participate in the hunt. The school has a definite equestrian tone — 40 percent of the girls are involved in its excellent riding program, using either the school's 35 horses or their own.

There are 126 boarders and about 35 day students representing 11 countries and 18 states; 19 percent of the students are international. The school is small but the program is extensive: more than 70 courses, including advanced placement and opportunities for independent study. Classes average 10 students to one teacher.

Tuition is $13,980 plus $400 in fees (riding is $500); room and board is $6,000.

NOTRE DAME ACADEMY
35321 Notre Dame Ln., off
U.S. 50 W. of Middleburg
Middleburg   (540) 687-5581

A 200-acre campus surrounds this coed college preparatory school for day students in grades 9 through 12. The school, founded in 1965, has a strong affiliation with the Roman Catholic Church. Of the 134 students, 55 percent are Catholic, and the faculty of 17 includes four Sisters of Notre Dame. Students in the upper grades wear uniforms.

Notre Dame offers advanced-placement courses in five test areas, accelerated programs, independent study and college credit through courses at local colleges. Intramural athletics are also an important part of a student's life here.

The 30 graduates in the class of 1994 were accepted at 11 different colleges, including the College of William and Mary, Radford University and the University of Virginia.

Tuition is $5,900; fees are $350.

RANDOLPH-MACON ACADEMY
Front Royal   (800) 272-1172, (540) 636-5200

This coed boarding school, which is affiliated with the United Methodist Church, is surrounded by a scenic 135-acre campus in the small town of Front Royal. The Upper School is an accredited prep school in grades 9 through 12, while the Middle School emphasizes a classical education in grades 6 through 8. Though the uniform school's structure is non-military, RMA is the only coed boarding school in the country with an Air Force Junior ROTC program. The FAA-certified flight program trains students from ground school to their first solo flight, with the option to become licensed pilots.

RMA's small class size — 10 students to one teacher — creates a good learning atmosphere, and faculty members emphasize the fundamentals and good study habits.

The campus has an outdoor track, five

tennis courts and fields for baseball, field hockey, football, lacrosse and soccer. Other sports facilities include a gymnasium and Nautilus room and indoor swimming pool.

Total enrollment is about 424 students from 28 states and 21 countries. Tuition is $4,295, plus $150 in fees; board is $5,200.

WAKEFIELD COUNTRY DAY SCHOOL
Washington   (540) 635-8555

The late William E. Lynn and his wife Pamela were so concerned about the erosion of education standards in public schools that in 1972 they founded Wakefield. Initially, their goal was to provide a good, classical education for their own six children. Since then, under headmistress Pamela Lynn, scores of students from pre-kindergarten through the 12th grade have benefited from the school's enriched curriculum. One hundred percent of the graduates have been accepted into their chosen colleges. Studies include two required years of Latin and two required years of French or Spanish. Homeric Greek is offered to students beginning in grade 9. The school offers advanced-placement courses in English, science, math and foreign languages.

Wakefield is 10 miles south of Front Royal on U.S. 522 in Rappahannock County. Tuition and fees range from $2,000 for pre-kindergarten to $5,200 for grades 8 through 12.

WOODBERRY FOREST
Woodberry Forest
Madison County   (540) 672-6008

This boarding prep school for boys sits on 1,400 acres in Madison County, about 30 miles north of Charlottesville and 70 miles south of Washington, D.C.

Independent and nondenominational, the school prepares students for successful performance at some of the best colleges and universities in the country.

Woodberry Forest offers a comprehensive advanced-placement program and a curriculum that includes rigorous requirements in English, math, foreign language, history and science, plus art, music and religion. About 400 boys from 31 states and 12 foreign countries attend the school, with the majority coming from Virginia and North Carolina.

The school was founded in 1889 by Robert S. Walker, a captain in the Confederate army who wanted a school to educate his six sons. Thomas Jefferson drew the floor plan for the headmaster's residence for his friend, William Madison, brother of James Madison.

The average class is 12 students. Professors also live on campus; more than two-thirds hold master's degrees and four have doctorates.

The campus is beautiful, as one would expect of a school with a $65 million endowment. Fine recreational facilities include an Olympic-size pool and a golf course. The school has many teams in every sport, so each student has a chance

The cost for a Blue Ridge college education differs widely. Some admissions offices quote a combined cost for tuition and room and board, while others list them separately. When comparing costs, be sure to ask which cost-quoting formula they use.

Insiders' Tips

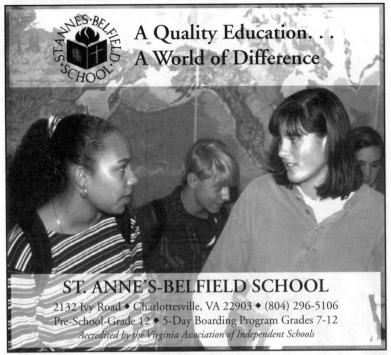

A Quality Education. . .
A World of Difference

ST. ANNE'S-BELFIELD SCHOOL
2132 Ivy Road ◆ Charlottesville, VA 22903 ◆ (804) 296-5106
Pre-School-Grade 12 ◆ 5-Day Boarding Program Grades 7-12
Accredited by the Virginia Association of Independent Schools

to compete against other boys of similar athletic ability.

Current annual tuition and fees are $16,900. One student in four receives tuition assistance.

THE MILLER SCHOOL OF ALBEMARLE
Charlottesville   *(804) 823-4805*

This is a college preparatory and academic military school on 1,600 beautiful acres 14 miles from Charlottesville. The student body is held to only about 94 students a year, with the majority enrolled in the Upper School, grades 9 through 12. The rest of the students are in grades 5 through 8. The Upper School is organized as a Cadet Squadron of the Civil Air Patrol, the official auxiliary of the U.S. Air Force. All students wear uniforms and are expected to conform to modified military procedures. Both girls and boys attend the school, but only boys board there.

The school's Victorian-style buildings are National Historic Landmarks, and the campus covers farmland, orchards, forests, a pond and a 12-acre lake for swimming, fishing and canoeing.

Eighty-three percent of the school's 1994 graduates were accepted by colleges and universities, with most entering schools in Virginia.

Day students pay $5,500 to $6,000 tuition; boarders pay $10,500 to $12,000. Uniforms are an additional $1,000. Financial aid is available; the average award is $4,500.

ST. ANNE'S-BELFIELD SCHOOL
Charlottesville   *(804) 296-5106*

Formed in 1970 by the merger of St. Anne's School, a girls' boarding school founded in 1910, with the Belfield School,

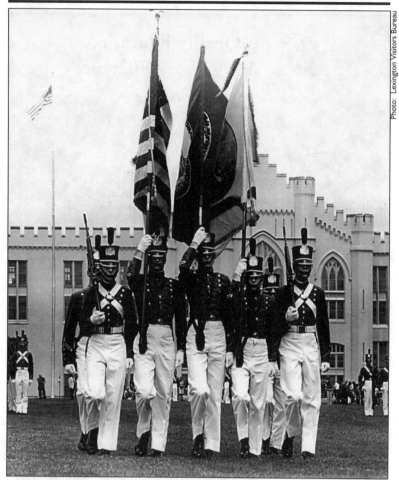

Photo: Lexington Visitors Bureau

Virginia Military Institute cadets on parade in front of Barracks, on the VMI post.

a coed elementary school established in 1955, St. Anne's-Belfield is in its third decade of educating youngsters. The accredited school is near the University of Virginia on two campuses totaling more than 60 acres.

The school offers a day program for preschool through grade 12, and a five-day boarding program for grades 7 through 12. The school's philosophy stresses personal and educational growth:

Although we expect our graduates to be prepared for the nation's finest colleges and universities, our true purpose is to create a challenging yet charitable atmosphere where students gain skills necessary for both creative and disciplined thought. . . . The transmission of knowledge, encouragement of curiosity and the development of responsible, honorable behavior are the great ends of education.

The school has a student body of

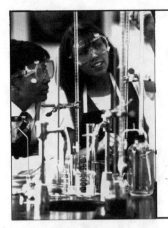

about 800 and limits the boarding program to 40 students in order to maintain a family-like atmosphere. A full range of advanced-placement and honors courses are offered for upper level students, while younger children study basic subjects, as well as French, art, drama, computers and physical education. Graduates advance to enroll in some of the nation's finest universities every year.

Annual tuition and fees range from $4,600 for a half-day session for preschoolers to $7,850 for grades 11 and 12. The five-day boarding fee is an additional $7,600. Financial aid is available to families who demonstrate need. About 28 percent of the students receive financial assistance.

NORTH CROSS SCHOOL
4254 Colonial Ave. S.W.
Roanoke   *(540) 989-6641*

North Cross is a coeducational day school enrolling 518 students ages 4 through 18 in prekindergarten through grade 12. Its goal since 1960 has been to prepare students "not just for college or a vocation, but for a full, rich and rewarding life." The school offers a program that accommodates a wide range of abilities and encourages personal accomplishment.

The school's 77-acre campus includes three academic buildings, including an art gallery, theater, greenhouse and 19,500-volume library. Athletics is an important focus with three playing fields and Carter Athletic Center, a 65,000-square-foot complex of three gymnasiums, racquetball and squash courts, an indoor track and a six-lane, 25-yard swimming pool. The 1994-95 tuition range was $2,915 for prekindergarten to $5,925 for grades 9 through 12.

ROANOKE CATHOLIC SCHOOL
621 N. Jefferson St., Roanoke (540) 982-3735

Roanoke Catholic, founded in 1889, is a coeducational college preparatory school enrolling 420 students ages preschool to grade 12. The school's state mission is to develop in students those characteristics and attitudes that will help them achieve full potential in all aspects of their lives. The school focuses on educating the whole child

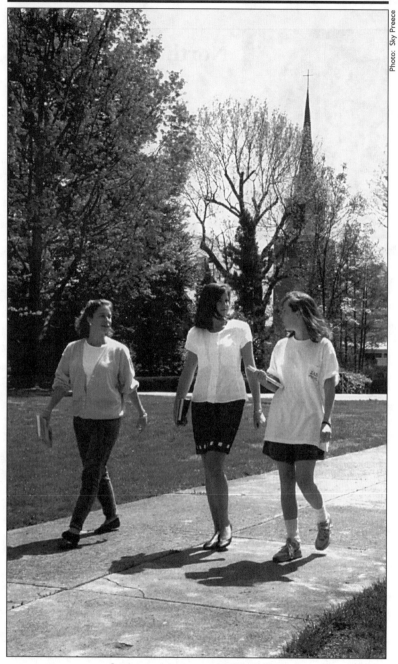

Photo: Sky Preece

Students on campus at Hollins College.

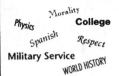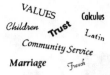
physically, intellectually, emotionally and spiritually.

The school has a strong academic program in a Christian atmosphere. The inclusion of Christian morals and values is an integral part of the entire curriculum. Athletics is also important, with the Athletic Association sponsoring and funding the Upper School sports program and sandlot soccer and basketball teams for the Lower School. The 1994-95 tuition range was $2,300 for kindergarten to $3,747 for Upper School.

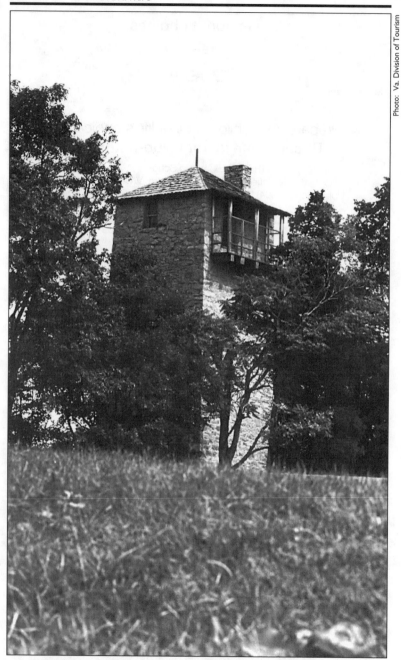

Photo: Va. Division of Tourism

The Shot Tower near Wytheville has been a Southwest Virginia landmark for a century and a half.

Inside
Southwest Virginia Daytrips

The mountain culture of Southwestern Virginia, comprised of 14 unique counties, is close to the Blue Ridge Mountains and offers such a refreshing cultural point of view for some outstanding daytrips. Time-wise, don't let the map of Southwest Virginia deceive you, however. A mountain mile can take considerably longer to navigate than the speedy miles on the efficient interstate highways of the Blue Ridge of Virginia. Besides, there's a lot of rugged mountain scenery to enjoy as you go, so leave ample time to get to your destination.

Mountains formed the culture of this land that has more miles of trout streams than roads. In the pioneer days, this beautiful mountainous country was the western frontier, romanticized with the legends of Daniel Boone. In 1775 Boone opened up the route to the west by carving out the Wilderness Road through the Appalachian Mountains.

Today, visitors can stand at various mountainous vantage points at 20,000-acre Cumberland Gap National Historical Park and see why Boone's route through the Gap soon caught on with so many adventurous spirits. Or, they may visit the Kentucky border's "Grand Canyon of the South," Breaks Interstate Park, where a 5-mile-long, 1,600-foot-deep gorge prevented even the trail-blazing Boone from selecting this particular passage as the gate to the promised land.

Hardy, adventurous souls still practice and cherish a culture born and nurtured by isolation from outside influences. This is evidenced by the area's famous bluegrass music and hallowed arts and crafts passed on by generations of self-sufficient natives who learned to eke out a living from the land, either by farming or coal mining.

The area's people, known for their genuine friendliness, are glad to share their culture with "outsiders" at special events throughout the region. Probably the most famous is the Old Fiddler's Convention, held for 59 years in the city of Galax on the second weekend in August, sponsored by Galax Moose Lodge 733. At this internationally known event, string music, folk songs and clogging entertain visitors from around the world while contestants compete for thousands of dollars in prizes.

The area's other major attraction is the world-famous Barter Theatre, the oldest professional repertory theater in America, in the Town of Abingdon (an attraction in itself). Founded during the Great Depression, the Barter began when a hungry young actor offered local residents theater tickets in exchange for food. Although the Barter now offers cash to its young actors, some of the country's best, for performances, it still continues its barter tradition, as well.

Another popular attraction, the outdoor drama, *Trail of the Lonesome Pine*, is also related to the mountains. Based on the famous novel of a proud mountain people by Big Stone Gap native John Fox Jr., the drama is performed here each summer to show how the coming of modern civilization changed life for the local mountain folks, especially a romantic young girl, June Tolliver.

As you may expect, the highest mountains in Virginia are here. The steepest peak is 5,730-foot-high Mount Rogers, which sets the scenic stage for the vast acreage of this remote area. Not far behind in stature is lofty 5,520-foot-high White Top, host to both maple and ramp festivals. Driving up either is an adventure you'll never forget, and don't be surprised to still see snow on the ground as late as April and May. When you're headed for the high country, expect at the least a 10-degree temperature drop.

Virginia's mountains are home to numerous state and national parks, including Hungry Mother, near Marion; Breaks Interstate on the Kentucky border in Coal Country; and Natural Tunnel, an 850-foot-wide limestone tunnel winding its way through the Southwest Blue Ridge Highlands. Hunting, fishing, swimming, hiking, canoeing and, of course, mountain climbing, are popular pastimes for adventurous visitors.

What some say is the most beautiful stretch of the Blue Ridge Parkway also winds along the western edge of Patrick County. The picturesque landmark, Mabry Mill, is nearby, with beautiful accommodations such as scenic Doe Run Lodge for the Parkway's many visitors.

The area's culture is carefully preserved by many institutions, among them the Southwest Virginia Museum and Historical State Park in Big Stone Gap and the Carter Family Fold, named for the famous Carter singing clan.

As you travel farther up the winding Appalachians, Coal Country is all around in the counties near the tip of Virginia. America's black gold grips not only the history but also the future of everyone living in the area. From the coke ovens of Buchanan County to the Harry Meador Coal Museum in Big Stone Gap, photos and equipment give you an understanding of a way of life that has long centered around a boom-or-bust economy. These days, tourism, happily, is quickly taking hold as the isolated land's alternative industry.

While sampling the best attractions the area has to offer, you won't be at a loss for places to eat, stay or shop.

With far too much interesting information to give ample justice to Southwest Virginia's unique culture, we offer you a sampling of the best and brightest of attractions, along with the names of tourism groups eager to send you enticing material so you'll visit and stay awhile.

Patrick County

Patrick County is home to one of the most beautiful sites on the Blue Ridge Parkway, **Mabry Mill**, at Milepost 176.1, made famous by artists and photographers the world over.

The eastern part of the county boasts **Fairystone State Park**, named for the small fairystone crosses found there. The crosses are much sought after as good-luck charms. Legend has it that the crystalline stones are teardrops that angels and fairies shed when Christ was crucified. Camping and cabins are available at the park, and there's a lake with a beach.

Dickenson County, Virginia
Rugged, Scenic, Different!

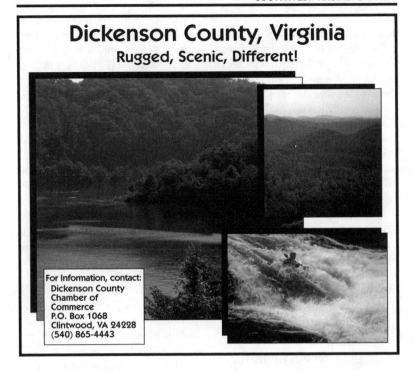

For Information, contact:
Dickenson County
Chamber of
Commerce
P.O. Box 1068
Clintwood, VA 24228
(540) 865-4443

With two-thirds of the county covered with woodlands, Patrick County is an outdoor lover's delight. The **Top of the Mountain**, a 3,000-foot plateau, is home not only to **Lovers Leap** and **Fred Clifton Park**, but to numerous shops in charming **Meadows of Dan**, with picnic spots and dining ranging from hot dogs to multicourse masterpieces at several fine restaurants, including **Chateau Morrisette Winery**, **Doe Run Lodge and Restaurant** and **Woodberry Inn** near Mabry Mill. Five minutes from the Meadows of Dan juncture is yet another restored, operating mill, **Cockram Mill**, where you can picnic beside the placid mill pond or browse through the souvenir shop.

Other scenic points of interest include **Mayberry Trading Post** at Milepost 180,

built in 1892. This white-frame general store is stocked with wonderful food and aromas, including apple butter, each fall. Nearby is **Mayberry Presbyterian Church**, founded in 1924 and a magnet to artists who come to paint or photograph the picturesque rock landmark.

Visitors also enjoy the **Reynolds Homestead**, the ancestral home of R.J. Reynolds, founder of the tobacco company bearing his name. It sits in restored elegance on the Reynolds Plantation in Critz. The original house and contemporary Continuing Education Center, now an extension of Virginia Tech, welcome visitors for numerous annual events.

Patrick County also is a sportsman's delight. It is known for **Primland Hunting Preserve**, a private, 10,000-acre hunting reserve stocked with thousands of game birds. Fishermen also will find the mountain streams sparkling with native and stocked trout at **Philpott Reservoir**, a man-made lake that stretches 15 miles and has a 100-mile shoreline with hundreds of campsites and a sandy beach.

The county has two of only a dozen covered bridges remaining in Virginia. **Bob White**, built in 1922, is off Va. 8 near Woolwine. **Jack's Creek Covered Bridge** was built in 1914 2 miles south of Woolwine on Va. 610. Both are beautiful examples of preserved Americana.

For more information on Patrick County, there are two groups to contact: the Blue Ridge/Piedmont Cultural Consortium in Martinsville at (540) 632-3221 and the Patrick County Chamber of Commerce at (540) 694-6012.

City of Galax, Carroll County and Grayson County

Carroll and Grayson counties and the City of Galax are bound together both by lay of the land and location.

An independent city, **Galax** is nestled in the Blue Ridge between Carroll and Grayson counties and serves as the commercial hub of the area. This Main Street community has a charming downtown and is home to the oldest (since 1935) and largest fiddlers' convention in the world the second week of August, sponsored by the Galax Loyal Order of Moose Lodge 733. Each year, about 30,000 people gather in Felts Park to enjoy the original music of pure American culture performed by a wide variety of nearly 2,000 talented artists who compete for thousands of dollars in prize money. The program includes folk song, fiddle, guitar, bluegrass banjo, clawhammer banjo and mandolin.

Outside of the big festival, you can enjoy the **Galax Mountain Music Jamboree** the third Saturday of each month (except August) at 7 PM. May through October, the jamboree is held outdoors at Grayson Street Stage; November through April, it moves indoors to the Rex Theatre on Grayson Street.

For shopping, don't miss **Rooftop of Virginia Cap Crafts**, where you'll find everything from a cake of lye soap to the finest of handmade quilts. In this cathedral-type setting at 206 N. Main Street, the local community action agency and native craftspeople cooperate to bring to the public a wide selection of authentic handmade crafts. The center is open year round.

Carroll County has numerous facilities for camping, swimming, fishing, horseback riding and hiking. You'll find an 18-hole golf course, **Olde Mill**, just off the Blue Ridge Parkway.

The county's most famous event is the annual **Hillsville Gun Show and Flea Market**, in its 27th year, conducted each Labor Day Weekend by VFW Grover King Post 1115. Join the 250,000 people who drive every year to this show. You'll spot cars lined up for miles before you get to the 100-acre-plus site, where more than 2,000 vendors offer every type of collectible imaginable. It's called the "Best Show in the South" — where the collectors collect. Call Melvin Webb about the guns at (540) 728-9810 and Ernest Martin about the flea market at (540) 728-7188.

Grayson County is rapidly becoming the recreational destination of Southwest Virginia. It is home to **Mount Rogers**, the highest peak in Virginia, with its 60-mile-long Mount Rogers National Recreation Area, Grayson Highlands State Park and New River Trail State Park,

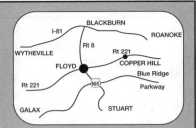
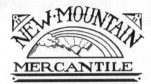
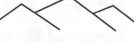
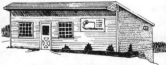

Virginia's only linear state park (a continuous park 57 miles long), offering hiking, bicycling and horseback riding.

Mount Rogers National Recreation Area is the real draw, with 154,000 acres of unspoiled land in the Jefferson National Forest. People, many hiking the **Appalachian Trail**, come to the area, isolated by altitude and climate, to return to another era and see a fragile ecosystem through its alpine meadows and spruce-crowned summits. The town of Damascus is famous for its mid-May party during **Appalachian Trail Days**, when hikers are invited to join in a parade with the townspeople, indulge in barbecued chicken at the fire station and square dance in the post office parking lot.

The Mount Rogers park stretches from the New River near Ivanhoe westward along the south side of I-81 to Damascus. Major access is off I-81 to Va. 16 south from Marion and Va. 600 south from Chilhowie. Headquarters for the area is on Va. 16, south of Marion; call (540) 783-5196. Maps are available here for $3.

Grayson Highlands State Park has 5,000 acres with facilities for camping, picnicking, swimming, horseback riding, hiking and nature study. To the delight of visitors, several hundred ponies roam freely through the park. On the last weekend of September each year, the ponies are herded up and auctioned off at the park.

The New River Trail State Park, the state's linear park, offers 57 miles of trails, much of it paralleling the scenic New River, the second-oldest river in the world.

For more detailed information, directions, points of interest, brochures and maps of the area, contact: the Galax-Carroll-Grayson Chamber of Commerce, (540) 236-2184); Mount Rogers National Recreation Area, (540) 783-5196; or Virginia's Division of State Parks, (804) 786-2132.

Town of Wytheville, Wythe County and Bland County

The town of Wytheville and Wythe and Bland counties pride themselves on being the Crossroads of America, being situated at the intersection of I-81 and I-77, which brings in thousands of tourists for shopping and dining.

Wytheville is known for its **Chautauqua Festival**, based on the historical tours featuring lectures, plays and concerts originating from the Chautauqua Institution near Buffalo, New York. An important forum for adult education, the tent Chautauquas flourished until the development of radio, which made them a thing of the past. Events take place in the **Elizabeth Brown Park**. Wytheville's charming downtown offers several walking tours in an old-fashioned and thriving business district with shops offering local crafts and outlet bargains. Another popular shopping site is **Snooper's Antique and Craft Mall**, where 50 local craftspeople display their work: antiques, quilts, hand-blown glass and pottery. Snooper's is on the I-81 frontage road 8 miles north of Wytheville. Ten miles north at Fort Chiswell is **Factory Merchants Outlet Mall**, featuring an array of discount shopping for everything from kitchenware to toys.

The most unique shop in the Wytheville area is **P.J.'s Christmas Carousel**, where children can ride a carousel of Christmas animals. P.J.'s offers handcrafted holiday decorations and gifts. It's next to Snooper's. While you're shopping, remember that there are 14 motels and 35 restaurants in Wytheville.

Wythe County is home to one of the most unique landmarks in the world, the shot tower at **Shot Tower Historical Park**, where U.S. 52 crosses the New River at the Poplar Camp Exit on I-77. The 70-foot tower, the only one of its kind known in the world, was built in the early 1800s to make shot for the firearms of frontiersmen and settlers. The tower is now the center of Virginia's newest state park, most of which is located in Wythe County. Its **New River Trail** offers the outdoor enthusiast opportunities for hiking, biking, horseback riding, canoeing and primitive camping.

Another great outdoor site is **Big Walker Lookout**, between Wytheville and Bland on U.S. 52. It has a chairlift, swinging bridge, cabin, gift shop and an observation tower 3,600 feet up that offers a view of five states.

Big Walker Mountain and Bland County offer a recreational activity unmatched in the Blue Ridge: llama hiking! With advance reservations, Bob and Carolyn Bane of **Virginia Highland Llamas**, (540) 688-4464, will lead you and your party, along with a herd of llamas, up Big Walker's old Appalachian Trail section. On special saddles, the llamas will carry your picnic lunch through lush green meadows up to a beautiful vista, about a three-hour journey. Listen for the eerie sound of the llamas humming. Why do they hum?

"Because they don't know the words," says Carolyn Bane. Actually, humming is how the llamas communicate.

For more information on Wytheville and Bland and Wythe counties, contact: the Wytheville Convention & Visitors Bureau, (540) 228-3211. For regional tourism information, you also may call (800) 446-9670 or write the Virginia Highlands Gateway Visitor's Center at Drawer B-12, Max Meadows, Virginia 24360.

Smyth County

If you love the outdoors, breathtaking scenery and retracing the steps of soldiers in one of the most important counties in the Civil War, by all means visit gorgeous Smyth County and enjoy all the natural

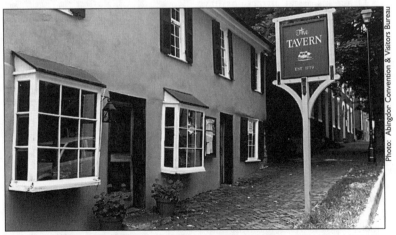

Imagine the people who have passed through this door at The Tavern, Abingdon's oldest building.

beauty and rich history it has to offer, along with a host of good country restaurants and inexpensive places to stay. The town of **Saltville** was known as the salt capital of Virginia, providing table salt and salt for animals, as well as salt necessary for preserving meat in the days before refrigeration.

Saltville's copious salt production brought an attack from the North on October 2, 1864. You still can see the trenches and fortifications from which the outnumbered Confederates nevertheless successfully defended the town's saltworks. Battle relics are on display in the **Saltville Museum** and at Virginia Highland Community College. Visitors also can see a reconstruction of the historical, rough-hewn **Madam Russell House**, home of Patrick Henry's sister.

The week before Labor Day, Saltville residents observe **Salt-Making Week**. They heat up some of the town's old salt kettles and boil down the brine, just as their ancestors did several hundred years ago. Then, on Labor Day, they celebrate with four days of music and fun.

Other historical attractions have equally interesting origins. The area's leading recreational area, **Hungry Mother State Park**, was named for Hungry Mother Creek. The park, 5 miles from Marion, off I-81. As legend has it, pioneer Molly Marley and her small child were caught in an Indian raid in which her husband was killed. After eating only berries for many days, she collapsed at the foot of the mountain known as Molly's Knob. Her child, unable to rouse her, wandered down the creek and finally found a group of houses. The only words he could say were "hungry" and "mother." A search party found the child's dead mother, and the creek took its name from this sad tale.

On a more upbeat historical note, Smyth County's town of **Troutdale** was journey's end to the famous author Sherwood Anderson, who helped shape the modern short story and wrote the famous Winesburg, Ohio. The annual Sherwood Anderson Short Story Competition recognizes aspiring authors. **Ripshin**, Anderson's home, is open by appointment.

For more information, call the Smyth County Chamber of Commerce in Marion at (540) 783-3161.

Washington County and Abingdon

Washington County, home of historic Abingdon, the oldest town west of the Blue Ridge, is alive with history, arts, music, education and Southern hospitality. It is indisputably the cultural center of Southwest Virginia. For recreation, try the national **Virginia Creeper Trail**, a 34-mile-long former railroad bed that gently climbs from Abingdon to Whitetop Mountain. It once was a Native American trail and then a railway. The Virginia Creeper Trail Club will send you information; write them at P.O. Box 2382, Abingdon, Virginia 24210.

What truly makes Washington County a premier vacation destination is Abingdon, a vital community with attractions of nationally known theater, arts, music, shopping, trendy restaurants, a four-star hotel and historic bed and breakfast inns.

The two unequalled jewels in Abingdon's cultural crown are the Barter Theatre, celebrating its 62nd anniversary, and the Martha Washington Inn, a lovingly restored classic hotel known for hospitality, gourmet food and fine service. Traditionally, people from around the

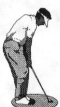

world come to see the Barter Theatre's
acclaimed plays, stay at the Martha Washington or an area bed and breakfast and
take their pick of the town's multitude of
cultural offerings.

In keeping with the system of barter,
Barter Theater exchanged Virginia's famous country hams for royalties to produce the works of such playwrights as
Noel Coward, Thornton Wilder and Bernard Shaw. Shaw, a vegetarian, returned
the ham and requested spinach. The Barter obliged him. As time passed, Barter
earned a reputation for top plays per-

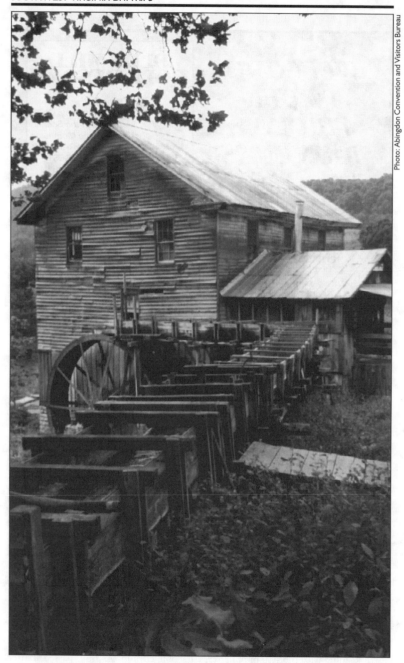

Photo: Abingdon Convention and Visitors Bureau

White's Mill is the oldest Water-powered, commercial grist and flour mill in Southwest Virginia.

formed by top professionals. For an up-coming schedule of playbills, call the Barter at (800) 368-3240.

The **Martha Washington Inn** matches the historical charm and elegance of the year it was founded, 1832. The home was built for Col. Francis Preston. After his death, it became the Martha Washington College for Women. After the college merged with Emory & Henry, the inn was used as a boarding house for actors at the Barter. In 1935, it opened as an inn. Its present owner, United Coal Company, spent more than $6 million on its renovation in 1992. The inn offers a restaurant, a nightclub, private club and gift shop.

For a descriptive brochure of area attractions, call the Abingdon Visitors & Convention Bureau at (540) 676-2282. You may want to take in the rest of Abingdon's sights on its scenic historic walking tour. A map is available by calling (540) 628-8141.

A very special shop that attracts a large following is the **Antique Orchid Herbary**, a few miles outside the town. You can experience everything from herbal barbecues to nature walks with an herbal picnic supper. For a list of delightful and unusual offerings, call (540) 628-1463.

The **King William Regional Arts Center** keeps art alive with exhibitions of national and regional interest, art camp, special events, and workshops and studios for adults and students. Call for a schedule of events at (540) 628-5005. If this interests you, you'll also want to go to **The Arts Depot**, where you'll see working artists in their studios, gallery exhibits, a performing arts series and an **Appalachian Center for Poets and Writers**. Call (540) 628-9091.

Each Christmas, Abingdon also conducts a charming candlelight tour of its historic homes. For information, call (540) 676-2282.

Tazewell County

Tazewell County, in the heart of mountainous Southwest Virginia, is known for scenic Burke's Garden. Stories abound about the fiercely proud, independent people here. The story goes that Cornelius Vanderbilt wasn't the only tycoon who didn't impress the locals when they wouldn't sell him land on which to build the now-famous Biltmore estate (eventually built in Asheville, North Carolina). Auto magnate Henry Ford, in the company of inventors Thomas Edison and Harvey Firestone, couldn't get a check cashed by the locals while on a camping trip.

Tazewell County became famous in 1842 when Dr. Thomas English wrote the poem, "Sweet Alice, Ben Bolt," while visiting the county. The poem later became a world-famous hit song inspired by Tazewell's beauty. The **Burke's Garden** area, about 50 square miles of rich, beautiful farmland encircled by a continuous mountain range, a National Historic District, is the largest rural historical district in Virginia. Those wishing to see the fabled area at its best, with produce, arts and crafts, should attend the September fall festival sponsored by the Burke's Garden Community Association, (540) 963-3385.

Other important towns are Richlands, Bluefield, Cedar Bluff and Pocahontas. One infamous town is Frog Level, so tiny, it's hardly on the map. But Frog Level Yacht Club T-shirts sell briskly around the world and at the Frog Level Service Station.

The history of Tazewell County and Southwest Virginia is chronicled from prehistoric to present times at the **Historic Crab Orchard Museum and Pioneer Park**, (540) 988-6755, in Tazewell. The park, with its eight log and two stone structures and a building housing horse-drawn equipment, depicts the pioneer lifestyle.

Another interesting historical area is **Paint Lick Mountain**, where Native Americans left their writing, pictures and artifacts.

Experience the area's history first hand at the **Cedar Bluff Heritage Festival** in September. Arts and crafts are center stage, along with a country store, antiques and vintage clothing. You can watch cider, apple butter and soap being made, while local historians and storytellers entertain. For more information call James K. McGlothlin at (540) 964-4889.

Historic **Pocahontas**, the most interesting town in the county, is designated a Virginia Historic Landmark. The first mine there was opened in 1882. You can tour the **Pocahontas Exhibition Mine**, showing a spectacular 13-foot-high coal seam. The mine is open May through October. For tour information, call (540) 945-5959. The **Coal Miner's Memorial** is in nearby Boissevain. If you get hungry, munch on the ribs at Cuz' Uptown Barbeque, a restored barn in Pounding Mill that features a "Cow and Elvis" decor. Or, if you're a tad fussier, shop and sip at the Tea and Sympathy gift shop and tea room on U.S. 19 S. in Claypool Hill.

For more about the area, call the Tazewell Area Chamber of Commerce & Visitors Center at (540) 988-5091, the Richlands Area Chamber of Commerce at (540) 963-3385, or Greater Bluefield Chamber of Commerce at (304) 327-7184.

Buchanan County

This is real coal country, on the Appalachian Plateau where nearly half of Virginia's coal — nearly 50 million tons — is produced. Despite an unstable employment picture, Buchanan County's residents know how to have a good time and have a great recreational area, **Breaks Interstate Park**, 4,200 acres nicknamed the "Grand Canyon of the South." The park has the largest canyon east of the Mississippi, carved by the Russell Fork River and guarded by sheer vertical walls. In a succession of waterfalls and rapids, the river lunges over and around massive boulders. Whitewater rafting is available, water conditions permitting. The coal exhibit at the visitors center is one of the most popular here. It hosts the annual, three-day **Autumn Gospel Sing Festival** on Labor Day weekend.

For more information, call the Buchanan County Chamber of Commerce at (540) 935-4147.

Russell County

Russell County, population 31,761, is famous for its coal mines, agriculture and incredible mountain scenery. Even the nomad, Daniel Boone, found Russell, "The Redbud Capital of the World," so beautiful that he put down roots here for a couple of years. One site to see is the House and Barn Mountain, a mountain named for these particular shapes.

For some of the best fishing east of the Mississippi, don't pass up the **Clinch River**, also a favorite with canoers. Lebanon's county park is home to a crystal clear waterfall. Camping is permitted.

The most popular festival here is the month-long **Honaker Redbud Festival**, named for the delicate Virginia budding tree that dots the mountains each spring. The county's fair in Castlewood each September is another fun event. The **Southwest Virginia Music Festival** in Belfast, held Labor Day weekend, is also well-attended.

For more information about Russell County, call the Russell County Chamber of Commerce at (540) 889-8041.

Dickenson County

Dickenson County is rich in history and mountain heritage. The Russell Fork provides world-class whitewater rafting, Class III to IV-plus, and some of the most breathtaking scenery east of the Grand Canyon. Hundreds of people each weekend brave the river, putting in at historic **Yellow Poplar Splashdam**. Call or write the Dickenson County Chamber at (540) 926-4328 for a rafting schedule. Part of Breaks Interstate Park reach into this county.

Each fall, **Pioneer Days** and the county fair celebrate a rich Appalachian heritage. The **Cumberland Museum and Art Gallery** in the county seat of Clintwood is dedicated to the preservation of the area's vanishing art and artifacts; call (540) 926-6632.

Another notable site is the historic **Fremont Train Station**, which has been restored near its original site at the intersection of Va. 63 and 83. And the homeplace of legendary bluegrass music duo Ralph and Carter Stanley, on Va. 643, is where Ralph holds his annual **Bluegrass Festival**.

If you're a railroad fan, don't miss Dennis Reedy's own railroad museum in Clinchco. He'll show you around by appointment; call (540) 835-9593.

For more information, call the Dickenson County Chamber at (540) 926-4326).

Wise County

Wise County, like others nearby, is a treasure trove of scenery, culture and attractions. However, it has more of them than most of its neighbors, with numerous recreational areas, a major outdoor drama and four museums.

Recreational opportunities abound in the Washington and Jefferson National Forest. Norton offers **Flag Rock Recreational Area** and **High Knob**, where you can see several states from one viewpoint. Another scenic overlook is Powell Valley. You can fish and camp at **North Fork Reservoir** in Point and **Oxbow Lake** in St. Paul.

Wise County's towns are also worth exploring. You'll know **Big Stone Gap** is special when you see that its visitors center is a restored railway car, Interstate Car #101, which has an illustrious history. For more information, call (540) 523-2060. The town is noted for its outdoor drama, *Trail of the Lonesome Pine*, staged during July and August at June Tolliver Playhouse, (800) TRAIL-LP. The play, based on the John Fox, Jr., novel, has been performed on the site of this historic event since 1964. The author's home is now a museum and national and Virginia Historical Landmark. Call (540) 523-2747.

Big Stone Gap has two other museums. Virginia Attorney General Rufus Ayers' 1893 three-story, native cut stone home houses the **Southwest Virginia Museum**. Call (540) 523-1322. And the **Harry Meador Coal Museum**, E. Shawnee Street and Shawnee Avenue, provides a peek at the history of this area's cornerstone industry. Admission is free. The department also oversees **Miners Park**, a monument to coal field workers in downtown.

Each October, Mountain Empire College in Big Stone Gap celebrates a **Home**

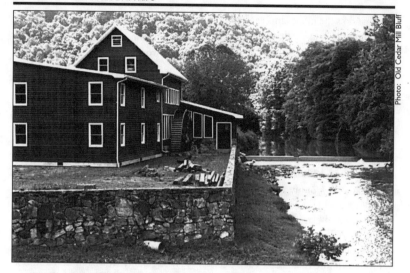

Photo: Old Cedar Mill Bluff

Old Cedar Bluff Mill is one of the region's major heritage tourist attractions.

Crafts Day, with traditional Appalachian crafts, demonstrations, storytelling, ethnic foods, dancing and music.

The town of Norton is another focal point of home crafts and historical preservation. **Country Cabin** is co-sponsored by Clinch Valley College and Appalachian Traditions, a nonprofit organization dedicated to preservation, promotion and perpetuation of traditional Appalachian culture. Each Saturday night, the public can attend performances of traditional mountain music. Appalachian Traditions also sponsors the annual **Dock Boggs Festival**, a one-day celebration of traditional mountain music, on the second Saturday in September.

Also be sure to see **Bee Rock Tunnel** on U.S. 23-Business. It's listed in *Ripley's Believe It or Not* as the "Shortest Railroad Tunnel in the World." Other attractions are the **Bullitt Mine Complex**, Westmoreland Coal dump train and the **Rotary Dump**, a machine that turns railroad cars upside down and empties the contents into a bin below.

For more sites to see, call the Wise County Chamber of Commerce at (540) 679-0961.

Scott County

Daniel Boone passed through this scenic wonderland on the Wilderness Road, and Scott County still prides itself on its gorgeous scenery, which inspired the country ballad, "Wildwood Flower." It's also home to the **Natural Tunnel State Park**. Since 1880, when statesman William Jennings Bryan declared it the "Eighth Wonder of the World," the million-year-old Natural Tunnel has attracted sightseers from all parts of the country. Daniel Boone was one of the first non-natives to see it. A video at the visitors center highlights historical and recreational attractions nearby. For more information, call the state park at (540) 940-2674.

Another major attraction is the **Carter Family Fold**, the homeplace of Sara and Maybelle Carter. Maybelle's daughter,

June, is the wife of singer Johnny Cash. It features a country music museum and live music every Saturday night. It's on A.P. Carter Highway in Hiltons. Call (540) 386-9480.

For more information, call the Scott County Chamber of Commerce at (540) 386-6665

Lee County

Last but certainly not least, at the tip of Virginia, triangle-shaped Lee County, bordering Kentucky and Tennessee, offers beautiful rolling hills and valleys nestled in the Tennessee River Basin. It is home to the Cumberland Gap, used by early settlers as the only means of passage during westward expansion. **Cumberland Gap National Historical Park** and the Washington and Jefferson National Park are also here.

The northern part of Lee has nearly 12,000 acres of the Jefferson forest for hiking, hunting, camping, picnicking, backpacking and sightseeing. **Lake Keokee**, a 92-acre waterway for fishing, boating and picnicking, and **Cave Springs Recreation Area**, a small lake for swimming and camping add other options. **Stone Mountain Trail**, 11 miles long, is a difficult but popular hiking trail here.

The **Cumberland Gap Park**, commemorating Daniel Boone and other early settlers, is in the extreme western portion of the county. On the edge of the park is **Cudjo's Caverns**, three levels of natural caves used by Native Americans

and Civil War soldiers. The camp features camping, hiking and the **Hensley Settlement**, a restored turn of the century mountain community that is a symbol of the determination and true grit of the early American pioneer. Shuttle bus service is provided, or you can go by horseback. Call (606) 248-2817.

The 26-acre **Cumberland Bowl Park** in Jonesville has swimming facilities, picnic tables and pavilions, a walking trail and children's playground. Plays are performed regularly in the amphitheater. **Leeman Field**, in Pennington Gap, has swimming, tennis courts and a horse ring and is the site of the annual **Lee County Fair** in August and **Tobacco and Fall Festival** in October. Another interesting site is the **African-American Historical Cultural Center**, (540) 546-5144, in Pennington Gap, housing a comprehensive collection of historical artifacts presided over by a full-time curator.

A mile north of Pennington Gap on Old Harlan Road, look for **Stone Face Rock**, a stone formation in the shape of an Indian's head that can be seen day or night. Widely believed to be a natural phenomenon, some theorists claim it is an ancient Cherokee Indian head carved by the Cherokees to mark the entrance to their holy grounds.

Lee is a few hours away from the Great Smokey Mountains and the Tennessee Valley Authority lakes. For more information, call the Lee County Chamber of Commerce at (540) 346-7766.

Index of Advertisers

"Go Pal" Bicycle Shop	260
200 South Street Inn	333
309 First Street	Insert
Afton Mountain Vineyards	Insert
Anchor House Resturant	409
Antique Fetish	265
Artists in Cahoots	Inside front cover
Arts and Valley Co-op	Insert
Arturro's	Insert
Awful Arthur's	385, Insert
Belle Meade B&B	317
Bizarre Bazaar	245
Bleu Rock Inn	318
Blue Ridge Brewing Co.	397
Blue Ridge Restaurant	469
Blue Wheel Bicycles	260
Boar's Head Inn	279
Books, Strings & Things	Insert
Brierley Hill	308
Brookside	295
C & O Restaurant	399
Carlos Brazilian International Cuisine	Insert
Cavalier Inn/Best Western	363
Center in the Square	Insert
Charcoal Steak House	Insert
Charlottesville Guide	11
Chateau Morrisette	141
Clifton Country Inn	325
College Inn	261
Comfort Inn-Airport	Insert
Cox Cable/Roanoke	24
Days Hotel - Charlottesville	364
Deer Lane Cottages	294
Dickenson Co. Chamber of Comm.	467
Dominion Lodging	Insert
Downtown Roanoke	Insert
Eastern Motor Inns, Inc.	Insert
Eastern Standard	400
English Inn	365
Fairview	336
Fancy Hill Motel	357
Fantasies Gift Shop	Inside front cover
For The Birds, Inc	Insert
Foster Harris House	318
Frederick House	301, Insert
Front Royal Canoe Co.	85
Gallery 3	Insert
Garment District	261
Gay Street Inn	Inside front cover
George C. Marshall Museum	
	Inside front cover
Ginger Hill	329
Graves Mountain Lodge	301
Green Fields	Insert
Greenskeeper/Baja Bean Co.	260, 261
Guests, Inc.	Insert
Hampton Inn - Charlottesville	365
Handcraft House	257
Hardware Store Restaurant	401
Hearth N' Holly Inn	297
Heartwood Books	260
Heritage House	318
Holiday Inn Express	Insert
Holiday Inn Airport	359
Holiday Inn Salem	360
Holiday Inn Tanglewood	Insert
Holiday Inn - Lexington	357
Honeysuckle Hill	Insert
Hotel Roanoke	Insert
Hotel Strasburg	352
House Unique Galleria, Inc.	Insert
Howard Johnson & Quality Inn	367
Hummingbird Inn	312
Inn at Keezletown Rd.	Index
Inn at Monticello	329
Inn at Narrow Passage	303
Inn at Sugar Hollow Farm	329
Inn at Union Run	308
Jefferson Vineyards	135
Jordon	255

Jordon Hollow Farm	303	River'D Inn	293
Joshua Wilton House	301	Roanoke Catholic School	463
Kathy's	Insert	Roanoke Marriott	Insert
Keswick Hall	281	Roanoke Regional Airport Comission	Insert
Knights Inn	366, Insert	Roanoke Valley Convention &	
La De Da	Insert	Visitors Bureau	Insert
La Maison Restaurant	Insert	Roanoker	Insert
Lexington Historical Shop	Inside front cover	Roccoco's	405
Little Chef	395	Rocklands	322
Little Shop of Madison	257	Ruby Rose Inn	295
Llewellyn Lodge at Lexington	307	Shenandoah Acres Resort	Insert
Longdale Bed & Breakfast	297	Shenandoah River Outfitters	294
Luigi's Resturant	Insert	Shenandoah Valley Travel Assoc.	7
Lynchburg College	451	Shenandoah Vineyards	143
Mac and Bobs	Insert	Sheraton Inn Charlottesville	367
Macado's	261	Sheraton Inn Airport	Insert
Market Street Wine Shop	136	Silver Linings	Insert
Mayne View	293	Silver Thatch Inn	332
McCormicks	Insert	South River Grill	Insert
Mediterranean Italian	Insert	Sperryville Emporium	149
Memory and Co.	403	Spring Farm Inn	294
Mill Mountain Coffee & Tea	Insert	St. Anne's Belfield School	459
Milton House B&B	295	Steeles Tavern Manor	309
Mincer's	260	Stonewall Jackson House	Inside front cover
Mountian Laurel Restaurant	469	Sugar Tree Inn	307
Museum of the American Frontier		Tanglewood Mall	Insert
	Inside front cover, Insert	The Colonnades	435
New Mountian Mercantile	469	The Gift Shop of Woodrow	
Northcross	461	Wilson's Birthplace	Insert
Oak Grove/The Park	427	The Inn at Meander Plantation	322
Oakencroft Vineyard	137	The Landing Restaurant	409
Olde Mill Golf Resort	473	The Mark Addy	334
Omni Charlottesville Hotel	366	Tivoli	322
Oregano Joe's	404	Virginia Born and Bred	Inside front cover
P. Buckley Moss Museum	147, Insert	Virginia Dare Cruise Boat	Insert
Palmer Country Manor	330	Virginia Metalcrafters	153
Pappagallo	Inside front cover	Virginia Military Institute	Inside front cover
Peaks of Otter Lodge	359	Washington And Lee University	449
Primland Hunting Reserve	473	Waynesboro Village Factory Outlets	Insert
Prince Michel De Virginia	139	Wayside Inn	352
Prospect Hill	331	Wertz's Country Store	249, Insert
Pulaski/ The Town of	33	Wilderness Canoe Co.	91
Radford University	446	Willies Hair Design	260
Radisson Patrick Henry	362	Willow Grove Inn	324
Ramada Inn	367	Willson Walker House	Inside front cover
Ramada Inn Lexington	357	Wintergreen Farm Sheepskin Shoppe	469
Random Row	404	Wong's	Insert
Rising Sun Bakery	261	Woodruff House	294
River House	303		

Index

Symbols

1740 House Antiques 258
1763 Inn and Restaurant 316, 393
1817 Antique Inn, The 327
1996 GOP Mock Election 165
200 South Street 333
309 First Street 391, 421

A

A Taste of Middleburg 171
Aberdeen Barn 396
Abingdon Visitors &
          Convention Bureau 474
Abram's Delight
          Candlelight Tour 190
Abram's Delight Museum 196
Affair in the Square 186
African American
          Heritage Festival 183
African-American Heritage
          Month 165
African-American Historical
          Cultural Center 478
Afton House Antiques 259
Afton Mountain 12
Afton Mountain Vineyards 142
Aileen Stores Inc. 245
Airports 440
Airshow 169
Airshow and Hot Air
          Balloon Festival 181
Albemarle County 31
Albemarle County Fair 183
Aldie Harvest Festival 186
Alexander's 383
Alleghany Cafe 424
Alleghany County 52
Alleghany Highlands Arts
          & Crafts Center 238
Always Roxie's 273
Alzheimer's Disease and Related

Disorders Support 438
American Association of
          Retired Persons 437
Amerind Gallery 252
Amherst County 34
An Evening of Elegance 172
Anchor House, The 409
Anchy's 411
Anderson Cottage 55
Andre Viette Farm
          and Nursery 12
Animal Farms 146
Annual Harvest Festival 182
Annual Hunt Country
          Stable Tour 174
Annual Kite Day 171
Annual Raft Race 179
Annual Zoo Boo 186
Antique and Classic
          Car Show 176
Antique Bottle and Collectible
          Show 166
Antique Car Show 170
Antique Collectors 258
Antique Mart, The 246
Antique Orchid Herbary 474
Antique Sale & Quilt Show 168
Antiques 5, 10, 164, 165, 176,
    185, 244, 246, 247, 250, 251,
    252, 256, 257, 258, 264, 267, 268
Antiques and Accents 255
Appalachia Coal and
          Railroad Days 181
Appalachian Center for
          Poets and Writers 474
Appalachian Mountain Christmas 191
Appalachian Traditions 477
Appalachian Trail 20, 84, 85, 470
Appalachian Trail Conference 176
Appalachian Trail Days 173, 470
Apple Barn 252
Apple Blossom Festival 121, 170
Apple Butter Making Festival 187
Apple Core Village Gift Shop 354
Apple Festival 184
Apple Harvest Arts
          & Crafts Festival 182

Appomattox 37
Appomattox Court House
        National Historical Park 69
Armory Art Gallery 233
Arnette's 262
Arnold's 424
Art Farm Galleries 205
Art Museum of Western Virginia 210
Art Show 170
Arthur's 248
Artists in Cahoots 205, 250
Arts & Crafts Festival 180
Arts and Crafts Bazaar 190
Arts and Crafts Festival 173
Arts and Culture 193
Arts Council of Central Virginia 227
Arts Council of the Blue Ridge 209
Arts Festival 177
Arturo's Italian Kitchen 383
Artworks 259
Ash Lawn-Highland 31, 223
Ash Lawn-Highland Spring Garden
        Week Wine Festival 168
Ashby Inn 316
Ashby Inn & Restaurant 392
Ashleys 274
Ashton Country House 300
Asian French Cafe 384
Augusta County 10, 247, 428
Autumn Gospel Sing Festival 475
Autumn Hill Vineyards/Blue
        Ridge Winery 140
Avenel 177
Awful Arthur's Seafood
        Company 384, 396, 421

B

Bacchanalian Feast 187
Back Creek Pump Storage Station 53
Back Street Cafe 392
Back to Berkeleys 361
Bacova Guild 248
Factory Outlet 274
Baja Bean Co. 396
Baldwin Park 437
Baldwin Place 429

Barboursville Ruins 30
Barboursville Vineyards 29, 140
Barr-ee Station 262
Barracks Road Shopping Center 263
Barter Theatre 465, 472
Baseball 25, 152
Bateau Festival, The 36
Bateau Landing 36, 407
Bath County 55, 417
Bath County Historical
        Society Museum 238
Battle of Cedar Creek 64
Living History and Reenactment 185
Battle of Cloyd's Mountain 63
Battle of Front Royal 66
Battle of New Market 62
Battle of Staunton River
        Bridge Reenactment 174
Battlefields Wilderness
        Battlefields 30
Bavarian Chef, The 395
Bay Pottery, The 247
Bayly Art Museum 220
Beale Treasure 42
Bear Mountain Outdoor School 239
Bed and Breakfast Inns 289
Bedford 40
Bedford City/County
        Museum 70, 230
Bedford County 266, 433, 434
Bedford House 41
Bedrooms of America Museum 198
Bee Rock Tunnel 477
Belle Boyd Cottage 66
Belle Grae Inn 247, 302, 420
Belle Grove Plantation 65, 196
Belle Meade Bed & Breakfast 317
Bent Mountain Lodge 344
Bernard's Landing
        Resort 39, 280, 369
Best Friend Festival 178
Best Seller, The 251
Best Western Cavalier Inn 364
Best Western Coachman 358
Best Western Inn at Hunt Ridge 356
Best Western Inn at Valley View 358
Best Western Keydet-General

Motel 355
Best Western Radford Inn 370
Best Western Red Lion 369
Best Western Staunton Inn 354
Beth Gallery and Press 221
Beverley, The 379
Bicycle Festival 179
Big Lots 269
Big Meadows Lodge 76, 79
Big Meadows Wayside 76, 79
Big Stone Gap 476
Big Stone Gap Country Fair 173
Big Walker Mountain
     and Lookout 471
Bikecentennial Trail 84
Billy's Ritz 385
Biltmore Grill 397, 422
Bisset Park 51
Bistro Bar 420
Bits, Bytes & Books 244
Black Orchid II Restaurant 364
Blacksburg 46, 267, 341, 411
Blacksburg Marriott 370
Bleak-Thrift House 256
Blessing of the Hounds 189
Bleu Rock Inn 317, 393
Blue Bend 55, 132
Blue Bird Cafe 397
Blue Grass Festival 173
Blue Ridge Board of Realtors 427
Blue Ridge Brewing
     Company, The 397, 422
Blue Ridge Dinner Theatre 199, 232
Blue Ridge Draft Horse and
     Mule Show 179
Blue Ridge Farm Museum 232
Blue Ridge Folklife Festival 188, 232
Blue Ridge Heritage Festival 180
Blue Ridge Homebuilders
     Association 433
Blue Ridge Institute 131, 233
Blue Ridge Institute
     Museums 130, 231
Blue Ridge Mountain Sports 264
Blue Ridge Music Festival 177, 228
Blue Ridge Parkway 73, 86
Blue Ridge Polo Club 160

Blue Ridge Pottery 29, 243, 258
Blue Ridge Restaurant 49, 413
Blue Stone Inn 377
Blue Wheel Bicycles 262
Bluefield 474
Bluegrass Festival 476
Bluemont Concert Series 174, 176
Blues Festival 182
Boar's Head Inn & Sports
     Club 162, 278, 279, 397
Boating 92
Bob Beard Antiques 252
Bogen's 411
Bonnie Blue National
     Horse Show 172
Bonsack 23
Book Gallery, The 264
Booker T. Washington
     National Monument 130
Books, Strings & Things 254
Bookstack, The 248
Bookstore, The 266
Bookstores 244, 247, 251,
     259, 263, 264
Boone's Country Store 43, 267
Boones Mill Apple Festival 43, 184
Botetourt County 17, 251, 252
Botetourt Museum 208
Bottle and Pottery Show
     and Sale 182
Bowling Green Golf Club 105
Boyd, Belle 5
Braford Antiques 250
Brandon Oaks 437
Brasa Restaurant and Tapas Bar 398
Breaks Interstate Park 475
Breckinridge, John C. 62
Bridge Club 423
Bridge Street Antiques 266
Bridgewater Air Park 443
Bridgewater College 448
Bridgewater Marina and Boat
     Rentals 40, 266
Bridgewater Para-Sail 266
Bridgewater Plaza 266
Brierley Hill 309
Brookfield Christmas Tree

Plantation 49
Brookneal-CampbellCounty
    Airport Authority 444
Brookside Restaurant, The 376
Brownsburg 250
Brush Mountain Arts and
    Crafts Fair 167
Brush Mountain Inn B&B 341
Bryce Resort 116, 122, 275, 427
Buchanan 17
Buchanan County 475
Chamber of Commerce 475
Buena Vista 250
Buena Vista Labor Day Festival 183
Buffalo Springs Herb Farm 251
Builders & Associates of
    Central Virginia 434, 435
Bullpasture Valley 273
Burke's Garden 474
Burnley Vineyards 140
Bus Lines 444
Byrd Visitor Center 76
Byrd's Walden Pond Products 49

C

C and O Restaurant 398
C&O Historical Society Archives 53
C&S Galleries 272
Cabins 76
Cabins at Brookside 353
Cafe Albert 417
Cafe France 407
Cafe Sofia 375
Cambria Emporium 48, 268
Cambria Whistlestop
    Arts Festival 177
Camp Gallery 228
Campbell County 434
Campgrounds 77
Camping 105
Candy Shop, The 250
Canoe Outfitters 92
Capt'n Sam's Landing 378
Car and Carriage Caravan 123
Car Flea Market and Corral 175
Car Rentals 441

Car Show 176
Carlos Brasilian International
    Cuisine 385
Carol Lee Doughnuts 424
Carolina Hosiery 265
Carousel Antiques 257
Carradoc Hall/Ramada Inn 364
Carriage Court 347
Carriage Outings, Inc. 30
Carroll County 468
Casanova Hunt Point-to-Point 165
Cascades 50, 98
Casey's Country Store 269
Casino, The 417
Cass Scenic Railroad 55
Castle Rock Recreation Area 50
Cat & Owl Steak and
    Seafood House 415
Catholic Church Museum 211
Cat's Meow Collectibles 252
Cave Mountain Lake 98
Cave Springs Recreation Area 478
Caverns 148
Cedar Bluff 474
Cedar Bluff Heritage Festival 475
Cedar Creek Battlefield Foundation
    and Re-enactment 64
Cedar Creek Relic Shop 66, 244
Cellar Restaurant 424
Celtic Festival 175
Cemeteries 65, 66, 68, 69, 70
Center in the Square 216
Chalet High 428
Chalot's Antiques 246
Champagne and Candlelight Tour 166
Champions Italian Eatery
    and Cafe 423
Charades 421
Charcoal Steak House 386
Charleys 407
Charlottesville 31, 258, 422, 431
Charlottesville and University
    Symphony Orchestra 219
Charlottesville Area
    Association of Realtors 433
Charlottesville Gamelan
    Ensemble 219

Charlottesville Transit Service 445
Charlottesville-Albemarle
        Airport 440
Chateau Morrisette Winery
        49, 144, 270, 467
Chatham 340
Chautauqua Festival in the Park 178
Chautauque Festival 470
Cheers 422
Cheese Shop, The 12, 249
Chermont Winery Inc. 143
Cherry Tree Players 229
Chesapeake & Ohio
        Historical Society 239
Chessie Nature Trail 15, 124
Chestnut Creek at Bernard's
        Landing 105, 113
Chihamba 219
Children's Day at the Market 172
Children's Parade 127
Chilhowie Apple Festival 185
Chili Cook-Off 180
Chili Cook-off and Community
        School Strawberry Fes 22
Christendom College 448
Christiansburg 47, 268, 343, 412
Christiansburg Depot Museum 48
Christmas and Flower Show 190
Christmas at the Manse 190
Christmas at the Market 189
Christmas Gallery 245
Christmas in Dixieland 151
Christmas in the Country 189
Christmas Store, The 249
City Market 253
Civil War 61
Civil War Living History Weekend 65
Civil War Re-enactment 170
Civil War Weekend 177
Claiborne House
        Bed and Breakfast 44, 340
Claire's 244
Classic Collections 266
Clayborne's 420
Clayton's 407
Claytor Lake 52, 97, 103, 131
Claytor Lake Arts and Crafts Fair 184

Clifton — The Country Inn 325, 399
Clifton Forge 52, 346
Clinch River 475
Clinch Valley College 477
Cline, Patsy 196
Clothes Line 247
Coal Miner's Memorial 475
Cockram Mill 467
Cockram's General Store
        49, 131, 236, 269, 424
Cocoa Mill Chocolates 251
Coffee Exchange, The 399
Collector Car Flea
        Market and Corral 175
Collector's Choice 248
Collector's Corner 271
College Inn 399
College Sports 152
College Square Shopping
        Center 250, 251
Colonial Art and Craft Shop 244
Colonnades, The 438
Colony House Motor Lodge 358
Colony of Virginia Ltd., The 272
Comfort Inn 354, 356,
        364, 368, 369, 371
Comfort Inn —
        Roanoke/Troutville 358
Comfort Inn Airport 358
Comfort Inn Radford 370
Commonwealth Park 156
Community Children's Theatre 129
Community Market 265
Concert Music Hall 423
Confederate Breastworks 59
Confederate Memorial Service 176
Confederate Museum 5
Confederate Winter Camp 165
Confetti's 421
Conservation Festival 176
Consolidated Shoe Store 265
Constitution Day Celebrations 183
Coopers Corner 410
Coors Concert Series 207
Copper Kettle Lounge 116
Corned Beef & Co. 386
Cornerstone Bed and Breakfast 315

Count Pulaski Bed & Breakfast and Gardens 344
Country Cabin 477
Country Fare 291
Country Garden Antiques 257
Country Goose Gift and Craft Shop 247
Country Manor 256
Country Mouse, The 258
Country Store Antique Mall 258
County Christmas House 270
County Records or County Sales 270
Coupe de Ville's 400
Court Days Festival 176
Court Square Tavern 399
Courthouse Antiques 255
Courtyard by Marriott 364
Covered Bridges 145
Covington 52, 346
Cowpasture River 56
Crab Orchard Museum and Pioneer Park 173
Craddock-Terry Shoe Factory Outlet 265
Crafters Fair 178
Crafter's Gallery, The 262
Crafts 243, 244, 245, 246, 248, 250, 251, 253, 256, 269
Craig County 18, 252
Craig County Museum 209
Creekside Village 244
Crestar 10-Miler 167
Crossroads Mall 254
Crows 55
Cudjo's Caverns 478
Culpeper County 256, 321
Culpeper Day 169
Cumberland Bowl Park 478
Cumberland Gap National Historical Park 478
Cumberland Museum and Art Gallery 476
Curiosity Shop 246

D

Daedalus Bookshop 259
Daleville 252
Damascus 470
Dancescape 219
Daniel Monument 69
Darby Needlecraft and Gifts 258
Days Inn 368
Dayton Autumn Celebration 187
Dayton Farmer's Market 246, 247
Dedmon Center 51
Deer Meadow Vineyard 134
Deerlane Cottages 353
Delaplane Strawberry Festival 172
DeLoach Antiques 259
Depot Antiques 10, 247
Depot Grille, The 10, 380
Derek's U-Spirit 262
Design Accessories 254
Diamond Hill 434
Diamond Hill Christmas Candlelight Tour 192
Dickens of a Christmas 191
Dickenson County 476
Dinner At Dusk 177
Dixie Caverns 151
Dixie Caverns Pottery 151
Dock Boggs Memorial Festival 184, 477
Doe Run Lodge Resort and Conference Center 79, 287, 371, 467
Dogwood Festival 167
Dominion Saddlery 255
Donkenny Fashion Outlet 269
Dooley's 367, 422
Douthat State Park 53
Down River Canoe Company 7, 93
Downtown Mall 263
Draft Horse and Mule Day 182
Draper Mercantile 272
Drapers Meadow 45
Dublin 52
Dudley Mart & Restaurant 410
Dulwich Manor 335
Durty Nelly's Pub 400, 422
Dusty's Antique Market 248

E

E.A. Clore Sons Inc. 243, 256
Eagle Nest Restaurant 416
Eagle Rock 18
Eagle's Nest Restaurant 55, 443
Early Time Antiques and
    Fine Art 258
Earth Gallery, The 256
East Coast Raw Bar 424
Easter Traditions 167
Eastern Mennonite College
    and Seminary 448
Eastern Standard Restaurant 400
Eastern Wine Festival at
    Morven Park 182
Edankraal 36
Edelweiss German Restaurant 380
Edgemont 432
Edgewood Farm Bed & Breakfast 323
Edgewood Farm Nursery 258
Edinburg 245
Edinburg Mill 66
Edinburg Ole' Time Festival 182
El Charro 377
El Dorado 375
El Rodeo Mexican Restaurant 386
Elder's Antique and
    Classic Autos 248
Elephant Walk, The 360, 421
Elizabeth Brown Park 470
Eljo's 262
Elks National Home 230
Elkton Autumn Days 186, 188
Elkwallow Wayside 77
Elm Park Estates 437
Elmer's Antiques 256
Elsie's Antique Shop 257
Emerson Creek Pottery 254, 267
Emil's 407
Emory & Henry College 456
Emporium, The 248
Enchanted Castle 30
Encore Gifts, Toys and
    Accessories Shop 271
Endless Caverns 150
English Inn, The 365

Estouteville 432
Eunice & Fester Antiques 257
Exchange Hotel 30
Executive Motel 370
Exhibition of Sporting Art 173

F

Factory Merchants Outlet Mall 470
Fairfax Hunt Steeplechase Races 183
Fairview Bed and Breakfast 336
Fairystone State Park 466
Faith Mountain Herbs and
    Antiques 256
Fall Fiber Festival & Sheep
    Dog Trials 186
Fall Foliage Festival 188
Fall Food Festival 184
Falwell Aviation Inc. 444
Falwell, Rev. Jerry 35
Family Folk Tale Festival 207
Fancy Hill Motel 357
Fantasies 251
Farfelu Vineyard 138
Farm Basket Shop, The 265
Farm Basket, The 408
Farmhouse, The 412
Fassifern 311
Fauquier County 255, 316
Fayerweather Gallery 221
Feed Mill, The 376
Ferrum College 43, 455
Festival Around Town 177
Festival by the James 177
Festival in the Park 22, 127, 172
Festival of Trees 189
Festival on the James 36
Festive Fare 404
Fete des Vendanges 139
Fifth Avenue Presbyterian
    Church Window 212
Fincastle 17, 251
Fincastle Festival 183
Fine Arts Center Shop 270
Finicky Filly, The 255
First Night Roanoke 191
First Night Virginia 191

Fishersville 12
Fishing 99, 284
Flag Rock Recreational Area 476
Flea Markets 244, 245
Fleetwood Farm 316
Fletcher Collins Theater 201
Flossie Martin Art Gallery 51
Floyd County 48, 269, 344
Flying Circus, The 128
Folk Arts and Crafts Festival 169
Foot Hunting 162
For the Birds 254
Forever Country 243
Fort Harrison 68
Fort Lewis Lodge 56, 113, 348
Fort Valley Riding Stable 108
Fort Young 53
Foster-Harris House 319
Fountain Hall Bed & Breakfast 321
Four & Twenty Blackbirds 394
Four County Players 218
Fox and Hounds Pub &
          Restaurant, The 378
Foxcroft School 457
Foxfield Races 161, 167, 168
Foxhunting 155
Frances Christian Brand
          Galleries 221
Franklin County 43, 267, 434
Franklin County Fall Arts and
          Crafts Festival 190
Fred Clifton Park 467
Frederick County Fair 179
Frederick House 302
Free Fishing Days 100, 101
Freeman, Dr. Douglas Southall 35
Freeman-Victorious Framing 262
Fremont Train Station 476
Friday Night Flatfooting
          Jamboree 269
Friendship Inn 359
Frog Level Yacht Club 474
From the Heart 267
Front Royal 5, 122, 244, 290, 426
Front Royal Canoe Company 92, 122
Front Royal-Warren County
          Airport 442

Frontier Festival 183
Full Moon Cafe 422
Fun Shop, The 255

G

Galax 468
Galax Mountain Music
          Jamboree 164, 468
Gallery 3 253
Gallery Cafe, Books and
          More 271, 412
Gallery of Mountain Secrets 274
Gamelan Ensemble 219
Gap Mountain 50
Garden Terrace Restaurant 118
Garland Hill 434
Garment District, The 262
Garth Newel Music Center 56, 239
Gatwick's Lounge 365
Gay Street Inn, The 319
General Store, The 250
George C. Marshall Museum 124
George Washington
          National Forest 124
Gift and Thrift Shop 246
Gifts Ahoy 266
Giles County 49, 270
Chamber of Commerce 50
Giles Little Theatre 50
Gilmore, Hamm and Snyder Inc. 264
Ginger Hill Bed & Breakfast 330
Ginseng Mountain Farm 274
Glass, Carter 36
Glen Maury Park 16
Glenmore 432
Glenmore Country Club 432
"Go Pal" Bicycle Shop 262
Golden Tub Bath Shop 248
Golf 103, 276, 279, 283, 285
Good Things On the Market 125
Gordonsville 30
Goshen Pass 13
Grady's Antiques 267
Grand Caverns 150
Grandin Movie Theatre 126, 215
Grandma's Bait Clothing Store 248

Grandma's Memories 271
Graves' Mountain Lodge 109, 321
Gray Ghost Vineyards 138
Grayson County 468
Grayson County Old Time
        Fiddler's Convention 178
Grayson Highlands State Park 468
Great American
        Duck Race 122, 180
Great Wagon Road 4
Greater Lynchburg
        Transit Company 445
Greater Piedmont Association
        of Realtors 431
Green Hill Equestrian Park 23
Green Tree, The 392
Green Valley Book Fair 247
Greenbrier Resort 52, 53
Greenbrier, The 284
Greene County 29, 258, 323
Greene House Shops 258
Greenfields 254
Greenskeeper Restaurant 401
Greenwood Antique Center 259
Grille, The 417
Guilford Ridge Vineyard 7, 135
Gun Show 165
Gunstock Creek Cooperative 41
Gypsy Hill Park 10

H

Hales Ford 266
Hales Ford Bridge 130
Hall of Valor Museum 6, 67, 122
Halloween Weekend 187
Hamiltons 266
Hamner, Earl Jr. 33
Hampton Inn 359, 365
Handcraft House 243, 257
Happy Birthday U.S.A. 178, 203
Harbortown Golf 266
Harbs' Bistro 381, 420
Hardware Store Restaurant, The 401
Harrison Heritage Museum 126
Harrison House 8
Harrison House (Fort Harrison) 201

Harrison Museum of African
        American Culture 210
Harrisonburg 8, 123,
        246, 300, 428
Harrisonburg-Rockingham
        Association of Realtors 428
Harry Meador Coal Museum 476
Harvest Festival on the Market 186
Haunted Caverns 186
Hearth N' Holly Inn 300
Heartwood Bookshop 259, 263
Heirloom Originals 267
Henry, Patrick 230
Henry Street African American
        Heritage Festival 183, 210
Henry Street Music Center 421
Hensley Settlement 478
Here and Now Art Gallery 270
Heritage Festival 7, 185
Heritage House 319
Heritage Repertory Theatre 218
Heritage Tourism Weeks 168
Herter Hall 239
High Country Restaurant 82
High Knob 476
High Valley Antiques and
        Collectibles 273
Highland County 56
Highland County Crafts 274
Highland County Maple Festival 57
Highland Inn 350, 372, 418
Highland Maple Festival 165
Highland County Arts Council 238
Highlands Arts & Crafts Center 273
Hiking 84
Hill High's Country Store 255
Hillsville Gun Show and
        Flea Market 468
Hilton — Lynchburg 368
Historic Car & Carriage
        Caravan 7, 150
Historic Crab Orchard Museum
        and Pioneer Park 475
Historic Fincastle Days 18
Historic Garden
        Week 159, 166, 207
Historic Old Newbern 238

Hockey 154
Hofauger Farmhouse 23
Holiday Inn Express 360
Holiday in Lexington 191, 207
Holiday Inn 351, 368, 416
Holiday Inn Airport 359
Holiday Inn Charlottesville/
        Monticello 366
Holiday Inn Covington 371
Holiday Inn Hotel Tanglewood 360
Holiday Inn Lexington 356
Holiday Inn of Blacksburg 370
Holiday Inn Salem 360
Holiday Inn Staunton 355
Hollins College 450
Holt's China 248
Holy Land USA 41
Holy Land USA Nature
        Sanctuary 230
Home Crafts Day 189, 476
Home Tour Gala 184
Homeplace, The 387
Homestead 56
Homestead Dining Room, The 418
Homestead Resort 111, 119,
        131, 283
Honaker Redbud Festival 168, 475
Hopkins Planetarium 126, 211
Horse Country 155
Horse Show 155, 174, 176
Horseback Riding 107
Horst Locher Ski School 116
Horton Cellars 140
Hospice of the Shenandoah Inc. 437
Hot Cakes 401
Hot Chilies Restaurant and Bar 412
Hot Springs 347
Hot-air Balloons 167
Hotel Roanoke & Conference
        Center 360
Hotel Strasburg 6, 352, 375
Hotels and Motels 351
Hottest Fun in the Sun
        Beach Day 180
House of Laird 340
House Unique Galleria 254
Howard Johnson

Lodge 356, 366, 369
Huckleberry, The 412
Hull's Drive-In 15, 207
Hume Ruritan Joust 159
Hummingbird Inn, The 312
Humpback Bridge 146
Hungry Mother Lake 103
Hungry Mother State
        Park 112, 180, 472
Hunt Country Tours 159
Hunt Country Winter
        Antiques Fair 164
Hunting 112
    Licenses 113
    Lodge 113
    Regulations 113
Hunting Hills 430
Hupp's Hill Battlefield Park &
        Study Center 66
Huyard's Country Kitchen 247, 377

I

Ice Cream Cottage 266
Ikenberry 252
Imperial Wok 416
Ingalls Field 444
Inn at Burwell Place, The 314
Inn at Gristmill Square 56
Inn at Keezletown Rd. 299
Inn at Little Washington,
        The 320, 394
Inn at Meander Plantation 321
Inn at Monticello 328
Inn at Narrow Passage, The 292
Inn at Sugar Hollow Farm, The 328
Inn at the Crossroads 328
Inn at Union Run, The 310, 382
Innkeeper Lynchburg 369
Innkeeper Motel 361
Innovations 262
International Bass Bonanza 172
International Gold Cup 187
Iris Inn, The 306
Iron Gate Gorge 53
Ironwood 429
Iroquois Club 421

Ivy Hill 434

J

J Rugles Restaurant 380
Jack Tale Players 43
Jack's Creek Covered Bridge 468
Jackson Statue 69
Jackson, Stonewall
        House 14, 68,124, 206
Jackson, Stonewall
        Memorial Cemetery 68
Jackson, Thomas J. "Stonewall" 62
Jackson's Headquarters 65
Jacob's Lantern 411
Jacob's Lounge 423
James Burke House Eatery 417
James Madison University 448
Dinner Theater 199
Life Science Museum 200
James River Basin
        Canoe Livery 15, 92, 94
James River Reeling and Rafting 94
James River Runners Inc. 94
Jasbo's at Ramada Inn 382
Jazz on the Lawn 144, 188
Jefferson Area Board for Aging 438
Jefferson Center 216
Jefferson Lodge, The 361
Jefferson, Thomas Visitors
        Center 224
Jefferson Vineyards Ltd. 33, 141
Jefferson's Tomato Fair 181
Jeff's Antiques 246
Jeweler's Eye, The 263
Johnny Appleseed Restaurant 354
Johnny Bull's Restaurant 368
Johnston, Andrew House 50
Johnston, Andrew Museum &
        Research Center 236
Jolly Roger Haggle Shop 247
Jones Memorial Library 35, 229
Jonesville 478
Jordan 258
Jordan Art Gallery 222, 259
Jordan Hollow Farm Inn 109, 296
Joshua Wilton House 377

Jousting 159, 187
Jousting Hall of Fame
        Tournament 175
J's Gourmet 244

K

Kafkafe 401, 423
Kaleidoscope 36, 184
Katie's Country Club 422
Keep Bed and Breakfast, The 310
Keller & George 264
Kenwood 304
Keswick Estate 432
Keswick Hall 278
Kids Kastoffs 267
Kidstuff 121
Killahevlin 290
Kimberly's Antiques and Linens 244
King William Regional
        Arts Center 474
Kinsinger's Kountry Kitchen 12, 249
Knights Court 371
Knight's Inn 361, 366
Knob Restaurant and
        Lounge, The 360
Krissia 264
Kurtz Cultural Center 3, 196

L

La De Da 254
La Maison Du Gourmet 387
Labor Day Spectacular 183
Lacey Springs 377
Lake Keokee 478
Lake Moomaw 53, 102
Lake Sherwood 55
Lakeview Restaurant at
        Douthat State Park 416
Lambsgate 306
Landing Restaurant, The 282, 409
Landmark Steakhouse and
        Lounge, The 408
Langhorne Manor 337
Lantern Tours 203
L'Arche 342
Latimer-Shaeffer Theatre 199

L'Auberge Provençale 374
Lavender Hill Farm 111, 313
Layman's 252
Le Chien Noir Restaurant 49, 414
League of Older
      Americans 437, 439
Lee Chapel 14, 68, 206
Lee County Chamber of
      Commerce 478
Lee Hi Truck Stop Restaurant 383
Lee, Robert E. 62, 68
Lee Statue 69
Leeman Field 478
Leesburg 217, 254
Leesburg Flower and
      Garden Festival 167
Leesburg Hauntings 186
Lenfest Center for the
      Performing Arts 206, 420
Les Fabriques 263
Levy's 264
Lewis Glaser Inc. 262
Lewis Mountain Cabins 76
Lewisburg 55
Lexington 12, 250, 309, 429
Lexington Historical Shop 250
Liberty Lake Park 41
Liberty University 454
Library, The 387
Lily's 388
Lime Kiln Theatre 15, 125,
      171, 207, 420
Limeton Pottery 243, 244
Lincoln Homestead 201
Linden Vineyards and
      Orchards 5, 137
L'Italia Restaurant and Lounge 378
Little Chef, The 395
Little Gallery, The 266
Little John's 402
Little Shop of Madison, The 256
Little Sorrel 68, 124, 206
Live Arts 218
Livestock Auction 170
Llewellyn Lodge at Lexington 311
Log Cabin Antiques 246
Lonesome Pine Arts and Crafts

Festival 168
Longdale Inn Bed & Breakfast 53, 346
Longdale Recreation Area 53
Longwood Cemetery 70
Looking Glass House 334
Loudoun County 254, 315
Loudoun County Civil
      War Roundtable 165
Loudoun Valley Vineyard 136
Loveladies Antiques 255
Lovers Leap 467
Lovingston Cafe 381
Lowell's Restaurant and Lounge 421
Lucy Selina Furnace 53
Luigi's 388
Luray 7, 123, 245, 293
Luray Caverns 123, 149
Luray Caverns Airport 443
Luray Caverns Car and
      Carriage Caravan 199
Luray Reptile Center and
      Dinosaur Park 7, 123
Luray Singing Tower 198
Lynchburg 34, 227, 264, 433
Lynchburg Association of
      Realtors 434
Lynchburg College 453
Lynchburg Fine Arts Center 227
Lynchburg Hillcats 152
Lynchburg Mansion Inn Bed
      and Breakfast 337
Lynchburg Museum at Old
      Court House 69, 228
Lynchburg Regional Airport 441

M

Mabry Mill 236, 466
Mabry Mill Blue Ridge Parkway
      Visitors Center 49
Mabry Mill Coffee Shop 82
Mac 'N' Bob's 388
Macado's 388, 402
Macado's Restaurant and
      Delicatessen 413
Madam Russell House 472
Madison County 256, 321

Madison Heritage Weeks 169
Madison House Bed & Breakfast,
   The 338
Madison, James Museum 220
Magic City Station 252
Magic Tricks 262
Maharaja 402
Maier Museum of Art 228, 454
Main Street Antiques 257
Main Street Program 436
Maintree Farm 107
Mallard Point 52, 436
Mama's Treasures 245
Manor at Taylor's Store, The 341
Maple Festival 57
Maple Hall 383
Maple Museum 239
March & Battle for Preservation 175
Mariner's Landing 40
Marion's Cafe 417
Mark Addy, The 334
Market Street Wineshop
   and Gourmet Grocery 263
Marriott Ranch 108
Marshall, George C.
   Museum and Library 205
Martha Washington Inn 472, 474
Martha's Cafe 402
Martin, Flossie Gallery 236
Mary Baldwin College 10, 448
Mary Bladon House, The 313
Massanutten 276
Massanutten Association
   of Realtors 428
Massanutten Homeowners
   Association 428
Massanutten Mountain Resort 123
Massanutten Resort 9, 117
Massanutten Trail Rides Inc. 107
Massanutten Village 428
Max 423
May Fest 173
Mayberry Presbyterian Church 467
Mayberry Trading Post 467
Mayfest 144
Mayne View, The 293
McCormick Farm 208

McCormick's Pub and
   Restaurant 304, 420
McDowell Battlefield 59
McDowell Presbyterian Church 71
McGuffey Art Center,
   The 32, 222, 259
McHone Antique Jewelry 246
McLean Falconer 425
Mead Associates, Realtors 425, 430
Meadow Lane Lodge 56, 349
Meadowridge 434
Meadows Farm Golf Course 105
Meadows of Dan 269, 467
Meadowwood 434
Meals on Wheels 438
Meander Inn at Penny Lane Farm 335
Mediterranean Italian &
   Continental Cuisine 388
Meems Bottom Bridge 145
Memory and Company 403
Mennonite 246, 249
Meredyth Vineyards 136
Merrie Olde England
   Christmas Festival 191
Michie Tavern 223, 403
Mid-Atlantic Chamber Orchestra 202
Middle Street Gallery 218
Middleburg 255
Middleburg Antiques Center 255
Middleburg Horse Trials 157
Middleburg Polo 159
Middleton Inn, The 320
Middletown 4, 122
Midsummer Eve 175
Miki Liszt Dance Company 219
Mill Mountain Coffee & Tea 25, 422
Mill Mountain Star 21
Mill Mountain Theatre 215
Mill Mountain Zoological
   Park 21, 125, 147
Mill Street Grill 420
Millboro 348
Miller Regional Art Center 235
Miller School of Albemarle, The 459
Miller's 422
Milmont Greenhouses 12
Milton Hall Bed & Breakfast Inn 347

Milton House Bed & Breakfast 298
Mincer's 263
Miners Park 476
Miniature Graceland 216
Mish Mish 268
Miss Virginia Pageant 179
Misty Mountain Vineyards Inc. 139
Monongahela National Forest 98
Montdomaine Cellars 142
Monterey 56
Montfair Stables 110
Montgomery Museum 235
Monticello 31, 224
Monticello Holiday Open House 190
Monticello Wine and
        Food Festival 187
Montpelier 30, 224
Montpelier Hunt Races 189
Montpelier Wine Festival 168
Morven Park 217
Morven Park Horse Trials 157
Moss, P. Buckley Museum 12
Mount Rogers 466, 468
Mount Rogers Naturalist Rally 173
Mount Rogers Ramp Festival 173
Mount Rogers
        Recreation Area 91, 468
    Mountain Biking 91
Mountain Biking 89, 276
    Tour Companies 91
Mountain Coffee and Tea 389
Mountain Cove Vineyards 143
Mountain Empire College 476
Mountain Inn 118
Mountain Lake 413
Mountain Lake Hotel and
        Resort 50, 286
Mountain Lake Symposium
        & Gallery 236
Mountain Springs Stables 108
Mountain Store 257
Mountain View Acres 436
Mountaintop Ranch 109
Mowing Day 175
Mt. Rogers High Country
        Outdoor Center 111
Mt. Solon 123

Mulligan's Pub & Eatery 420
Murray's Fly Shop 100
Museum of American Cavalry 198
Museum of American Frontier
        Culture 10, 124, 202
Museums 66
Music at Twilight 174
Music Festival 177, 178
Music for Americans 179

N

Naked Mountain Vineyard 137
National Jousting Championship 187
Natural Bridge of
        Virginia 16, 277, 357
    Caverns 151
    Restaurants 383
    Wax Museum 124
    Zoo 147
Natural Chimneys Jousting
        Tournament 9, 181
Natural Chimneys Park 123
Natural Tunnel State Park 477
Nature by Design 264
Neighborhood Art Show 171
Nellysford 262
Nelson County 33, 334
Nelson County Summer
        Festival 134, 176, 177
New Castle Mercantile 252
New London Airport 444
New Market 6, 245
New Market Airport 443
New Market Arts & Crafts Show 182
New Market Battlefield Days Inn 353
New Market Battlefield Historical
        Park 6, 62, 198
New Market Heritage Days 171
New Market Battlefield
        Historical Park 67
Military Museum 67
New Mountain Mercantile 49, 269
New Mountain Mercantile Here
        and Now Gallery 235
New Play Competition 215
New River 45

New River Canoe Livery 92, 95
New River Community College 52
New River Cruise Company 415
New River Fine Arts Gallery 272
New River Trail State Park 468, 471
New River Valley Airport 444
New River Valley Arts and
         Crafts Guild 236
New River Valley Arts Council 234
New River Valley
         Association of Realtors 436
New River Valley Home
         Builders Association 436
New River Valley Horse Show 180
New River Valley Mall 268
New River Valley Speedway 154
Newbern Fall Festival of
         Arts & Crafts 188
Newcomb Hall Arts Space 222
Newman Library 234
Newport 50
Newport Agricultural Fair 181
Nicholas & Alexandra Gallery,
         The 259
North Cross School 461
North Fork Reservoir 476
North Mountain Vineyard
         & Winery 134
North-South Skirmish 170, 185
Norton 477
Norwood Art Gallery 271
Notre Dame Academy 457

O

Oak Grove Players 201
Oak Manor Farms 110
Oakencroft Holiday Open House 189
Oakencroft Vineyard and
         Winery 141
Oakland Grove
         Presbyterian Church 53
Oaks, The 269, 343
Oasis Vineyard 5, 138
Oatlands 217
Oatlands Sheep Dog Trials 169, 217
Oktoberfest 186

Old Blue Equestrian
         Sports Center 156
Old Cabell Hall 220
Old Church Gallery 235
Old Country Store 266
Old Fincastle Festival 209
Old Hales Ford Country Store 266
Old Hardware Store 263
Old Michie Theatre 219
Old Post Office
         Restaurant & Lounge 375
Old Salem Days 25
Old South Antiques Ltd. 250
Old Time Fiddler's
         Convention 163, 181
Old Town Easter Egg Hunt 166
Old Town Gift Shop 258
Old Town Hoe Down 180
Old White Club 424
Olde Country Store 15, 250
Olde Mill 468
Olde Mill Golf Resort 105
Olde Salem Days 183
Olde Virginia Barbecue 410
Omni Charlottesville Hotel 366
Once Upon a Time Clock Shop 248
Opera Roanoke 213
Orange County 29, 257, 323, 431
Orchard Gap Deli 82
Orchards 252
Oregano Joe's 404
Orkney Springs 6
Orkney Springs Hotel 6
Orvis Factory Outlet 253
Oscar's Restaurant 362
Other Times LTD 267
Otter Creek Restaurant 82
Otters Den 41
Outdoor Art Show 170
Outdoor Skyline Arrow 122
Outlet Shopping 245, 249, 253,
         265, 267, 269, 270, 274
Outpost, The 412
Overnight Wilderness Outfitters 109
Oxbow Lake 476

P

P.J.'s Carousel Collection
      Christmas Stores 272, 470
Paddle Wheel Cruises 409
Page County 427
Paint Bank State Trout Hatchery 53
Paint Lick Mountain 475
Palais Royal 263
Palette Art Gallery 235
Palmer Country Manor 330
Palms, The 420
Pampered Palate Cafe 248, 380
Panorama Restaurant 77
Pano's 378
Paper Chase Farm 155
Paper Treasures 7, 245
Pappagallo 251
Park, The 422
Park-Oak Grove, The 438
Parkhurst Restaurant 377
Patrick County 466
Paula Lewis 259
Peaks of Otter Lodge and
      Restaurant 41, 79, 82, 369
Peddler Antiques, The 266
Peebles Department Store 268
Peking Palace Restaurant 411
Penn Laird 300
Pennington Gap 478
Personal Touch, The 274
Perspective Art Gallery 233
Pest House Medical
      Museum and Confederate
      Cemetery 70, 129, 228
Peter Kramer 256
Pewter Corner 263
Philpott Reservoir 468
Phoenix, The 262
Piedmont Vineyards and Winery 137
Pine Knoll Gift Shop 245
Pine Tavern Restaurant
      and Lodge 49, 414, 424
Pioneer Day 172
Pioneer Days 476
Plain Dealing 432
Plains Promenaders 196

Plantation Days Festival 179
Plow & Hearth 264
Plumb Alley Day 173
Pocahontas 474, 475
Pocahontas Exhibition Mine 475
Point of Honor 36, 130, 229
Polo 159
Polo in Middleburg 169
Poor Farmers Market 269
Poplar Forest 37, 40, 41, 231, 434
Poultry Festival 8
Primland Hunting Preserve 467
Prince Michel de Virginia
      Vineyards 138
Prince Michel Restaurant 395
Printer's Ink 254
Prism Coffeehouse 220, 422
Pritchett Museum 200
Prospect Hill 406
Prospect Hill Cemetery 66
Prospect Hill Inn 331
Pulaski 51, 344, 436
Pulaski Antique Center 272
Pulaski County 271, 415
Pulaski County Speedway 52
Pulaskifest 188
Pullman Restaurant, The 380
Purcell Oriental Rug Co. Ltd. 263

Q

Quality Inn - Roanoke/Salem 361
Quality Inn Shenandoah Valley 354
Quality Inn Skyline Drive 352
Quilts Exhibit 165
Quilts Unlimited 273

R

R.P. Collectibles 272
Race Car Driving 154
Radford 50, 271, 412
Radford University 237, 456
Radford's Gallery Underground 424
Radisson Patrick Henry Hotel 362
Ragged Mountain Running Shop 262
Rail Road Days 178
Railroad Festival 69

Rainbow Gap 53
Raines Real Estate 435
Ramada Inn 353, 357
Ramada Inn - Monticello 367
Ramada Inn Luray 353
Ram's Head Bookshop 254
Randolph-Macon Academy 457
Randolph-Macon Woman's
        College 454
Randolph's 367
Random Row 404, 405
Rapidan River Vineyards 139
Rappahannock County 28, 431
Rare Finds 256
Ray's 424
Real Estate 425
Rebec Vineyards 143
Red Fox Fine Art 255
Red Fox Tavern, The 393
Red Hill 230
Red Lobster Restaurant 408
Redcoat Antiques 264
Remington's 389
Renaissance Gallery 259
Renaissance, The 415
Rendezvous 177
Resorts 275
Retirement 425
Retirement Communities 437, 439
Reynolds Homestead 467
Richard's Antiques 246
Richlands 474
Ripshin 472
Rising Sun Bakery 404
River Farm 7
River House, The 290
River Rental Outfitters 94
River Ridge Mall 264
River Ridge Ranch 110
River Run and Bicycle Ride 168
River'd Inn 293, 376
Riverfest 122, 180
Riverside Park 70
Rivianna Reservoir 102
Road to Antietam 170
Roanoke 21, 252
Roanoke Airport Marriott 362

Roanoke Catholic School 461, 463
Roanoke College 451
Roanoke Comedy Club 421
Roanoke County 23
Roanoke Express 154
Roanoke Railway Festival 186
Roanoke Regional Airport 441
Roanoke Regional Home Builders
        Association 430, 435
Roanoke Symphony Orchestra 214
Roanoke United
        Methodist Home 438
Roanoke Valley 16
Roanoke Valley Association
        of Realtors 430
Roanoke Valley Historical Society
        and Museum 126, 210
Roanoke Valley Horse Show 25, 176
Roanoke Weiner Stand 389
Roanoker Restaurant, The 389
Roanoke Symphony Polo Cup 160
Roanoke Valley Horse Show 156
Roaring Run Furnace 18
Roaring Run Recreation Area 53
Robertson, James I. 61
Rockbridge 309
Rockbridge Baths 250
Rockbridge County 13
Rockbridge Restaurant 357
Rockbridge Vineyard 135
Rockingham County 8, 246, 428
Rockingham County Fair 181
Rockingham Fairgrounds 123
Rocklands 323, 396
Rocky Knob Cabins 79
Rocky Knob Recreation Area 87
Rocky's Antique Mart 248
Rococo's 405
Rodes Farm Inn 34, 381
Rodes Farm Stables 110
Rooftop of Virginia Cap Crafts 468
Rose River Vineyards and
        Trout Farm 138
Rose Street Interiors 247
Rosemont 432
Rotunda, The 225
Round Hill 255

Rowe's Family Restaurant 248
Royal Oak Bookshop 244
Ruby Rose Inn Bed and
        Breakfast, The 299
Ruffled Grouse Society 56
Rugby Road 433
Rush River Company 256
Russell County 475
Russell's Yesteryear 252
Ryan's Fruit Market 247

S

Saigon Cafe 405
Salem 24
Salem Avalanche 25, 152
Salem Civic Center 25
Salem Fair and Exposition 25, 179
Salem Museum, The 211
Sal's Pizza Restaurants 410
Salt-Making Week 472
Saltville 472
Saltville Museum 472
Sam Snead's Tavern 418
Sampson Eagon Inn, The 304
Sam's On the Market 254
Sand Trap Tavern 354
Sandra's Cellar 252
Sani-Mode Barber Shop 271
Santa at the Lake 190
Sawhill Gallery 201
Scarpa 263
Schoolhouse Fabrics 49, 270
Science Museum of
        Western Virginia 126, 211
Scooch's 421
Scott County 477
Scotto's Italian Restaurant
        and Pizzeria 379
Scottsville on the James 227
Scrooge Day 192
Scruples 420
Second Story 251
Sedalia Center 41, 231
Sedalia Coffeehouse 231
Sedalia Country Fair 188
Seminole Square 264

Senior Corps of
        Retired Executives 437
Septemberfest 184
Seven Bends Gallery 245
Seven Hills Inn 310
Sevier Gallery 199
Shakin' 202
Sharks 420
ShenanArts Inc. 202
Shenandoah Acres Resort 12, 124
Shenandoah Apple
        Blossom Festival 170
Shenandoah Area Agency
        on Aging 437
Shenandoah Caverns 149
Shenandoah Cloggers 202
Shenandoah County 427
Shenandoah County Homebuilders
        Association 428
Shenandoah National Park 108
Shenandoah River
        Outfitters Inc. 7, 94
Shenandoah Summer Music
        Theatre 195
Shenandoah University 448
Shenandoah Valley Music
        Festival 178, 197
Shenandoah Valley Art Center 204
Shenandoah Valley Bach Festival 174
Shenandoah Valley Builders
        Association 428
Shenandoah Valley Country Club 105
Shenandoah Valley
        Crafts and Gifts 245
Shenandoah Valley Heritage
        Museum 8, 201
Shenandoah Valley Music Festival 6
Shenandoah Valley Regional
        Airport 443
Shenandoah Valley Travel
        Association 107
Shenandoah Vineyards 135
Shenanigans 264
Shenvalee Golf Resort 354
Sherando Lake State Park 12, 98, 124
Sheraton Inn 354
Sheraton Inn Charlottesville 367

Sheraton Inn Roanoke Airport 362
Sherwood Anderson Short Story
        Competition 472
Shot Tower Historical Park 471
Showalter's Orchard and
        Greenhouse 247
Silver Linings 248
Silver Thatch Inn 332, 405
Simonpietri's Gift Shop 244
Sinking Creek Bridges 146
SIRIUS 48
Ski Lessons 116
Skiing 115, 276, 284
Sky Bryce Airport 442
Skyland 128
Skyland Lodge 75, 77
Skyline Caverns 5, 122, 149
Skyline Drive 5, 73, 122
Skyline Village Shopping Center 246
Sleep Inn Tanglewood 363
Sleepy Hollow Farm 325
Smith & Thurmond Inc. 433
Smith Mountain Flowers 266
Smith Mountain Lake 38, 97, 102,
        266, 423, 434
    Fall Festival 188
    Airport 444
    State Park & Visitors Center 89
Smithfield Plantation 177, 234
Smyth County 471
    Chamber of Commerce 472
Snooper's Antique and Craft Mall 470
Snowshoe Ski Resort 55
Somerset Shop, The 258
Sorghum Molasses Festival 188
Sounding Knob 88
South River, An American Grill 379
Southern Culture 405
Southern Inn 382
Southern Kitchen 377
Southern Lamp & Shade
        Showroom 267
Southern Soldier Statue 70
Southwest Virginia 465
    Museum 476
    Music Festival 476
Southwestern Virginia Pioneer

Festival 173
Special Olympics 164
Spectator Sports 151
Spencer, Anne 36
Spencer, Anne House
        and Garden 229
Sperryville 28, 256, 317
Sperryville Emporium 256
Sporting Gallery, The 255
Spring Balloon Festival 167
Spring Farm Inn 296
Spring Fly-In 122, 170
Spring Garden Show 167
Spring Hill Cemetery 70
Spring House, The 376
Spring in the Valley Arts
        & Crafts Show 166
Spring Wildflower Symposium 171
Springhouse Antiques 256
Spurs 422
St. Anne's-Belfield School 460
St. Maarten Cafe 405
Stanardsville 323
Stanley 296
Stanley Blue Grass Festival 173
Star City Diner 421
Starkey's Bistro 360
Starr Hill Café 406
Statler Brothers Complex 204
Staunton 9, 124, 247, 300, 428
Staunton-Augusta Art Center 204
Staunton-Augusta Association
        of Realtors 429
Steeles Tavern 305
Steeles Tavern Manor 305
Steeplechase Races 160
Stepping Out 181
Stone Face Rock 478
Stone Mountain Trail 478
Stone's Cafeteria 412
Stonewall and National
        Cemeteries 65
Stonewall Brigade Band 202
Stonewall Vineyards 144
Stony Mountain Fibers 259
Strasburg 5, 244
Strasburg Emporium 5, 244

Strasburg Museum 5, 66, 198
Stuarts Draft 249, 428
Studios on the Square 253
Sugar Tour 57
Sugar Tree Country Store and
         Sugar House 273
Sugar Tree, The 306
Summer Festival of the Arts at
         Ash Lawn-Highland 177
Sun and Sand Beach Weekend 176
Sun Bow Trading Company 259
Sunnybrook Inn Restaurant 390
Sunrise House
         Chinese Restaurant 411
Super 8 Motel 371
Suter's 246
Swannanoa 204
Swannanoa Marble Palace
         and Sculpture Garden 34
Swedenburg Winery 136
Sweeney's Curious Goods 264
Sweet Adelines 220
Sweet Briar College 453
Sweet Things 125
Swimming 95
Swimming Pools 96
Swoope 306
Sycamore Tree, The 342

T

T.G.I.F. 251
   Outlets 267
T.S. Eways 263
Tack Box 255
Talbots 263
Tanglewood Mall 24
Tarara Vineyard & Winery 135
Taste of the Mountains
         Main Street Festival 182
Tastings 406
Tazewell County 474
Tea Room Cafe at the 1817, The 406
Tea Room Cafe, The 327
Tennis 276, 284, 286
Terrace Lounge, The 422
Texas Steak House 408

Texas Tavern 390
Thanksgiving at Wintergreen 189
Theatre at Washington, The 217
Theda's Studio 271
Third Street Coffeehouse 421
Thornrose House at Gypsy Hill 305
Three Legged Cow Cafe 414
Threshing Time 189
Tingler's Mill 20
Tivoli 324
To the Rescue National
         Exhibition 212
Tomahawk Mill Winery 144
Top of the Mountain 467
Top Rail, The 422
Totier Creek Vineyard 142
Touch the Earth 247
Tourist Information
   Alleghany Highlands Chamber
         of Commerce 55
   Augusta-Staunton-Waynesboro
      Travel Information
         Center 10, 12
   Bath County Chamber of
         Commerce 56
   Bedford Area Chamber of
         Commerce 41
   Blacksburg Chamber of
         Commerce 47
   Botetourt County Chamber of
         Commerce 18
   Chamber of Commerce of Front
         Royal and Warren Coun 5
   Charlottesville/Albemarle
         Convention & Visitors Bu 33
   County of Craig 21
   Floyd County Chamber of
         Commerce 49
   Franklin County Chamber of
         Commerce 45
   Greater Lynchburg Chamber of
         Commerce 37
   Harrisonburg-Rockingham County
         Convention and Visi 9
   Highland County Chamber of
         Commerce 59
   Historic Fincastle Inc. 17

Jerry's Run Virginia
   Visitor's Center 55
Lexington Visitors Center 14
Loudoun County Conference/
   Visitor Bureau 28
Luray-Page Chamber of
   Commerce 8
Lynchburg Convention &
   Visitors Bureau 35
Nelson County Department
   of Tourism 34
New Castle Ranger Office 21
Orange County Visitors Bureau 30
Pulaski County Chamber
   of Commerce 52
Radford Chamber
   of Commerce 51
Roanoke County-Salem
   Chamber of Commerce 24
Roanoke Valley Convention &
   Visitors Bureau 22
Shenandoah County
   Travel Council 6
Smith Mountain Lake Chamber of
   Commerce/Partnership 39
Virginia Division of Tourism 2
Winchester-Frederick County
   Visitor Center/Chamber 4
Tours of Historic Avenel 177
Traditional Frontier Festival 183, 203
Traditions of Christmas 190
Travelodge — Roanoke North 363
Trebark Outfitters 253
Treehouse, The 129
Treetop 367
Trillium House 335
Trinity Episcopal Church
   Annual Stable Tour 159
Troutdale 472
Troutville 17, 251
Troutville Antique Mart 17, 251
Trudy's Antiques 252
Tuckahoe Antique Mall 259
Tuesday Evening Concert Series 220
Tultex Mill Outlet 265
Tuttle & Spice General
   Store Museum 199

Twin Porches 343

U

Uncle Bill's Treasures 271
University of Virginia 225
University Cemetery 69
University Corner 262
University of Virginia 451
   Sports 153
University Transit Service 445
Upperville Colt and
   Horse Show 156, 174
Upstairs, Downstairs 272

V

V Magazine 419
Valley Country 422
Valley Crafters 244
Valley Framing
   Studio & Gallery 204, 250
Valley Green Art and
   Craft Co-op 262
Valley Metro Greater Roanoke
   Transit Company 444
Valley Pike Inn 51, 415
Valley Program for Aging
   Services Inc. 437
Valley View 438
Verona Flea Market 248
Vicker's Switch 412
Village Accents 266
Village Inn, The 378
Village Square 266
Villager Antiques 246
Vinegar Hill Theater 32
Vinifera Wine Festival 182
Vinifera Wine Growers
   Association Festival 136
Vintage Virginia Wine Festival 174
Vinton 23, 26
Vinton Dogwood Festival 172
Vinton Folklife Festival 183
Vinton July 4th Celebration 179
Vinton Old-Time Bluegrass Festival
   and Competition 181
Virginia Apparel Outlet 267, 268

Virginia Beef Expo 167
Virginia Blues Festival 182
Virginia Born and Bred 243, 251
Virginia Center for the
            Creative Arts 228
Virginia Chili Cook-off 172
Virginia Commonwealth Games 179
Virginia Creeper Trail 472
Virginia Discovery Museum 128, 221
Virginia Division of Tourism 2, 107
Virginia Explore Park 126
Virginia Fall Foliage Festival 186
Virginia Fall Races 185
Virginia Festival of
            American Film 187, 227
Virginia Garlic Festival 143, 188
Virginia Gold Cup Races 161, 169
Virginia Handcrafts Inc. 264
Virginia Heritage Weekend 187
Virginia Highland Llamas 471
Virginia Highlands Festival 181
Virginia Highlands Gateway
            Visitor's Center 471
Virginia Horse Center 156
Virginia Horse Festival 157
Virginia Institute for the
            Deaf and the Blind 10
Virginia Kentucky District Fair 181
Virginia Made Shop 243, 248
Virginia Metalcrafters 12, 124, 249
Virginia Military Institute
            and Museum 68, 450
Virginia Mountain
            Outfitters 15, 100, 111
Virginia Mountain Peach Festival 181
Virginia Museum of
            Transportation 126, 213
Virginia Mushroom Festival 5, 170
Virginia Polo Center 160
Virginia Poultry Festival 170
Virginia School of the Arts 230
Virginia Shop, The 264
Virginia State Parks 107
Virginia Tech 45, 455
   Airport 443
   Duck Pond 234
   Hokie Basketball 154

   Sports 154
Virginia Wine Festival 134
Virginia's Explore Park 212
VMI Museum 124, 206

W

Waccamaw Pottery 254
Wades Mill 251
Wakefield Country Day School 458
Walker, Gary C. 63
Walnuthill 314
Walton House, The 424
Walton's Mountain Museum 33, 221
Ward's Rock Cafe 391, 421
Warm Hearth Village Retirement
            Community 439
Warm Springs 56, 348
Warm Springs Spa 71
Warren County 426
Warren Rifles Confederate
            Museum 66, 197
Warren-Sipe Museum 67
Warrenton 255
Warrenton Farmers Market 171
Warrenton Horse Show 156, 185
Warwickton Mansion
            Bed and Breakfast 55
Washington 255, 317
Washington and
            Lee University 68, 449
Washington, Booker T. National
            Monument 39, 232
Washington County 472
Washington's Office Museum 196
Waterwheel Restaurant, The 418
Wax Museum 151
Waynesboro 12, 249, 306, 428
Waynesboro Board of Realtors 429
Waynesboro Outlet Village 12
Waynesboro Players 202
Waynesboro Village Factory
            Outlet Mall 249
Wayside Inn 352, 375
Wayside Theatre 4, 122
Weasies Kitchen 379
Westminster Canterbury 438

Westminster Organ
          Concert Series 220
Weyers Cave 299
Whetstone Ridge 80
Whimsies 264
White Elephant 255
White Horse Antiques 270
White Post 374
White Top 466
Whitehouse Antiques 259
Whitetop Mountain 472
   Maple Festival 166
   Sorghum and Molasses Festival 189
Whitey Taylor's Franklin County
       Speedway 44
Wilderness Battlefields 30
Wilderness Road Regional
          Museum 51, 70, 165, 238
Wildflour Cafe and Catering 391
Wildflower Weekend 170, 171
Wildnerness Canoe Company 15, 95
Wildwood 434
Williams Corner Bookstore 263, 423
Willie's Hair Design 263
Willow Grove Inn 324, 396
Willowcroft Farm Vineyards 136
Willson-Walker House 382
Wilson, President Woodrow 9
Wilson Warehouse 18
Wilson, Woodrow Museum
          and Birthplace 203
Wilton House,
          Inn and Restaurant 300
Winchester 2, 243, 426
Winchester Regional Airport 442
Winchester's Handworks Gallery 243
Windy Gap Mountain 43
Wine and Cheese Festival 173
Wine Festival 168, 182, 184
Wineries 133
Winridge Bed & Breakfast 339
Wintergreen 118, 280, 381
Wintergreen Farm
          Sheepskin Shoppe 270
Wintergreen Four Seasons Resort
          34, 100, 105, 423, 433
Wintergreen Vineyard & Winery 142

Winton Country Club 38
Wise County 476
Wonderful World of Miniature Horses
          Theme Park 128, 146
Woodberry Forest 458
Woodberry Inn 467
Woodland 270
Woodlane Craft Shop 273
Woodruff House 296
Woods Creek Park 124
Woodstock 6, 245, 291, 376
Woodstock Museum 199
Woodstone Meadows Stable 109
Wool Days 170
Wythe County 471
Wytheville 470

X

XYZ Cooperative Gallery 234

Y

Yellow Poplar Splashdam 476
Youth Orchestra 220

ORDER FORM
Fast and Simple!

Mail to:
Insiders Guides®, Inc.
P.O. Drawer 2057
Manteo, NC 27954

Or:
for VISA or
Mastercard orders call
1-800-765-BOOK

Name _____

Address _____

City/State/Zip _____

Qty.	Title/Price	Shipping	Amount
	Insiders' Guide to Richmond/$14.95	$3.00	
	Insiders' Guide to Williamsburg/$14.95	$3.00	
	Insiders' Guide to Virginia's Blue Ridge/$14.95	$3.00	
	Insiders' Guide to Virginia's Chesapeake Bay/$14.95	$3.00	
	Insiders' Guide to Washington, DC/$14.95	$3.00	
	Insiders' Guide to North Carolina's Outer Banks/$14.95	$3.00	
	Insiders' Guide to Wilmington, NC/$14.95	$3.00	
	Insiders' Guide to North Carolina's Crystal Coast/$12.95	$3.00	
	Insiders' Guide to Myrtle Beach/$14.95	$3.00	
	Insiders' Guide to Mississippi/$14.95	$3.00	
	Insiders' Guide to Boca Raton & the Palm Beaches/$14.95	$3.00	
	Insiders' Guide to Sarasota/Bradenton/$12.95	$3.00	
	Insiders' Guide to Northwest Florida/$14.95	$3.00	
	Insiders' Guide to Lexington, KY/$14.95	$3.00	
	Insiders' Guide to Louisville/$14.95	$3.00	
	Insiders' Guide to the Twin Cities/$12.95	$3.00	
	Insiders' Guide to Boulder/$12.95	$3.00	
	Insiders' Guide to Denver/$12.95	$3.00	
	Insiders' Guide to Civil War in the Eastern Theater/$14.95	$3.00	
	Insiders' Guide to North Carolina's Mountains/$14.95	$3.00	
	Insiders' Guide to Atlanta/$14.95	$3.00	
	Insiders' Guide to Branson/$14.95 (12/95)	$3.00	
	Insiders' Guide to Cincinnati/$14.95 (9/95)	$3.00	
	Insiders' Guide to Tampa Bay/$14.95 (12/95)	$3.00	

Payment in full (check or money order) must
accompany this order form.
Please allow 2 weeks for delivery.

N.C. residents add 6% sales tax _____

Total _____